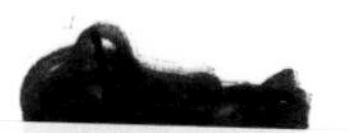

# Biomedical Engineering Series

*Edited by* Michael R. Neuman

*Medical Imaging: Techniques and Technology,* Martin Fox

*Artificial Neural Networks in Cancer Diagnosis: Prognosis and Treatment,* R.N.G. Naguib and G.V. Sherbet

*Biomedical Image Analysis,* Rangaraj M. Rangayyan

*Endogenous and Exogenous Regulation and Control of Physiological Systems,* Robert B. Northrop

# Electromagnetic Analysis *and* Design *in* Magnetic Resonance Imaging

**Jianming Jin**
Department of Electrical and Computer Engineering
University of Illinois at Urbana-Champaign
Urbana, Illinois

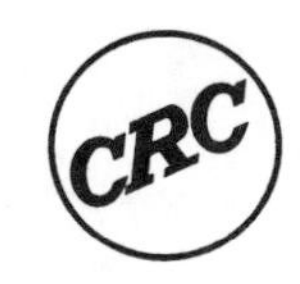


**CRC Press**
**Boca Raton London New York Washington, D.C.**

**Library of Congress Cataloging-in-Publication Data**

Jin, Jian-Ming, 1962–
Electromagnetic analysis and design in magnetic resonance imaging / Jianming Jin.
p. cm. -- (CRC Press series in biomedical engineering)
Includes bibliographical references and index.
ISBN 0-8493-9693-X (alk. paper)
1. Magnetic resonance imaging. 2. Electromagnetism. I. Title.
II. Series: Biomedical engineering (Boca Raton, Fla.)
QC762.6.M34J56 1998
616.07'548—dc21 98-21867
CIP



Direct all inquiries to CRC Press LLC, 2000 Corporate Blvd., N.W., Boca Raton, Florida 33431.


International Standard Book Number 0-8493-9693-X
Library of Congress Card Numb 98-21867
Printed in the United States of America 1 2 3 4 5 6 7 8 9 0
Printed on acid-free paper

# Preface

This book presents a comprehensive treatment of electromagnetic analysis and design of three key devices used in a magnetic resonance imaging (MRI) system, namely, the magnet, the gradient coils, and the radiofrequency (RF) coils. It also includes the analysis and characterization of the interactions of electromagnetic fields with a biological subject.

Because of the importance of MRI, a large number of scientists and engineers have been working in this fast-growing field. As a result, many books on MRI have been published. However, most of these books deal with the principles of MRI and imaging techniques. Few of them provide a detailed treatment on the analysis and design of the hardware of an MRI system from the engineering perspective. The lack of a reference book on this topic has been an inconvenience for a growing number of MRI engineers for many years. This work is intended to remove this inconvenience. Although the materials covered here can be found in electromagnetics textbooks and MRI literature, it is a rather time-consuming task to search and organize them in an easy-to-understand format. Therefore, what is contained in this book is the result of my study of other people's work combined with my understanding of electromagnetics and some of my own work.

In 1994, our department started to offer a new course entitled "Magnetic Resonance Principle and Instrumentation" to the graduate students in bio- and electrical engineering at the University of Illinois at Urbana-Champaign. The course covers topics such as RF and gradient coil design, nuclear magnetic resonance (NMR) coherence excitation and detection, NMR signal analysis and processing, design of biological studies, and MRI safety hazards. I was asked to cover the analysis and design of magnets, gradient coils, and RF coils. Since there was no textbook available on these topics, I prepared a set of course notes to be distributed in class. These course notes now form the basis of this book.

This book contains five chapters. The first chapter is a simple introduction to MRI, which is intended for students who do not have any knowledge about MRI. The second chapter is on the basic concepts of electromagnetics and the emphasis is on the topics that are closely related to MRI. These include Helmholtz and Maxwell coils, inductance calculation, and the magnetic fields produced by some special cylindrical and spherical surface currents that form the foundation for birdcage and magnet designs. Chapter 3 deals with the basic principles for the analysis and design of gradient coils for MRI applications. It includes the design of gradient coils using discrete wires and the target field method for the design of gradient coils, including shielded coils, using distributed currents. The analysis of RF coils is covered in Chapter 4. The methods of analysis described include a simple one based on the equivalent lumped-circuit model and a rigorous one based on the integral equation formulation. The chapter also includes a brief survey of some special-purpose RF coils. The final chapter describes analytical and numerical methods for analysis of the electromagnetic field in biological objects, a problem that is important for high-frequency MRI.

To help readers understand some basic electromagnetic phenomena and RF coil characteristics, I wrote a software program called MRIEM that can be downloaded from my home page. It can be used to analyze a variety of RF coils and to calculate the RF fields in the human head. To supplement and reinforce the concepts and ideas presented and to facilitate the use of this book in the classroom, I have also designed a number of exercise problems which are included.

This book is written for engineers, physicists, and graduate students working in the field of MRI. It can also be read by electrical engineers who wish to understand the hardware of an MRI system. The readers are assumed to have the basic knowledge (undergraduate level) of vector algebra, circuits, and electromagnetics.

JIANMING JIN
*Urbana-Champaign, Illinois*
*December 1997*

# About the Author

**Jianming Jin** joined the faculty of the Department of Electrical and Computer Engineering at the University of Illinois at Urbana-Champaign (UIUC) in 1993, after serving as a Senior Scientist at Otsuka Electronics (USA), Inc., Fort Collins, CO. Currently, he is an Associate Professor of Electrical and Computer Engineering and Associate Director of the Center for Computational Electromagnetics at UIUC. He is also an affiliate member of the Magnetic Resonance Engineering Laboratory in the Beckman Institute of UIUC. He serves as an Associate Editor of the *IEEE Transactions on Antennas and Propagation* and as a member of the Editorial Board of *Electromagnetics Journal.* His name is listed in the university's *List of Excellent Instructors.* He has published over 70 articles in refereed journals and several book chapters, authored the first comprehensive textbook on the finite element method for electromagnetic analysis, *The Finite Element Method in Electromagnetics* (New York: Wiley, 1993), and co-authored another book on applied mathematics, *Computation of Special Functions* (New York: Wiley, 1996). His current research interests include computational electromagnetics, magnetic resonance imaging, gradient and RF coil design, bioelectromagnetics, scattering and antenna analysis, and electromagnetic compatibility. He has published papers on RF coil analysis, design, and optimization and RF field computation in the human body in MRI and co-taught a course on "Magnetic Resonance Principle and Instrumentation."

Dr. Jin is a member of the U.S. National Committee of the International Radio Science Union, Tau Beta Pi, Applied Computational Electromagnetics Society, International Society of Magnetic Resonance in Medicine, and a Senior Member of the Institute of Electrical and Electronics Engineers (IEEE). He served as the Symposium Co-Chairman and Technical Program Chairman of the 1997 and 1998 International Symposia on Applied Computational Electromagnetics, respectively. He is a recipient of a 1994 National Science Foundation Young Investigator Award and 1995 Office of Naval Research Young Investigator Award. He also received a 1997 Junior Xerox Research Award from the UIUC College of Engineering. In 1998, he was appointed as the Henry Magnuski Scholar in the Department of Electrical and Computer Engineering.

Dr. Jin received the B.S. and M.S. degrees in applied physics from Nanjing University, Nanjing, China, in 1982 and 1984, respectively, and the Ph.D. degree in electrical engineering from the University of Michigan, Ann Arbor, in 1989.

# Acknowledgments

I wish to thank Professors R. L. Magin, A. Webb, and Z. P. Liang for their collaboration on a graduate MRI course offered in the Department of Electrical and Computer Engineering at University of Illinois at Urbana-Champaign. Professor Liang and Dr. A. C. Wright provided useful comments on the first draft of Chapter 1. My appreciation also goes to my graduate students, Mr. J. Chen, Miss Z. Feng, and Mr. M. Kowalski, for their assistance. Mr. Chen and Miss Feng calculated some numerical results in Chapters 4 and 5. Mr. Kowalski wrote a report, which became the first draft for Chapter 1. He and Dr. G. X. Fan have also checked some of the formulas. All remaining errors are, of course, my responsibility. The head model in Chapter 5 was provided by Dr. P. J. Dimbylow of National Radiological Protection Board, U.K., whose generosity is greatly appreciated. The measured data on a ladder coil were provided by Dr. Wright. My early collaboration with Dr. G. X. Shen and Dr. T. Perkins was very enjoyable. The support for my research from the National Science Foundation (NSF) is also gratefully acknowledged. Finally, I would like to thank my wife, Yanqing, for her love and support. This book is dedicated to her and our children, Angela, David, and Joy (who was born just after I finished the manuscript).

JIANMING JIN
*Urbana-Champaign, Illinois*

# Contents

# Chapter 1

# Introduction to Magnetic Resonance Imaging

## 1.1 Introduction

Magnetic resonance imaging, commonly known as MRI, is a powerful non-invasive imaging technique that has played and will continue to play an important role in the medical community. In clinical practice, it can assist physicians in both diagnosis and presurgical planning with limited risk to the patient. In laboratory research, it can help neurologists and other biological scientists to discover novel basic anatomical structures and physiological principles. Unlike some other imaging techniques like x-ray computed tomography (CT), MRI does not require exposure of the subject to ionizing radiation and hence is considered safe. It also provides more information than other imaging modalities since MR signals are sensitive to several tissue parameters.

MRI belongs to a larger group of techniques which are based on the phenomenon of nuclear magnetic resonance (NMR). This phenomenon was discovered in bulk materials by Bloch and Purcell in 1946. As we will see later, certain atomic nuclei, when placed in a static magnetic field, will assume one of the two states: one has a higher energy level and the other has a lower energy level (Fig. 1.1). The energy difference between the two states is linearly proportional to the strength of the applied magnetic field. This is known as the Zeeman effect. In thermal equilibrium, the number of nuclei in the higher energy state is slightly less than the number of nuclei in the lower energy state. A nucleus in the higher energy state can fall to the lower energy state by emitting a photon with energy equal to the energy difference between the two states. A nucleus in the lower energy state can jump to the higher energy state by absorbing a photon with energy matching the

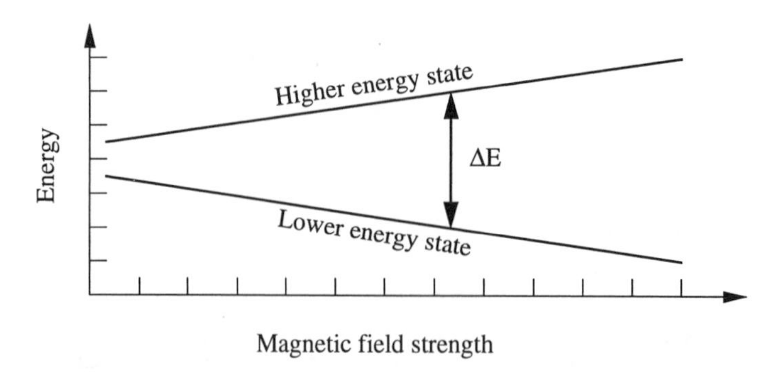


**Figure 1.1.** Splitting of energy level caused by the application of a static magnetic field.

energy difference between the two states. Therefore, when the nuclei in the applied magnetic field are irradiated by such photons, which are actually electromagnetic fields of certain frequency generated by a radiofrequency (RF) probe, some nuclei in the lower energy state will absorb the photons and jump to the higher energy state. This destroys the thermal equilibrium. Immediately after the irradiation of photons, the excess nuclei in the higher energy state will return to the lower energy state to recover the equilibrium, emitting photons or electromagnetic fields which can be detected by an RF probe. Since the frequency of the emitted electromagnetic signals is determined by the energy difference of the two states of the nuclei and the decay of the signals in time depends on the molecular environment of the nuclei, the NMR signals received by an RF probe can be analyzed to study the properties of the nuclei and their environment.

For many years, NMR was primarily used for spectroscopic analysis before Lauterbur (1973) proposed using it for imaging purposes. The basic principle of using NMR for imaging is simple. Since the energy difference between the two states of certain nuclei in an external field depends on the strength of the external field, this energy difference at each point in the object to be imaged can be made different by varying the magnetic field from point to point. As a result, the energy of the photons and, consequently, the frequency of the electromagnetic fields absorbed or emitted by the nuclei are also different from point to point. After signals from all nuclei are received, their frequency may be used to determine spatial information about the nuclei. This simple phenomenon provides a basic foundation for all NMR imaging although the actual imaging methods are more complicated. The number of imaging techniques has blossomed since Lauterbur's pioneering work. Technological developments have also increased the quality of NMR images. For example, the advent of superconducting magnets has made possible higher signal-to-noise ratio (SNR) and higher image resolution than were possible with resistive or permanent magnets. Modern computers have made possible whole volume imaging techniques which offer increased SNR and decreased image acquisition times. So-called "artifacts," which are the distortions of the image due to unwanted effects such as motion, can be controlled using complex RF pulse sequences. Advances in coil technology have improved image quality and made techniques such as surface and microscopic imaging possible.

In this chapter, we first describe the physical principles of NMR and then the hardware of a basic MRI experiment. After that, we describe some basic pulse sequences and imaging methods. This chapter is intended for the readers who do not have any knowledge about MRI. More comprehensive treatment of the subject can be found in Chen and Hoult (1989), Hornak (1996), Mansfield and Morris (1982), Morris (1986), Parikh (1991), Rinck (1993), Sigal (1988), Stark and Bradley (1992), Vlaardingerbroek and den Boer (1996), and Young (1984).

## 1.2 Physical Principles of Nuclear Magnetic Resonance

To understand MRI, we first have to understand the basic physical principles of nuclear magnetic resonance which describe the behavior of certain nuclei in an applied magnetic field. The description below is based on a classical mechanical model, although NMR can be more accurately treated by quantum mechanics.

### 1.2.1 Property of Spin

Modern quantum mechanics reveals that certain atomic nuclei possess a property known as spin. In order to visualize spin, one may imagine a proton as being a small sphere of distributed positive charge that rotates at a high speed about its axis. Since the proton has mass, the rotation generates an angular momentum. Particles such as electrons also have an angular momentum associated with their orbital motion. Since the charge of the proton is distributed in the small sphere, some net charge is circulating about its axis, as illustrated in Fig. 1.2. This current, in turn, produces a small magnetic field. Neutrons can also be thought of as a sphere of distributed positive and negative charges. Because these charges are not uniformly distributed, the neutron also generates a magnetic field when it spins. These small magnetic fields are called "magnetic moments,"

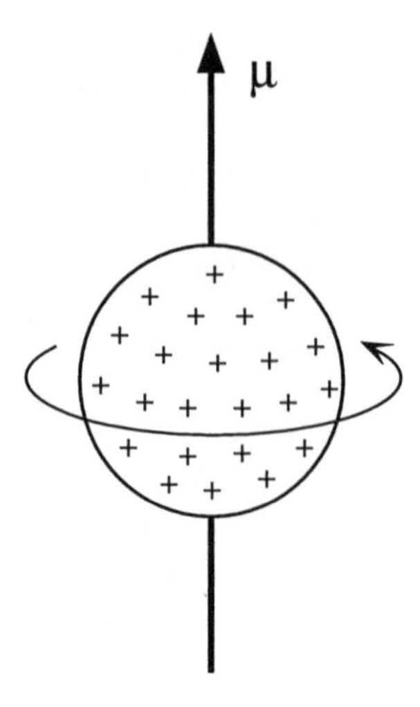


**Figure 1.2.** The distributed charge in a proton generates a magnetic moment when the proton spins about its axis.

symbolized by $\boldsymbol{\mu}$. The relationship between the angular momentum $\mathbf{J}$ and the magnetic moment $\boldsymbol{\mu}$ of a nucleus is given by (Gadian 1995, Slichter 1996)

$$\boldsymbol{\mu} = \gamma \mathbf{J} \tag{1.1}$$

where $\gamma$ is a proportionality constant characteristic of a given nucleus known as the "gyromagnetic" or "magnetogyric" ratio.

Now consider a nucleus with two protons as an isolated system. The Pauli exclusion principle indicates that the angular momentum of each proton must assume opposite spin states, to avoid creating a degeneracy. One can understand this effect classically by considering the interaction of two magnetic moments. There are two possible arrangements for the angular momentum and, consequently, for the magnetic moment of each proton, leading to two distinct possibilities for the nucleus. Either the magnetic moments can be aligned in the same sense, which results in a higher energy configuration, or in an opposite sense, resulting in a lower energy configuration. Since the opposite sense has a lower energy, this will be the more stable arrangement. In such a configuration, the net momentum of the nucleus is zero, and no magnetic moment is generated. Such nuclei are of little interest in NMR because they do not interact strongly with external magnetic fields.

For nuclei with an odd number of protons or an odd number of neutrons, it is impossible to arrange the spins to produce a zero net angular

**Table 1.1.** Gyromagnetic ratio of some nuclei.

| Nucleus | $^1$H | $^{13}$C | $^{19}$F | $^{23}$N | $^{31}$P |
|---|---|---|---|---|---|
| $\gamma/2\pi$ (MHz/T) | 42.58 | 10.71 | 40.08 | 11.27 | 17.25 |

momentum. All such nuclei are said to have nuclear spin. These include $^1$H, $^{13}$C, $^{19}$F, $^{23}$N, and $^{31}$P, whose gyromagnetic ratios are given in Table 1.1. Henceforth, we will limit our discussion to a single proton ($^1$H) for simplicity.

The $^1$H species is, in fact, the most significant nucleus for most MRI studies because of its high natural concentration in the human body as part of the water molecule and its high NMR "sensitivity." The high sensitivity of the $^1$H species can be intuitively understood by considering the fact that there is typically only one electron shielding the magnetic moment that the nucleus produces. This lack of shielding is even more pronounced for hydrogen in water, where the nature of the O-H bond is ionic. This tends to remove the shielding electron from the $^1$H nucleus. The effect of this is to make the nucleus' state more easily permutable from external influences. In NMR, we are interested in our ability to make the nucleus "resonate" between energy states by applying external magnetic fields.

### 1.2.2 Behavior of Nuclei in an External Magnetic Field

We now consider the effect of applying an external, uniform magnetic field, which is usually referred to as the $B_0$ field, to an isolated proton. By convention, we allow the magnetic "field" (notice that we are actually talking about a magnetic flux density $B_0$) to point in the $z$ direction. The proton may assume one of two equilibrium positions: either with its $z$-component of magnetic moment aligned with the external field, referred to as the "parallel" state, or with its $z$-component of magnetic moment opposed to the external field, referred to as the "anti-parallel" state (Fig. 1.3). Both states are considered stable, although the energy associated with the former state is clearly lower than that of the latter. The angle $\theta_0$ in Fig. 1.3 can be determined by the value of the magnetic moment $\mu$ and its $z$-component $\mu_z$, which are given by quantum mechanics as

$$\mu = \frac{\gamma h\sqrt{3}}{4\pi}, \qquad \mu_z = \frac{\gamma h}{4\pi} \tag{1.2}$$

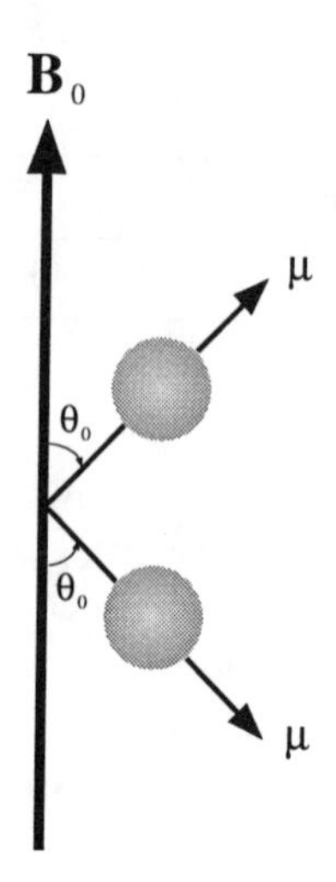


**Figure 1.3.** A proton in the presence of a magnetic field may align itself in one of two ways—the parallel or anti-parallel state.

where $h$ is called Planck's constant, given numerically by $6.629 \times 10^{-34}$ J · s (Canet 1996). Hence,

$$\theta_0 = \cos^{-1}\left(\frac{\mu_z}{\mu}\right) = \cos^{-1}\frac{1}{\sqrt{3}} \approx 54.7°. \tag{1.3}$$

The difference in energy between the two states is

$$\Delta E = 2\mu_z B_0. \tag{1.4}$$

Therefore, if a proton "flips" (changes from one energy state to the other), it will either emit or absorb a photon of frequency $\nu$. This frequency can be found from the Bohr relation

$$\Delta E = h\nu. \tag{1.5}$$

Combining Eqs. (1.4) and (1.5), we have

$$\nu = \left[\frac{2\mu_z}{h}\right] B_0. \tag{1.6}$$

Notice that the quantity in the brackets is constant, demonstrating that the frequency is directly proportional to the magnetic field strength. For protons, the bracketed quantity is given numerically by 42.58 MHz/T (Price *et al.* 1988).

Now consider the effect of the impressed magnetic field on the motion of the nuclear magnetic moment. Assume that at some initial time, which can be taken to be zero without loss of generality, the magnetic moment $\boldsymbol{\mu}$ is given by

$$\boldsymbol{\mu}(0) = \hat{x}\mu_{x0} + \hat{y}\mu_{y0} + \hat{z}\mu_{z0}. \tag{1.7}$$

The torque acting on the magnetic moment is

$$\boldsymbol{\tau} = \boldsymbol{\mu} \times \mathbf{B}_0. \tag{1.8}$$

The torque on any object is related to its angular momentum $\mathbf{J}$ by the definition of angular momentum

$$\boldsymbol{\tau} = \frac{d\mathbf{J}}{dt}. \tag{1.9}$$

Recall that the angular momentum of a nucleus is linearly related to its magnetic moment by Eq. (1.1). Combining this with Eqs. (1.8) and (1.9) gives

$$\frac{d\boldsymbol{\mu}}{dt} = \gamma(\boldsymbol{\mu} \times \mathbf{B}_0) \tag{1.10}$$

which represents three scalar equations

$$\frac{d\mu_x}{dt} = \gamma\mu_y B_0 \tag{1.11}$$

$$\frac{d\mu_y}{dt} = -\gamma\mu_x B_0 \tag{1.12}$$

$$\frac{d\mu_z}{dt} = 0. \tag{1.13}$$

Combining the first two equations gives, for the transverse components,

$$\frac{d^2}{dt^2}\begin{pmatrix}\mu_x \\ \mu_y\end{pmatrix} + (\gamma B_0)^2 \begin{pmatrix}\mu_x \\ \mu_y\end{pmatrix} = 0. \tag{1.14}$$

Solving differential equations (1.13) and (1.14) with the initial condition (1.7), we obtain

$$\boldsymbol{\mu}(t) = \hat{x}(\mu_{x0}\cos\omega t + \mu_{y0}\sin\omega t) + \hat{y}(\mu_{y0}\cos\omega t - \mu_{x0}\sin\omega t) + \hat{z}\mu_{z0} \tag{1.15}$$

where $\omega = \gamma B_0$. This solution represents the precession of the magnetic moment about the axis of the applied field, as shown in Fig. 1.4. The frequency of this precession is

$$f = \frac{\omega}{2\pi} = \frac{\gamma B_0}{2\pi} \tag{1.16}$$

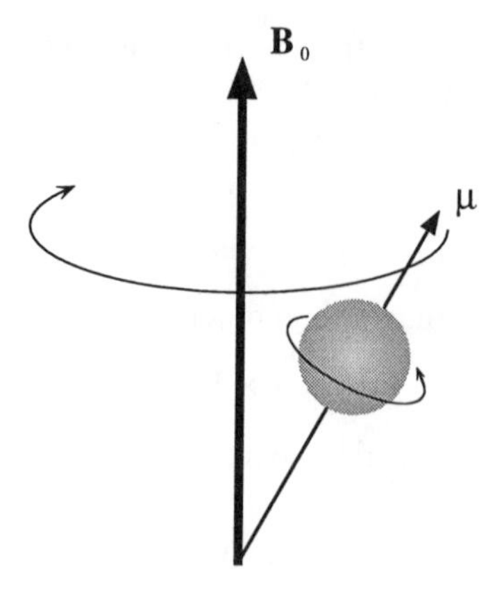


**Figure 1.4.** A proton will precess about the axis of an applied magnetic field.

which is the so-called Larmor or resonant frequency of the nucleus.

We now wish to examine the relationship between the frequency of stimulated radiation given in Eq. (1.6) and the precessional frequency of the magnetic moment in Eq. (1.16). From Eq. (1.2), we obtain the gyromagnetic ratio as

$$\gamma = \frac{4\pi \mu_z}{h}. \tag{1.17}$$

The above result, when substituted into Eq. (1.16), shows that

$$f = \frac{\gamma B_0}{2\pi} = \frac{2\mu_z}{h} B_0 \tag{1.18}$$

which is the same as the frequency of the radiation exchanged in the transition between the parallel and anti-parallel states.

### 1.2.3 Bulk Magnetization

We now consider the effect of an external magnetic field on a bulk sample of non-magnetic material. Before the field is impressed, all the nuclei of the material are oriented in random directions, resulting in zero net magnetic moment (Fig. 1.5). Since we are interested in only $^1$H nuclei, we will neglect the effect of other nuclei on the magnetization of the sample, which may be justified by recalling that most other nuclei that have net spin are heavily "shielded" by their electronic orbitals. Once the magnetic field is applied, each individual magnetic moment must align itself either with or against the external field. Again, we refer to the former, lower energy state as the

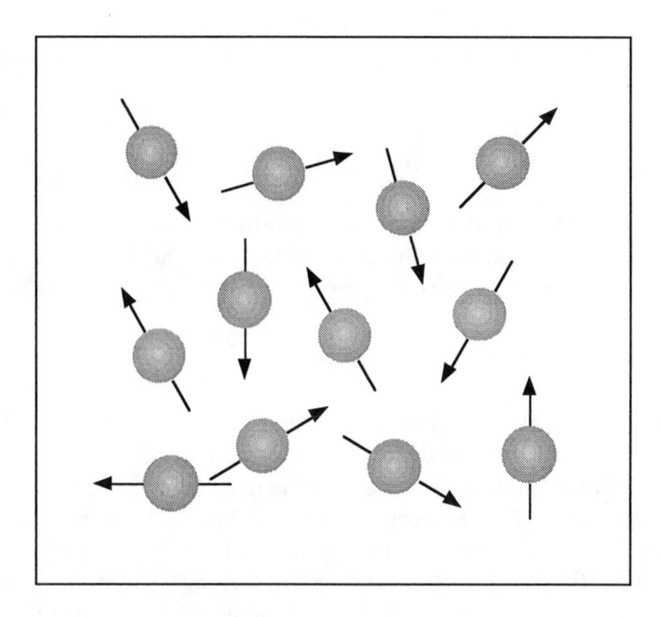

**Figure 1.5.** A bulk sample of ideal material has no net magnetic moment in the absence of an applied magnetic field because of the random orientation of the nuclei's individual magnetic moments.

parallel ($\alpha$) state and the latter, higher energy state as the anti-parallel ($\beta$) state. Let $N_\alpha$ denote the probability that a given nucleus will be found in the $\alpha$ state and $N_\beta$ denote the probability that it will be in the $\beta$ state. Then, since a given proton must assume one state or the other, we have

$$N_\alpha + N_\beta = 1. \tag{1.19}$$

If the system is in thermal equilibrium, the probabilities are also governed by Boltzmann's law (Canet 1996)

$$\frac{N_\alpha}{N_\beta} = \exp\left(\frac{\Delta E}{k_B T}\right) \tag{1.20}$$

where $k_B$ is Boltzmann's constant ($k_B = 1.3806 \times 10^{-23}$ J $\cdot$ K$^{-1}$), $T$ is the absolute temperature of the sample, and $\Delta E$ is the energy difference between the two states. For protons at 20°C, $\Delta E$ is on the order of $10^{-26}$ J and $k_B T$ is on the order of $10^{-21}$ J (Gadian 1995). Therefore, Eq. (1.20) may be approximated as

$$\frac{N_\alpha}{N_\beta} \approx 1 + \frac{\Delta E}{k_B T} \tag{1.21}$$

which is the so-called "high temperature approximation." Taking $N_\alpha \approx N_\beta \approx 1/2$ gives

$$N_\alpha - N_\beta \approx \frac{\Delta E}{2k_B T}. \tag{1.22}$$

The above equation represents an estimation of the net percentage of protons that are aligned with the external magnetic field. The net magnetic moment per unit volume, also known as magnetization, is therefore

$$\mathbf{M} = (N_\alpha - N_\beta) n \mu_z \hat{z} \approx \frac{\Delta E}{2k_B T} n \mu_z \hat{z} \tag{1.23}$$

where $n$ denotes the number of protons per unit volume. This net magnetization is time invariant despite random thermal interactions. However, as the temperature increases, the net magnetization is destroyed. In addition, since $\Delta E$ is proportional to $B_0$, it follows that the net magnetization is proportional to the applied field strength. In NMR, the returned RF signal is obtained by "observing" the precession of this magnetic moment. A stronger $B_0$ field is therefore almost always desirable since it increases the magnitude of the magnetization.

### 1.2.4 Effects of a Radiofrequency Pulse

We would now like to examine the effect of RF radiation on the magnetization of the sample in a uniformly applied field. To do so, we need to develop the equations that govern the behavior of the magnetization in the presence of magnetic fields. Since the net magnetization is directly proportional to the magnetic moment of an individual proton, we expect that $\mathbf{M}$ obeys the same differential equations as $\boldsymbol{\mu}$, assuming that the individual magnetic moments are not mutually coupled.

When a sample is placed in a uniform magnetic field oriented in the $z$ direction, it develops a net magnetization in the $z$ direction. Assume that at the moment $t = 0$ this magnetization is somehow tipped into the direction such that

$$\mathbf{M}(0) = \hat{x} M_{x0} + \hat{z} M_{z0}. \tag{1.24}$$

We would expect from our experience with magnetic moments that the magnetization would begin to precess about the applied field. Consider this initial value problem with the initial condition in Eq. (1.24) and the governing differential equations

$$\frac{dM_x}{dt} = \gamma M_y B_0 \tag{1.25}$$

$$\frac{dM_y}{dt} = -\gamma M_x B_0 \tag{1.26}$$

$$\frac{dM_z}{dt} = 0. \tag{1.27}$$

The solution to these equations is

$$\mathbf{M} = M_{x0}(\hat{x}\cos\omega t - \hat{y}\sin\omega t) + \hat{z}M_{z0} \tag{1.28}$$

where $\omega = \gamma B_0$ is the angular frequency of precession. Notice that the magnetization vector is rotating in a left-handed sense relative to the applied field. That is, if you point the thumb of your left hand in the direction of the magnetic field, the magnetization precesses in the same sense in which your other fingers curl.

The trajectory of the magnetization vector in the "laboratory" (stationary) frame is depicted in Fig. 1.6(a). We would like to find a reference frame in which the magnetization vector is stationary. To accomplish this, we choose a set of basis vectors $(\hat{x}', \hat{y}', \hat{z}')$ to span three-dimensional space. Since the $z$ component of the magnetization is already stationary, we let $\hat{z}' = \hat{z}$. We know that our frame must rotate in a left-handed sense to keep up with the magnetization. To accomplish this, let

$$\hat{x}' = \hat{x}\cos\omega_r t - \hat{y}\sin\omega_r t \tag{1.29}$$

$$\hat{y}' = \hat{x}\sin\omega_r t + \hat{y}\cos\omega_r t \tag{1.30}$$

where $\omega_r$ is the angular frequency of the frame. If we let $\omega_r = \gamma B_0$, the magnetization appears in our "rotating frame" as

$$\mathbf{M} = \hat{x}' M_{x0} + \hat{z}' M_{z0} \tag{1.31}$$

which is a constant, indicating that the magnetization vector is stationary in the rotating frame, as illustrated in Fig. 1.6(b).

We are now prepared to examine the effects of an oscillating RF magnetic field, linearly polarized in the $x$ direction, on the magnetization vector. By convention, this field is called the $B_1$ field. We consider the situation where $\mathbf{B}_0$ is again $z$ directed and the initial state of $\mathbf{M}$ is given by

$$\mathbf{M}(0) = \hat{z}M_0. \tag{1.32}$$

We notice first that the RF magnetic field may be written as

$$\mathbf{B}_1 = \hat{x}B_{10}\cos\omega t = \mathbf{B}_{\mathrm{CW}} + \mathbf{B}_{\mathrm{CCW}} \tag{1.33}$$

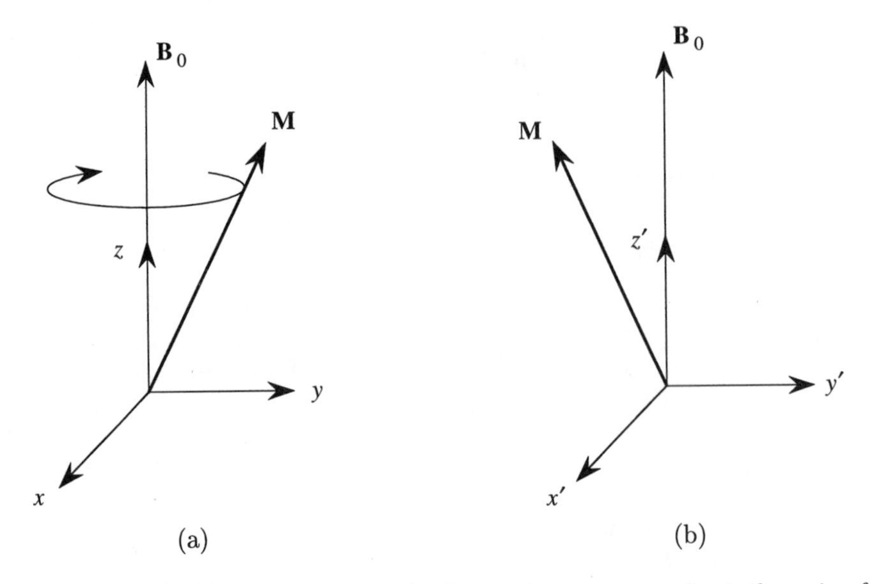


**Figure 1.6.** (a) The net magnetization vector precesses about the axis of an applied magnetic field as viewed from the laboratory frame. (b) The net magnetization vector under the influence of an applied magnetic field is stationary in the rotating frame.

where

$$\mathbf{B}_{\mathrm{CW}} = \tfrac{1}{2}B_{10}(\hat{x}\cos\omega t - \hat{y}\sin\omega t) \tag{1.34}$$
$$\mathbf{B}_{\mathrm{CCW}} = \tfrac{1}{2}B_{10}(\hat{x}\cos\omega t + \hat{y}\sin\omega t) \tag{1.35}$$

with $B_{10}$ being the magnitude of the magnetic field. This indicates that $\mathbf{B}_1$ in Eq. (1.33) can be considered as the sum of two rotating magnetic fields: one, $\mathbf{B}_{\mathrm{CW}}$, is rotating clockwise and the other, $\mathbf{B}_{\mathrm{CCW}}$, is rotating counterclockwise (Fig. 1.7). Such rotating fields are called circularly polarized fields. If the field $\mathbf{B}_1$ oscillates at the same frequency with which our frame rotates, then

$$\mathbf{B}_{\mathrm{CW}} = \tfrac{1}{2}B_{10}\hat{x}' \tag{1.36}$$
$$\mathbf{B}_{\mathrm{CCW}} = \tfrac{1}{2}B_{10}(\hat{x}'\cos 2\omega_r t + \hat{y}'\sin 2\omega_r t). \tag{1.37}$$

The linearity of the system guarantees that the total effect of the RF field can be found as the sum of the effects of its components. For now we will consider only the effect of $\mathbf{B}_{\mathrm{CW}}$, since it can be shown later that $\mathbf{B}_{\mathrm{CCW}}$ has no appreciable effect on the magnetization vector.

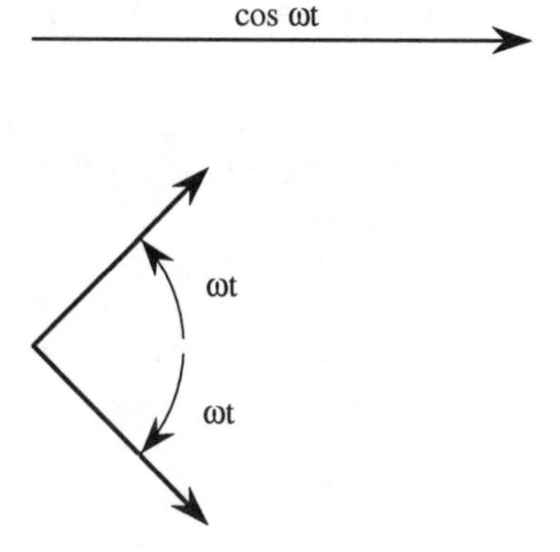


**Figure 1.7.** A linearly polarized field may be decomposed into two oppositely rotating fields.

To consider the effects of $\mathbf{B}_{\text{CW}}$, we now recast the equation of motion

$$\frac{d\mathbf{M}}{dt} = \gamma \mathbf{M} \times \mathbf{B} \tag{1.38}$$

in our rotating frame. Notice that

$$\begin{aligned}\frac{d\mathbf{M}}{dt} &= \frac{d}{dt}(\hat{x}' M_{x'} + \hat{y}' M_{y'} + \hat{z}' M_{z'}) \\ &= M_{x'} \frac{d\hat{x}'}{dt} + M_{y'} \frac{d\hat{y}'}{dt} + \hat{x}' \frac{dM_{x'}}{dt} + \hat{y}' \frac{dM_{y'}}{dt} + \hat{z}' \frac{dM_{z'}}{dt}.\end{aligned} \tag{1.39}$$

Since, from Eqs. (1.29) and (1.30),

$$\frac{d}{dt}\begin{pmatrix}\hat{x}' \\ \hat{y}'\end{pmatrix} = \mathbf{\Omega} \times \begin{pmatrix}\hat{x}' \\ \hat{y}'\end{pmatrix} \tag{1.40}$$

where $\mathbf{\Omega} = -\omega_r \hat{z}$, we can write Eq. (1.39) as

$$\frac{d\mathbf{M}}{dt} = \mathbf{\Omega} \times \mathbf{M} + \frac{\delta \mathbf{M}}{\delta t} \tag{1.41}$$

where $\delta\mathbf{M}/\delta t$ represents the time derivative of $\mathbf{M}$ as viewed from inside the rotating frame. Combining Eqs. (1.38) and (1.41) gives

$$\begin{aligned}\frac{\delta \mathbf{M}}{\delta t} &= \frac{d\mathbf{M}}{dt} - \mathbf{\Omega} \times \mathbf{M} = \gamma \mathbf{M} \times \mathbf{B} - \mathbf{\Omega} \times \mathbf{M} \\ &= \gamma \mathbf{M} \times \left(\mathbf{B} + \frac{\mathbf{\Omega}}{\gamma}\right) = \gamma \mathbf{M} \times \mathbf{B}_{\text{eff}}.\end{aligned} \tag{1.42}$$

The value of the effective magnetic field, $\mathbf{B}_{\text{eff}}$, in the rotating frame is given by

$$\mathbf{B}_{\text{eff}} = \hat{z}\left(B_0 - \frac{\omega_r}{\gamma}\right) + \hat{x}'\frac{B_{10}}{2} \tag{1.43}$$

where, once again, we are considering only the effect of $\mathbf{B}_{\text{CW}}$. Since we have chosen the frequency of rotation of the frame to be the Larmor frequency, $\omega_r = \gamma B_0$, the $z$ component of the effective magnetic field disappears. From our familiarity with equations of the form of Eq. (1.42), we may predict that the magnetization vector will precess about the effective magnetic field in the rotating frame, which is now simply

$$\mathbf{B}_{\text{eff}} = \hat{x}'\frac{B_{10}}{2}. \tag{1.44}$$

The rotation has an angular frequency

$$\omega_{\text{rot}} = \gamma B_{\text{eff}}. \tag{1.45}$$

The resultant motion, usually termed nutation, is depicted in Fig. 1.8. It should be clear that we may now rotate the magnetization vector to any desired angle away from its equilibrium position by applying an oscillating magnetic field in the transverse plane. Applying an RF pulse for a duration $T$ seconds results in an angular deflection

$$\theta = \gamma B_{\text{eff}} T. \tag{1.46}$$

Notice that a large gyromagnetic ratio would allow us to more quickly perturb the magnetization vector away from its equilibrium position. In practice, it is frequently important to be able to rotate $\mathbf{M}$ by 90° and 180°. This is accomplished by the so-called "90° pulse" and "180° pulse," the durations of which may be theoretically predicted from Eq. (1.46). Solving for time, we have

$$T_{90} = \frac{\pi}{2\gamma B_{\text{eff}}} \tag{1.47}$$

and

$$T_{180} = \frac{\pi}{\gamma B_{\text{eff}}}. \tag{1.48}$$

Following a 90° pulse, the magnetization vector precesses in the transverse plane as viewed from the laboratory reference frame. If an RF coil is properly placed around the sample, an electromotive force (emf) will be induced by the rotating magnetization vector.

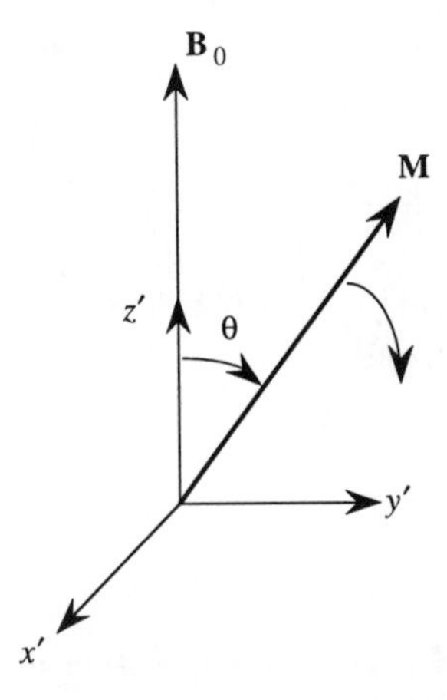


**Figure 1.8.** Under the influence of an $x'$ directed RF magnetic field, the magnetization can be rotated away from its equilibrium position.

Let us consider the effect of $\mathbf{B}_{\text{CCW}}$. This effect can be seen clearly if we establish a new rotating frame $(x'', y'', z)$ that rotates with $\mathbf{B}_{\text{CCW}}$. In this rotating frame, $\mathbf{B}_{\text{CCW}}$ is a constant: $\mathbf{B}_{\text{CCW}} = \frac{1}{2}B_{10}\hat{x}''$. Following a similar procedure described earlier, we find that the effective magnetic field in the new rotating frame is given by

$$\mathbf{B}_{\text{eff}} = \hat{z}\left(B_0 + \frac{\omega_r}{\gamma}\right) + \hat{x}''\frac{B_{10}}{2} = \hat{z}2B_0 + \hat{x}''\frac{B_{10}}{2}. \tag{1.49}$$

This indicates that the magnetization vector will precess about $\mathbf{B}_{\text{eff}}$ at an angular frequency $\omega_{\text{rot}} = \gamma\sqrt{4B_0^2 + \frac{1}{4}B_{10}^2}$. The direction of $\mathbf{B}_{\text{eff}}$ deviates from the $z$ axis by an angle $\theta = \tan^{-1}(B_{10}/4B_0)$. Since the value of $B_{10}$ is several orders of magnitude lower than that of $B_0$, $\omega_{\text{rot}} \approx 2\gamma B_0$ and $\theta \approx 0$; hence, the effect of $\mathbf{B}_{\text{CCW}}$ is negligible. Therefore, only $\mathbf{B}_{\text{CW}}$ has a significant effect on the magnetization vector.

Using the same procedure, we can also show that the effect of frequencies other than the Larmor frequency is also negligible when the frequency is far away from the Larmor frequency. Of course, when the frequency is close to the Larmor frequency, the effect becomes appreciable.

Finally, we would like to compare the effectiveness, in terms of rotating the magnetization vector to a specified angle $\theta_0$, of a linearly polarized $\mathbf{B}_1$ field to that of a circularly polarized $\mathbf{B}_1$ field. The circularly polarized field having a magnitude of $B_{10}^{\text{cir}}$ may be written, as viewed from the rotating

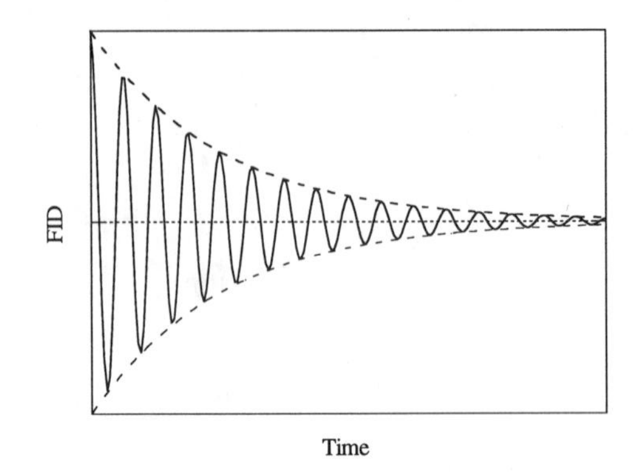


**Figure 1.9.** The received FID after application of a 90° pulse. Because of relaxation, the received NMR signal exhibits exponential decay.

frame, as

$$\mathbf{B}_1^{\text{cir}} = \hat{x}' B_{10}^{\text{cir}} \tag{1.50}$$

and hence the effective magnetic field $B_{\text{eff}} = B_{10}^{\text{cir}}$. This value is twice that realized with a linearly polarized field of the same magnitude. This indicates that it takes twice as much energy input into the system for linear polarization to deflect the magnetization by a given angle. Later, it will be clear that the choice of polarization affects the efficiency of RF reception, which has important implications for SNR.

### 1.2.5 Phenomenological Relaxation—the Bloch Equations

After the application of a 90° RF pulse, our model predicts that the magnetization vector will perpetually rotate in the transverse plane. This is inconsistent with experimental observations, which show a free induction decay (FID) in the received RF signal, as illustrated in Fig. 1.9. In order to explain this effect, we will first examine the phenomenological NMR model due to Bloch and then revise our heuristic model to provide a physical basis for relaxation (decay) of magnetization.

The Bloch equations, as they are commonly known, provide one of the simplest models for the behavior of a nuclear spin system after pulse excitations. The only limitation the model has is that it is based on classical principles, and, as such, cannot explain the finer details of NMR spectra, since these are typically due to complex quantum effects. According to

Canet (1996), the Bloch equations may be written

$$\frac{dM_{x,y}}{dt} = \gamma(\mathbf{M} \times \mathbf{B})_{x,y} - \frac{M_{x,y}}{T_2} \tag{1.51}$$

$$\frac{dM_z}{dt} = \gamma(\mathbf{M} \times \mathbf{B})_z + \frac{M_0 - M_z}{T_1} \tag{1.52}$$

where $T_2$ and $T_1$ are the so-called transverse and longitudinal relaxation times, respectively, and $M_0$ denotes the equilibrium value of magnetization which is assumed to lie in the $z$ direction. Notice that the form of Eqs. (1.51) and (1.52) is very similar to that of the equations we developed based on the behavior of an isolated magnetic moment. We will see that, in fact, the physical causes of relaxation are related to the mutual influence of magnetic moments and their interaction with their environment, factors which we did not consider in the development of the previous model.

For a general solution to the Bloch equations, the reader is referred to Abragam (1978). We wish to examine the special case where the magnetization has been deflected by a 90° pulse. After the pulse, we allow $\mathbf{B}_0$ to persist, and we are interested in the behavior of the magnetization. As we will see, the effect of the relaxation process is the return of the magnetization vector to its equilibrium state. We consider the situation where the RF field has been applied in the transverse plane so that, initially,

$$\mathbf{M}(0) = \hat{x}M_0. \tag{1.53}$$

Solving Eq. (1.51), which may be written as

$$\frac{dM_x}{dt} = \gamma M_y B_0 - \frac{M_x}{T_2} \tag{1.54}$$

$$\frac{dM_y}{dt} = -\gamma M_x B_0 - \frac{M_y}{T_2}, \tag{1.55}$$

we obtain

$$M_x(t) = M_0 \exp\left(-\frac{t}{T_2}\right)\cos(\gamma B_0 t) \tag{1.56}$$

$$M_y(t) = -M_0 \exp\left(-\frac{t}{T_2}\right)\sin(\gamma B_0 t). \tag{1.57}$$

If one uses a properly aligned coil to detect the RF signal thus generated, the received signal, which is often called the FID, appears as in Fig. 1.9.

Turning our attention to the longitudinal component, we notice that since $\mathbf{B}$ lies entirely in the $z$ direction, the quantity $\mathbf{M} \times \mathbf{B}$ never has a non-zero $z$-component. Therefore, the second Bloch equation (1.52) becomes

$$\frac{dM_z}{dt} = \frac{M_0 - M_z}{T_1} \tag{1.58}$$

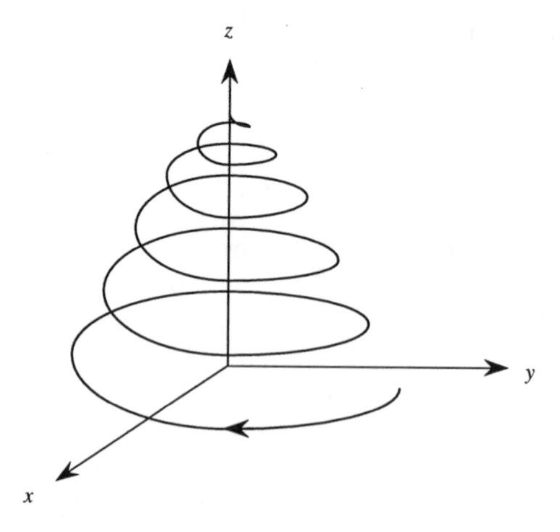


**Figure 1.10.** The path of the tip of the magnetization vector as it returns to equilibrium as viewed from the laboratory frame.

with an initial value

$$M_z(0) = 0. \tag{1.59}$$

The solution of this equation is also well known, and is given by

$$M_z(t) = M_0 \left[ 1 - \exp\left( -\frac{t}{T_1} \right) \right] \tag{1.60}$$

which gradually re-establishes the magnetization in the $z$ direction. From Eqs. (1.56), (1.57), and (1.60), we may now visualize the return of the magnetization vector to equilibrium, as illustrated in Fig. 1.10.

### 1.2.6 Physical Origins of Relaxation

In order to understand the physical origin of relaxation, it is necessary to revise our heuristic model for the behavior of bulk magnetization in the presence of magnetic fields. The classical explanation for relaxation (Bradley *et al.* 1983) starts by considering a sample of material under the influence of no magnetic field. In such a situation, the magnetic moments of the nuclei are randomly oriented, resulting in no net magnetic moment. When the $B_0$ field is applied, all nuclei precess about the $z$-axis at the Larmor frequency with a precessional angle $\theta_0$. However, some of the nuclei precess about the $+z$ axis and the remaining precess about the $-z$ axis (Fig. 1.11). This forms two "cones" of precession, the "upper"

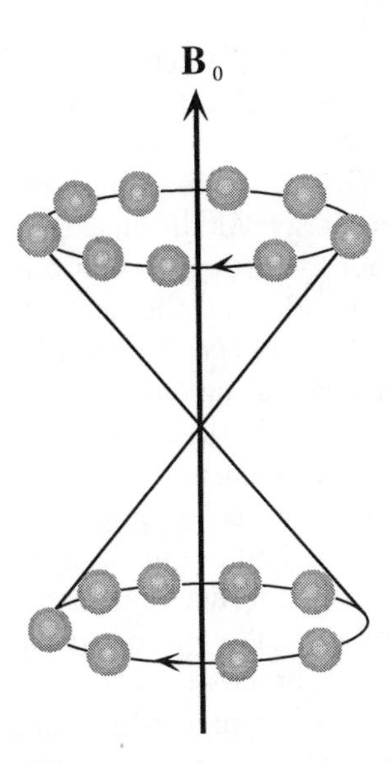


**Figure 1.11.** Nuclei in bulk material under the influence of an applied magnetic field may be imagined as precessing into two cones corresponding to the parallel and anti-parallel states.

cone and "lower" cone, representing the parallel and anti-parallel states of the quantum model, respectively. In most materials at room temperature, more protons precess in the upper cone, resulting in paramagnetic bulk magnetization. It is critical to notice that the phase of nuclei in the upper and lower cones is random, so no net transverse magnetization is produced, despite the fact that each nucleus has a transverse component to its magnetic moment. Upon application of an RF pulse, phase coherence is established in both cones. Since the RF pulse is at the resonant frequency, it also stimulates flipping between the two cones. This allows energy to be imparted into the system. As a result, nuclei, in a net sense, migrate to the anti-parallel cone. Once the population of nuclei in each cone is the same, there is no net axial magnetization. If the pulse were to stop then, it would be a 90° pulse.

After a 90° pulse, as the magnetization precesses in the transverse plane, two types of relaxation occur. "Longitudinal" or "spin-lattice" relaxation brings the axial magnetization back to equilibrium and is quantified by $T_1$, which, therefore, is called the "longitudinal relaxation time." "Transverse" or "spin-spin" relaxation reduces the transverse magnetization to zero and is quantified by $T_2$, which is called the "transverse relaxation time." Most materials of interest have $T_2 < T_1$.

In longitudinal relaxation, nuclei, under the applied $B_0$ field, gradually migrate back to the parallel cone to re-establish their equilibrium population distribution. When a nucleus "flips" back to the parallel cone, it experiences a change in its energy. As shown earlier, this energy difference is characterized by the Larmor frequency. Radiation at the Larmor frequency will stimulate this emission and bring the nuclei back to equilibrium more quickly. The return to equilibrium is called spin-lattice relaxation since the "lattice" is responsible for stimulating and absorbing this release of energy. The "lattice" refers to the matrix in the material to which the nuclei belong. Obviously, positions in the lattice are not static for liquids or gases. The lattice may provide radiation at the resonant frequency through random thermal motions of nuclei. In liquids, molecules are more free to rotate, translate, and collide with one another than they are in solids. Therefore, the chance that stimulated emission will occur is, in general, greater and, consequently, $T_1$ is shorter for liquids than for solids (Young 1984).

In transverse relaxation, the precessing nuclei gradually "de-phase" (that is, lose coherence) until no net transverse magnetization remains. Due to variations in the lattice's composition, which are natural even for a "homogeneous" material since we are thinking on the atomic scale, the magnetic field strength may vary from nucleus to nucleus. These variations are most often due to the motion of other charged particles in the lattice, especially other nuclei (hence the name "spin-spin" relaxation). These types of disturbances are both transient and random. Nuclei precess more quickly in regions of stronger local magnetic fields, while those in weaker fields precess more slowly. As a result, the nuclei lose coherence and de-phase. In liquids, these local fields are very transient and tend to average to zero over short periods of time, while in solids, these fields may persist for much longer periods of time. Therefore, $T_2$ is generally greater for liquids than for solids (Canet 1996). In either type of material, these field fluctuations are random. As a result, the nuclei gradually return to a state of random phasing, where there is no net transverse magnetization.

In reality, however, FIDs received in an RF coil do not have an envelope that decays with time constant $T_2$. Even in the most homogeneous external fields that can be generated today, there are inhomogeneities, especially in human MRI, where the size of the sample is close to that of the magnet. Such inhomogeneities are usually much greater than the inhomogeneities caused by local, microscopic fields. This accelerates the decay of the FID, which is traditionally modeled as having an exponential decay with a new, shorter time constant $T_2^*$. It is important to notice, however, that the envelope of the FID is no longer truly exponential. Nevertheless, this does not prevent one from measuring $T_2$ as long as one is willing to use more

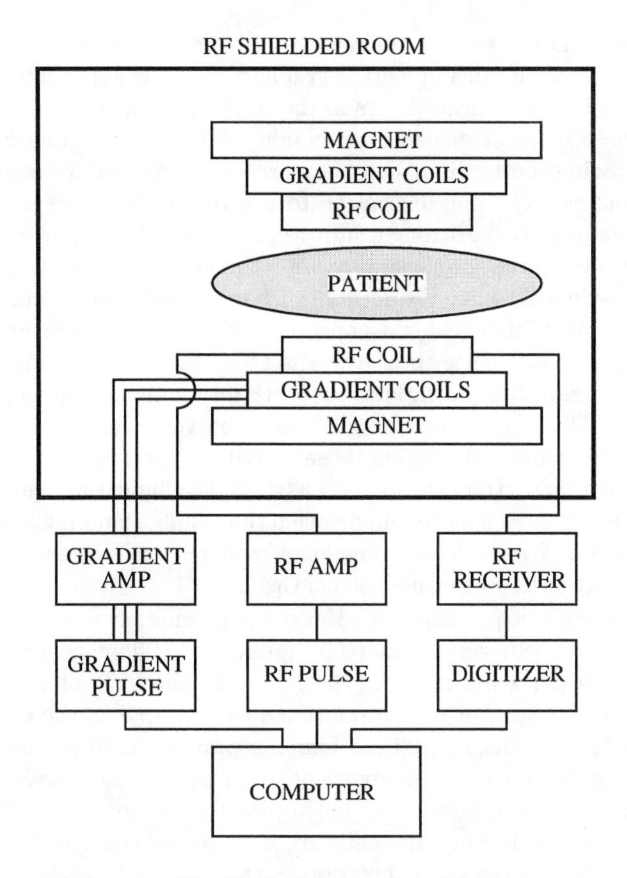


**Figure 1.12.** Block diagram of an MRI system.

elaborate pulse sequences than a simple 90° pulse.

## 1.3 Hardware of Magnetic Resonance Imaging

This section describes the key hardware components in a basic MRI experiment. As illustrated in Fig. 1.12, the key components in an MRI system include a main magnet, a set of gradient coils, an RF coil, a transmitter, a receiver, and a computer.

### 1.3.1 The Main Magnet

In all NMR experiments, it is necessary to generate a strong magnetic field—the $B_0$ field, which is uniform over the volume of interest. Even when field gradients are desired, a main magnet is used to generate a primary field while "gradient coils" create a gradient which is superimposed upon the main field. It is almost always in the interest of the experimenter that the main field be as strong as is economically feasible. A high main field strength provides better SNR and better resolutions both in frequency and spatial domains. The only exception to the rule that "more is better" is when the main field is so strong that it requires RF radiation of a frequency high enough to interact undesirably with the subject under test. This is often a factor in MRI when the effect of such radiation on the human subject is of concern. Very high field NMR spectroscopic systems, however, tend not to be limited by this since these systems typically have very small sample sizes, which diminishes the importance of RF interaction phenomena at high frequencies. This also allows the RF coil to be very close to the majority of the sample volume, enhancing its sensitivity. Spectroscopic systems are available with field strengths as high as 17.5 T. Clinical imaging systems typically have field strengths no stronger than 2 T. Some functional MRI systems have 3 T or 4 T main magnets, and research systems are being developed with even higher field strengths.

The primary requirement for the main magnet, however, is that its field be uniform. In clinical imaging applications, homogeneities on the order of a few parts per million (ppm) over a spherical volume 50 cm in diameter are typical. For high resolution spectroscopy, on the other hand, homogeneities as high as 1 part per billion over a spherical volume 5 mm in diameter may be required. In any event, the main magnet rarely produces a field of sufficient uniformity by itself. For this reason, "shim" coils are frequently employed. The shim coils are a set of coils designed to produce a field, polarized in the same direction as the main field, of known spatial dependence. In the case of a coil-type main magnet, such as a resistive or superconducting magnet, there will typically be several coaxial shim coils: one with $z$ dependence (linear), one with $z^2$ dependence (quadratic), and so on, where $z$ is the axial direction of the coil. In this way, if the main magnet's non-uniformity is known, the shims can be set to carry gradients which cancel (by superposition) the inhomogeneous components of the main field. More frequently, however, less direct empirical procedures are used to adjust the shims since the main field's inhomogeneity is generally difficult to characterize.

Depending upon the application, permanent, resistive, or superconducting magnets may be used. Permanent magnets offer the advantages of simplicity and affordability. They also typically have very weak fringe fields, which makes site planning easier since the apparatus does not need to be heavily shielded to avoid unwanted interactions that might result from a magnetic field extending outside of the room of the experiment. Permanent magnets may also be very small, which has recently generated interest in their possible use in microfluidic NMR spectroscopy (NMRS), where very small samples are used. In MRI applications using permanent magnets, the subject is placed between the two poles of the magnet. It is not easy, however, to shape the pole faces to provide a very uniform magnetic field over the volume of interest. The temperature drift of permanent magnets is also a non-trivial problem since the RF frequency is usually not controlled by any type of feedback and would therefore not remain at the Larmor frequency if the temperature were to change after calibration.

Resistive magnets are based on the principle of the Helmholtz coil pair. As such, they use currents in "imperfect" conductors to produce magnetic fields. This causes subsequent heat loss of the system which is often the limiting factor in how strong the field may be. Cooling systems are often required to dissipate the heat. MRI systems using resistive magnets typically have field strengths from 0.05 to 0.4 T, with the upper limit primarily due to the difficulty associated with heat dissipation. The lower limit is dominated by a complicated trade-off among resolution, imaging quality, and acquisition time. In addition to not being very strong, resistive magnets are extremely inefficient. However, they are easy and inexpensive to fabricate and maintain, and can be easily turned off.

Superconducting magnets are becoming very common in MRI and high resolution NMRS applications. Any desired field strength over 0.5 T practically requires the use of superconducting magnets despite their high cost and complexity. The coil windings, made from an alloy such as niobium-titanium, are cooled to temperatures below 12 Kelvin by immersion in liquid helium, whose boiling point is 4.2 K (Gadian 1995). The consequent loss of liquid helium can be very expensive (Olendorf 1988). In addition, the magnet may "quench" if it gets too hot and stops superconducting. However, the fields produced by a properly designed superconducting magnet can be very strong, homogeneous, and stable.

### 1.3.2 The Gradient Coils

All MRI modalities and many localized spectroscopic techniques require deliberate inhomogeneities to be introduced into the $B_0$ field. As noted previously, the Larmor frequency depends on the magnetic field strength. This being the case, known inhomogeneities can be used to frequency encode spatial information about the returned signal. For such schemes to be successful, the known, applied gradient must not be dominated by the unknown, undesired fluctuations in the field produced by the main magnet. Many clinical imaging systems are capable of producing 10 $\mathrm{mT{\cdot}m^{-1}}$ gradients to this end.

In addition to strong gradients, some imaging techniques require gradient pulsing. The duration of these pulses must typically be on the order of $T_2$ to be effective. Since gradient coils have a natural self-inductance, they cannot be switched on or off instantaneously. Coils with large inductances may be driven to their desired steady state quickly at the expense of power by using compensating driver circuitry, which adds complexity to the system. The switching of gradient coils induces undesirable eddy currents in the surrounding structures, especially the magnet, which may distort gradient uniformity. To compensate for this, so-called "pre-emphasis" pulse shaping may be used or some form of passive or active shielding may be employed.

In addition, desired gradients are typically linear, since the mathematics of most imaging schemes depends on this simple type of gradient. At the very least, the shape of the gradient must give unambiguous spatial information about the sample. That is to say that, given the local field strength, there should be only one point in space that may be inferred from knowledge of the gradient's spatial dependence. This is not a significant problem for most coils in their field-of-view (FOV).

Gradients for most modern imaging schemes can be produced in any of the three spatial directions without physically rotating the gradient coils. Notice that, although the variation of the field may be in the transverse plane, the only component of interest in the produced field is oriented in the axial direction since this is the direction of the main field.

### 1.3.3 The Transmitter

As we have seen, it is necessary to irradiate the sample under test with an RF field—the $B_1$ field, in order to tip the magnetization away from its equilibrium position and generate a detectable NMR signal. In practice, RF fields are produced by a transmitter and an RF coil. The transmitter is responsible for pulse shape, duration, power, and timing (repetition rate). The RF coil is responsible for coupling the energy generated by the transmitter to the nuclei of the sample.

To generate an RF pulse, the transmitter first uses a frequency synthesizer to generate an oscillation of a user-defined frequency. Then, a waveform generator creates a user-defined pulse shape which is subsequently mixed (multiplied) with the pure tone; thus, an RF pulse is created. Once this is done, the pulse, or a sequence of various pulses, is repeated at a user-defined repetition rate.

Modern transmitters typically use digital pulse shape generators. As such, their minimum time resolution may be an important consideration. However, most experimental concerns regarding transmitters relate to pulse sequence and shape design, which are often not considerably encumbered by the hardware employed.

There are two fundamental types of pulses employed in NMR: "hard" and "soft" pulses. Hard pulses are typically rectangular pulses which are broadband. The name "hard" refers to the lack of frequency selectivity employed with this type of pulse. In fact, in order to get the spectrum of the pulse to be uniform over the range of interest, one must often shorten the pulse, which further extends the bandwidth. Recall the fact that the Fourier transform of a rectangular pulse is a sinc function whose center, if the original pulse is sufficiently short, may be considered as flat over a small band.

Soft pulses, on the other hand, are often sinc-shaped in order to provide frequency selectivity. This is frequently desirable in imaging and localized spectroscopy techniques. However, a good sinc shape requires some "lead-in" time before the peak of the pulse. This may be a limiting factor in how selective the pulse can be. In soft pulsing, one must also be sure that the center frequency is close to the actual Larmor frequency of the system. Since such a pulse is usually narrowband, one may lose a good deal of efficiency from a relatively small frequency error. More complicated pulses other than the sinc shaped pulse can also be designed for improved frequency selectivity.

### 1.3.4 The RF Coils

In all NMR, it is necessary to excite the nuclei into coherent precession. This requires coupling between the nuclei and some source of RF power (the transmitter). To receive a meaningful signal, one also needs a device to couple the nuclei to some external circuitry. These devices are called RF coils.

The RF coil, also known as an RF resonator or RF probe, is responsive to frequencies in the general band defined by the Larmor frequency of interest. It is desirable for the FOV of the coil to be filled by the sample and little else so that no unnecessary noise is introduced into the received signal, or equivalently, so that little power is wasted from the transmitter. This often requires that the probe have dimensions comparable to the sample. For sample sizes much smaller than the corresponding wavelength, a solenoidal coil may be an efficient resonator. This is usually the case in spectroscopic experiments.

In human imaging, the wavelength is generally the same order of magnitude as the sample. To build an effective "coil" in this case is very difficult. Traditionally, saddle coils have been preferred over solenoids as they allow better patient access when the main magnet is also of a solenoidal shape. Increasingly, however, a design called the "birdcage coil" is being used. This coil cleverly combines lumped capacitors with distributed "leg" inductance to form a volume resonator. The resonance, if the coil is designed correctly, increases the efficiency of the coil at operating frequencies. The lumped capacitors provide a way for the resonator to store electrical energy without storing an electrical field in the patient. This is very desirable since electric fields typically lead to conduction currents in any type of sample, which introduces some loss of efficiency. In humans, the heating generated by conduction currents is often a safety concern for the patient.

It is also very important that the coil generates a very uniform $B_1$ magnetic field, since the tip angle is a function of field magnitude. By reciprocity, a coil which generates an inhomogeneous field will also have an inhomogeneous sensitivity in its FOV. Any inhomogeneities will introduce distortions into images. Although mathematical techniques and certain pulse sequences can overcome this, inhomogeneity is generally undesirable. Unfortunately, the requirement for a sharp FOV and a uniform field distribution are fundamentally in direct conflict, so a trade-off is always necessary. One approach to resolving this conflict is to use two RF coils: one for transmitting and the other for receiving.

It is also desirable to have a coil which permits "quadrature" excitation and detection. Electromagnetically, this is equivalent to being able to generate and receive circularly polarized fields. Recall that we have previously argued that the most effective way to couple energy into the nuclei (and, by reciprocity, out of them) is by using circularly polarized fields that rotate at the Larmor frequency. For this, a circuit is needed to split equally the transmitting power into two channels and introduce a 90° phase delay in one of the channels. These two channels are then fed to the two inputs of the RF coil to produce two fields perpendicular to each other. For receiving, a circuit is also needed to introduce a 90° phase delay in one of the two output signals so that both signals are in phase and can be combined coherently. The two circuits can actually be combined into one (Fig. 1.13).

### 1.3.5 The Receiver

To convert the received RF signal from the RF coil into a form suitable for an analog-to-digital converter (ADC) or digitizer, some receiver circuitry is often employed. The use of ADCs is pervasive in modern NMR as it allows digital signal processing. The first stage of the receiver is often a so-called "low noise amplifier" (LNA) which prevents the weak received signal from being dominated by noise as it travels down a transmission line to the main

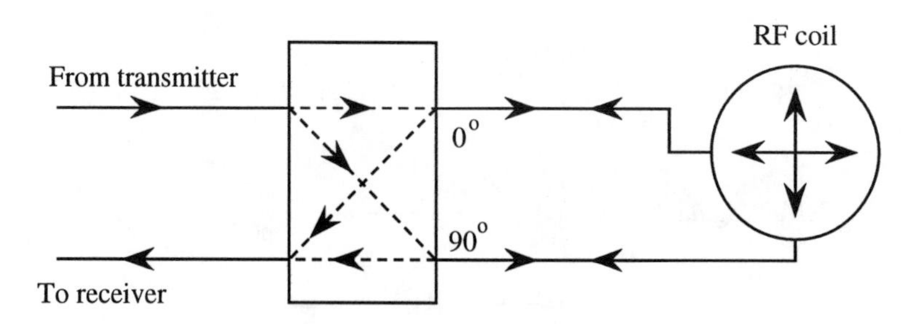


**Figure 1.13.** A 3-dB coupler splits the transmitting power into two channels and introduces a 90°-phase shift in one of the channels to provide quadrature excitation. During reception, it combines two signals with a 90°-phase correction.

receiver. The second stage of the receiver is a transmission line to carry the RF signal from the RF coil to a remote location where it is more convenient to have bulky circuitry.

The rest of the receiver is often a superheterodyne style circuit used to demodulate the signal from the RF band into a low frequency band which the ADC or other data analyzing equipment can handle. This demodulation is usually done with respect to a reference frequency set to the same frequency as the emitted RF radiation.

## 1.4 Basic Pulse Sequences and Imaging Methods

This section describes briefly the basic RF pulse sequences to measure $T_1$ and $T_2$ and basic imaging methods to obtain MR images. Again, for a more comprehensive treatment of the topic, the reader is referred to other books, such as Chen and Hoult (1989), Parikh (1991), Rinck (1993), and Vlaardingerbroek and den Boer (1996).

### 1.4.1 RF Pulse Sequences

The simplest pulse sequence used in NMR imaging and spectroscopy is known as "partial saturation." This sequence consists of repeated 90° pulses with the interval $T_R$, as illustrated in Fig. 1.14.

The first pulse tips the equilibrium magnetization vector into the transverse plane. The FID generated immediately after this pulse has a maximum value that we will call $\text{FID}_0$. It is customary to make $T_R > 5T_2^*$, so that the transverse magnetization will decay to zero before the next pulse is applied. Since most materials have $T_1 >> T_2$, the axial magnetization may not necessarily have recovered. Therefore, upon application of the

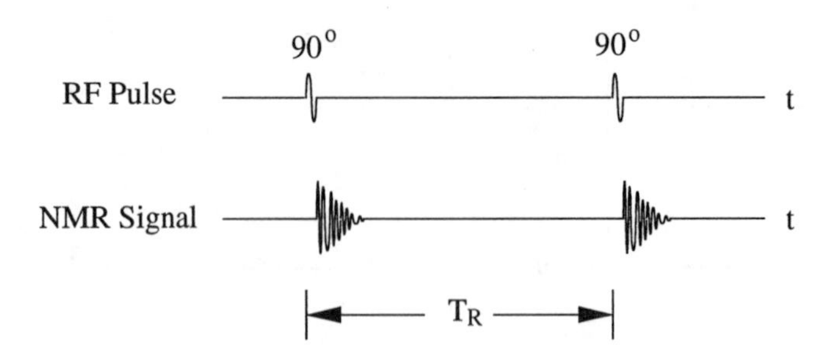


**Figure 1.14.** Partial saturation sequence.

second pulse, the initial value of the new FID is given by

$$\mathrm{FID}_1 = \mathrm{FID}_0 \left[1 - \exp\left(-\frac{T_R}{T_1}\right)\right]. \tag{1.61}$$

Apparently, for a fixed $T_R$, $\mathrm{FID}_1$ is greater for a shorter $T_1$ and weaker for a longer $T_1$. Therefore, the partial saturation sequence can be used to distinguish materials of different $T_1$ when the materials have the same hydrogen density. More commonly, the partial saturation sequence is used to measure the density or concentration of one chemical species in the presence of another NMR sensitive species, using so-called $T_1$ discrimination. It should be clear that since $\mathrm{FID}_0$ depends upon the equilibrium value of magnetization $M_0$, it, in turn, depends linearly upon the concentration of the species in question. If the species to be measured has a shorter $T_1$ than the other species, one may suppress the undesired FID by selecting $T_R$ so that the undesired species' magnetization does not recover fully between sequence repetitions. If the repetition rate can be chosen so that the desired species still fully recovers, then the undesired species may be suppressed to any degree, by simply acquiring enough repetitions since the undesired FID gets smaller and smaller each time.

Another common sequence used in practice is called the "inversion recovery" sequence, which is primarily used to measure $T_1$ and/or species concentration. Notice that it is necessary to measure longitudinal relaxation in such roundabout ways since we cannot observe the return of the axial magnetization to equilibrium with an RF coil. In inversion recovery, a 180° pulse is applied, followed by a latent time $T_I$, and a 90° pulse, as shown in Fig. 1.15. The total frame repetition time is denoted as $T_R$.

After the application of a 180° pulse, the magnetization vector is rotated down to the $-z$ axis and, hence, no FID is observed since the magnetization has no transverse component. During the first lag time, the magnetization in the axial direction is recovering. Application of a 90°

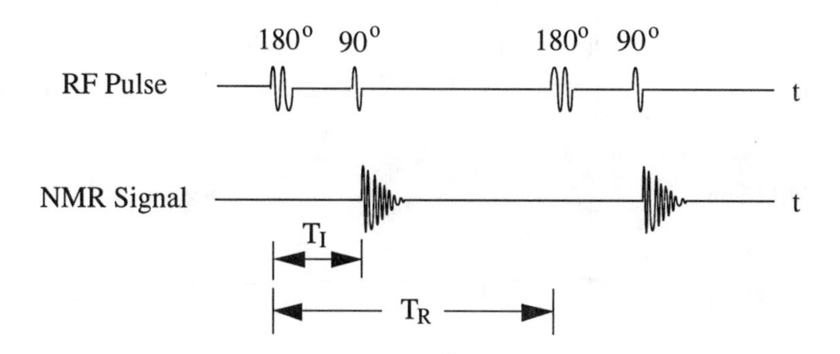


**Figure 1.15.** Inversion recovery sequence.

pulse at this point causes the unrecovered magnetization vector to fall into the transverse plane. This generates an FID whose initial value is related to the equilibrium magnetization by

$$\mathrm{FID}_0 \propto M_0 \left[1 - 2\exp\left(-\frac{T_I}{T_1}\right)\right]. \tag{1.62}$$

From this equation, we can see that the proper choice of the time delay, $T_I$, may annihilate the FID altogether. This is one way to use inversion recovery for $T_1$ discrimination. This technique is advantageous since it allows an arbitrary relationship to exist between the $T_1$ values of the desired and undesired species.

So far, however, we have not discussed a technique to measure $T_2$. One may get a rough estimate of $T_2^*$ simply by observing points on the envelope of the FID; but, since this parameter depends on external field inhomogeneities, it is rarely of interest. The so-called "spin echo" sequence provides a way to measure $T_2$. This sequence consists of a 90° pulse, followed by a time delay $T_E/2$, a 180° pulse, and another time delay (Fig. 1.16). As usual, let $T_R$ denote the length of a frame.

To understand this sequence, it is essential to recognize that the static inhomogeneities of the external field, creating different Larmor frequencies for different regions, are time independent and, thus, the spin dephasing caused by these is reversible. After the 90° pulse, the magnetization lies wholly in the transverse plane. Here it is instructive to consider the positions of individual magnetic moments in the rotating reference frame. To this end, let the 90° pulse be applied along the $x'$ axis, which results in the magnetization being aligned with the $y'$ axis, where coherence has been established [Fig. 1.17(a)]. Now, those nuclei which are under the influence of slightly stronger fields will rotate faster and, hence, have some net rotation in the frame that rotates at the "mean" Larmor frequency.

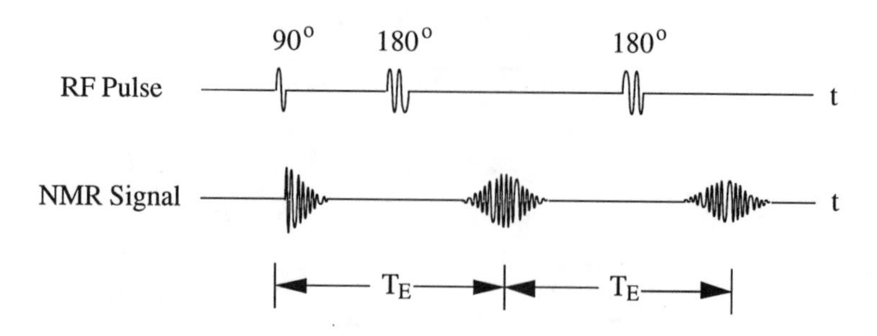


**Figure 1.16.** Spin echo sequence.

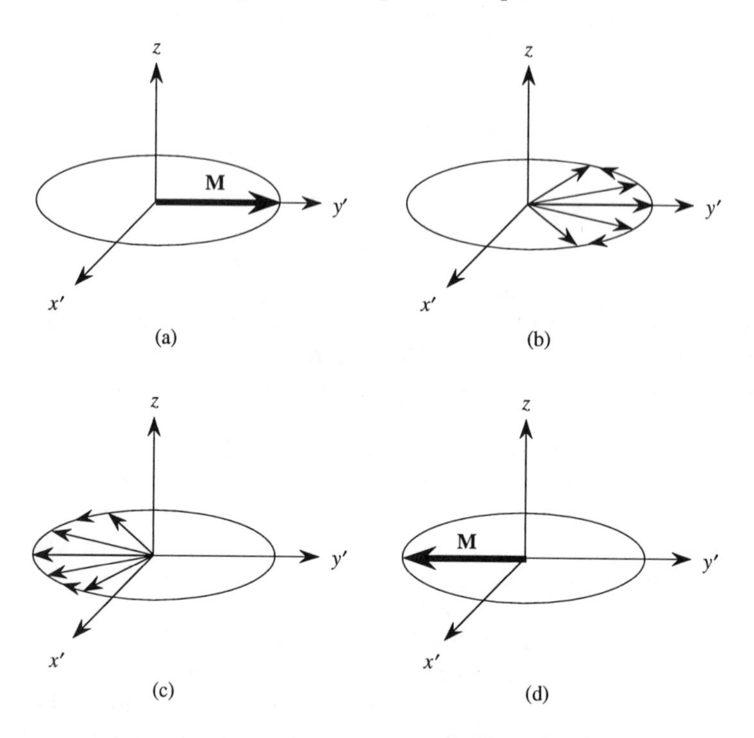


**Figure 1.17.** (a) After a 90° pulse, the magnetization lies along the $y'$ axis. (b) Because of field inhomogeneity, the nuclei start to lose coherence. (c) Application of a 180° pulse rotates the magnetization. (d) The coherence is re-established.

Those under the influence of weaker fields will rotate slowly, lag behind, and experience a negative-sensed net rotation in the frame [Fig. 1.17(b)]. Coherence is quickly destroyed by this action, and the FID decays to zero.

However, if we now apply a 180° pulse, also along the $x'$ axis, each

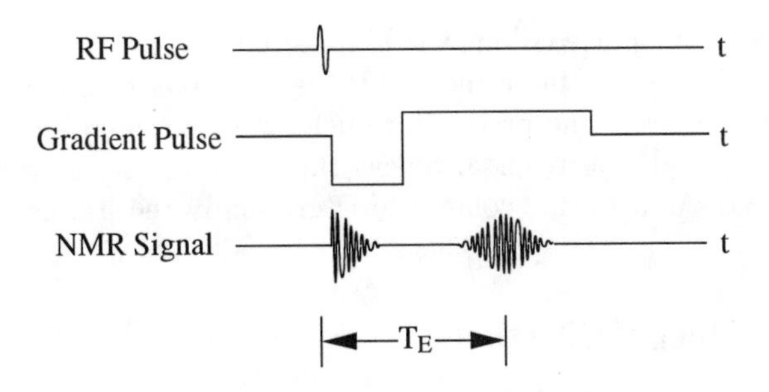


**Figure 1.18.** Gradient echo sequence.

individual magnetic moment will be rotated 180° about the $x'$ axis [Fig. 1.17(c)]. Notice that now the faster nuclei are behind the mean nuclei and the slower nuclei are ahead. Therefore, the faster nuclei will eventually cross the paths of the slower nuclei and coherence is again temporarily established [Fig. 1.17(d)]. At this point, however, the peak value of the so-called "echo" signal will not be equal in magnitude to the initial value of the FID, because spin-spin relaxation effects also degrade the spin phase coherence in a random way which is not reversible by the 180° pulse. The peak value of the echo ($E_0$) is related to the initial value of the $\mathrm{FID}_0$ by

$$E_0 = \mathrm{FID}_0 \exp\left(-\frac{T_E}{T_2}\right). \tag{1.63}$$

One measurement, then, suffices to infer the value of $T_2$. Often, however, one may apply additional 180° pulses to generate additional echoes for the sake of increased accuracy. It is seen that $T_2$ discrimination may be accomplished by suppressing the spin echo of a species with a short $T_2$ through the use of a relatively long $T_E$.

A technique of importance for $T_2^*$ measurement is called the "gradient echo" sequence. Since $T_2^*$ is shorter for regions of poor field homogeneity, its value may be used to find areas such as tissue-air interfaces where one would expect poor homogeneity. In functional neuroimaging, one is often interested in the field gradients that occur naturally around deoxyhaemoglobin molecules (Gadian 1995). A $T_2^*$ weighted image may therefore be used to provide a map of deoxyhaemoglobin concentration, which can be correlated to neural activity.

In the gradient echo sequence, a 90° pulse is applied followed by a deliberate gradient, generated by superimposing a gradient field on the $B_0$ field. The field gradient is then reversed at a later time (Fig. 1.18). To understand this sequence, we again examine the situation as viewed from the rotating frame. The 90° pulse, applied along the $x'$ direction, causes the magnetization to be placed along the $y'$ direction. Nuclei found in stronger fields begin to precess in the frame and those in weaker field regions precess in the opposite sense. The precessing nuclei start to de-phase. When the gradient is reversed, the reversal places the "fast" nuclei in weaker fields and vice versa. As a result, coherence is gradually re-established at time $T_E$.

### 1.4.2 Basic Imaging Methods

The basic principle behind all imaging methods is the resonance equation given by $\omega_r = \gamma B_0$. One of the first such techniques to develop historically was "back projection" imaging. For simplicity, we consider the problem of imaging a slice of a three-dimensional object. This slice can be frequency selected by applying a steep gradient in the direction perpendicular to the slice. To describe this process, let the imaging plane lie in the $xy$-plane. This plane is chosen simply for convenience and does not mean that the slice must lie transverse to the $B_0$ field. Assume that we wish to select a slice located at $z_0$ with thickness $\Delta z$. We apply a $z$ gradient so that the magnetic field is given by $B_0 + zG_z$. To excite the nuclei within the slice, we irradiate the object with an RF sinc pulse whose center frequency is given by $\omega_0 = \gamma(B_0 + z_0 G_z)$ and frequency bandwidth by $\Delta\omega = \gamma \Delta z G_z$. Since the sinc pulse contains only frequencies within the band, only nuclei in the slice are excited and those outside the slice are not affected.

Now, return to the back projection imaging method, whose RF and gradient pulse sequences are shown in Fig. 1.19. First, we apply a $z$ gradient and irradiate the subject with an RF sinc pulse to excite the nuclei in the slice. This is followed by a smaller negative $z$ gradient to re-phase the nuclei across the thickness of the slice. As soon as the RF pulse and the $z$ gradient are turned off, an $x$ gradient ($G_x$) is turned on and the FID is recorded. The frequency of the FID is given by $\omega = \gamma(B_0 + xG_x)$, which provides a unique relationship between position along the $x$-axis and frequency of the returned NMR signal. Such a relationship is known as "frequency encoding." Since the $x$ gradient is applied during the recording of FID, this gradient is also called the read-out gradient, in addition to the frequency encoding gradient. Then, we repeat the process with the read-out gradient at an angle $\phi$ from the $x$-axis. The required read-out gradient ($G_f$) can be generated using the $x$ and $y$ gradients with

$$G_x = G_f \cos\phi, \qquad G_y = G_f \sin\phi. \tag{1.64}$$

This process can be repeated for many different angles, from which many projections are obtained. The data can then be transformed by a computer to form a two-dimensional image.

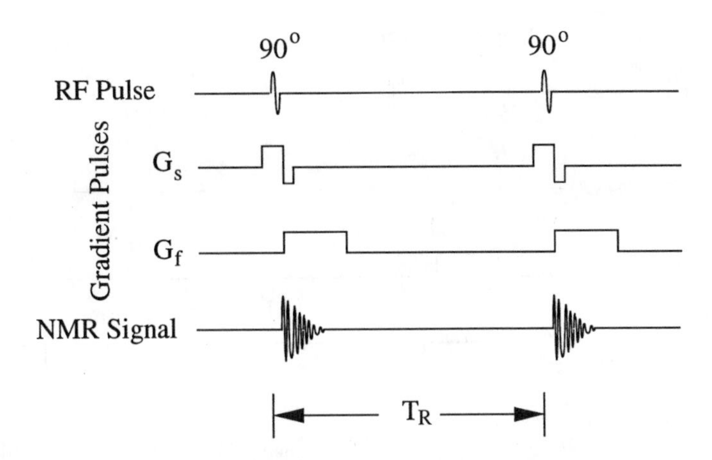


**Figure 1.19.** Back projection imaging sequence.

The back projection technique is really a form of computed tomography, and, as such, can be computationally intensive. There is usually some distortion left in the image as a consequence of taking an insufficient number of such projections for complete reconstruction. The type of distortion introduced by taking a finite number of projections is blurring of sharp corners and other features. Also, field inhomogeneities are detrimental to this technique.

Historically, one of the next imaging techniques to arise was called the two-dimensional Fourier transform (2DFT) technique. Again, consider the imaging of a slice of a 3D object. For this, one first defines the slice to be imaged by applying a steep gradient perpendicular to this slice. Let us assume that the slice is parallel to the $xy$-plane and, therefore, the steep gradient to be applied is the $z$ gradient. Next, it is necessary to "phase-encode" the $y$-axis. This is accomplished by applying a $y$ gradient pulse. During the application of the pulse, nuclei in regions of stronger magnetic field strength will precess faster than those in regions of weaker field strength. As a result, after some finite time, there will be an accumulated phase difference among the nuclei. Usually, for the first acquisition, the pulse is halted once nuclei on the edges of the sample have accumulated a phase difference of 180°. When the cycle is repeated, progressively larger phase shifts are deliberately induced in each cycle. This is done in order to increase the resolution in the $y$ direction, which, for this technique, depends on the number of such acquisitions.

A read-out gradient is then applied in the $x$ direction. It is during this gradient that NMR signals are actually acquired by the instrumentation.

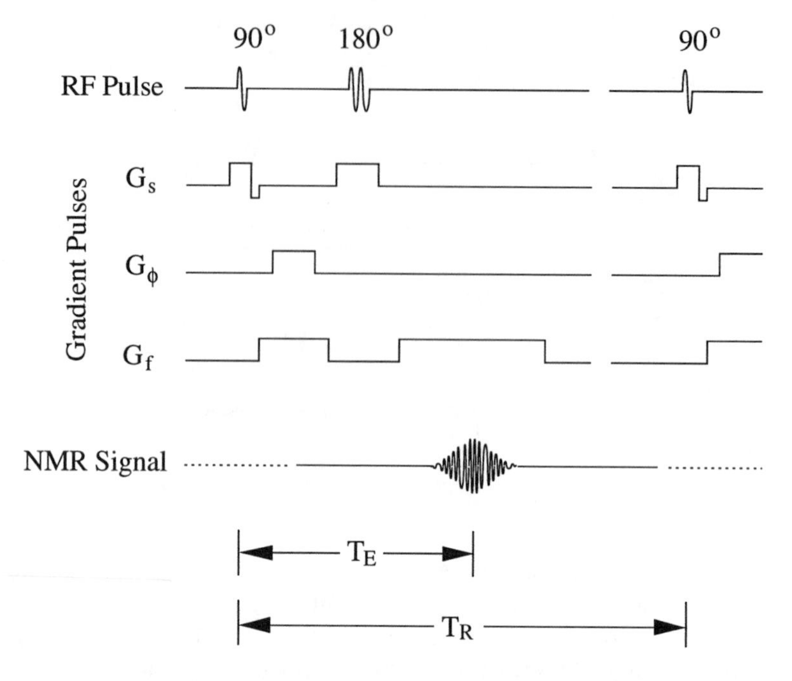


**Figure 1.20.** Spin echo imaging sequence.

The result of this gradient is to frequency encode the $x$-axis in much the same way as encoding was done in projection reconstruction.

This technique can be used in conjunction with spin echo, inversion recovery, and gradient echo pulse sequences. Figure 1.20 shows the spin echo imaging sequence. First, a slice selective 90° RF pulse is applied together with a slice selection gradient. The FID found immediately after the 90° RF pulse is not used. A phase encoding gradient ($G_\phi$) is then applied together with a frequency encoding gradient to de-phase the spins. The frequency encoding gradient is applied here so that the spins will re-phase by the center of the echo. After that, a slice selective 180° RF pulse is applied in conjunction with the slice selection gradient to re-phase the spins. Finally, the frequency encoding gradient is applied and the echo is recorded. The entire sequence is repeated with different phase encoding gradient amplitudes.

The inversion recovery imaging sequence that uses the spin echo is given in Fig. 1.21. The sequence starts with a slice selective 180° RF pulse in conjunction with a slice selection gradient. The remainder of the sequence after a time $T_I$ is the same as the spin echo imaging sequence.

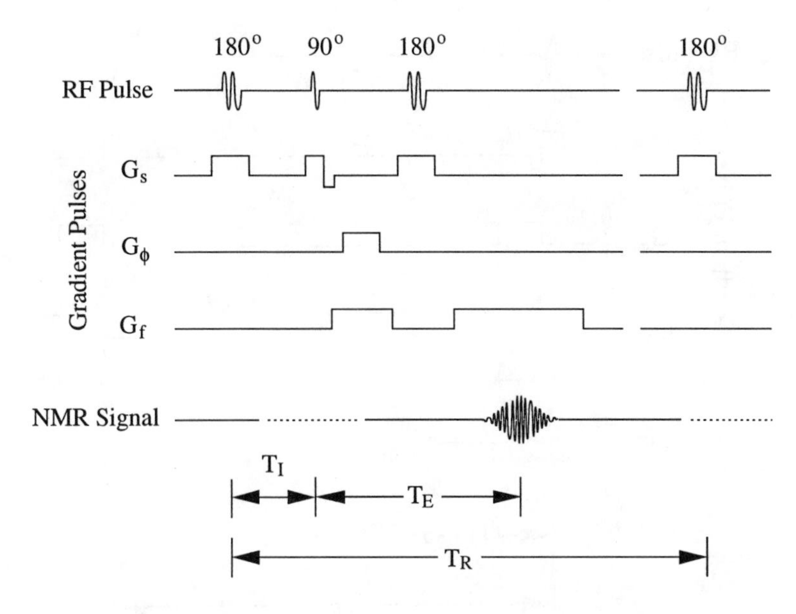


**Figure 1.21.** Inversion recovery imaging sequence.

Both spin echo and inversion recovery sequences employ 90° and 180° RF pulses. The imaging method using the gradient echo sequence, depicted in Fig. 1.22, however, does not require 90° RF pulses. In this sequence, a slice selective RF pulse is applied in conjunction with a slice selection gradient to rotate the magnetization vector away from the $z$-axis with an angle between 10° and 90°. A phase encoding gradient is then applied together with a negative frequency encoding gradient. When the phase encoding gradient is turned off, the frequency encoding gradient is reversed, producing the gradient echo. The entire sequence is repeated with different phase encoding gradient amplitudes.

The main advantage of the 2DFT imaging methods is that they produce sharper images and introduce less natural distortion. Also, 2DFT is much less sensitive to field inhomogeneities than projection reconstruction. Field inhomogeneities produce feature size distortions in 2DFT images rather than blurring as in projection reconstruction. It turns out that for most medical purposes, the former type of distortion is more tolerable. For this reason, 2DFT is one of the most commonly used imaging techniques (Gadian 1995).

Finally, we mention that since NMR signals depend on several parameters such as $T_1$, $T_2$, $T_2^*$, and spin density, the NMR images depend on these parameters as well and thus can be given different contrast by

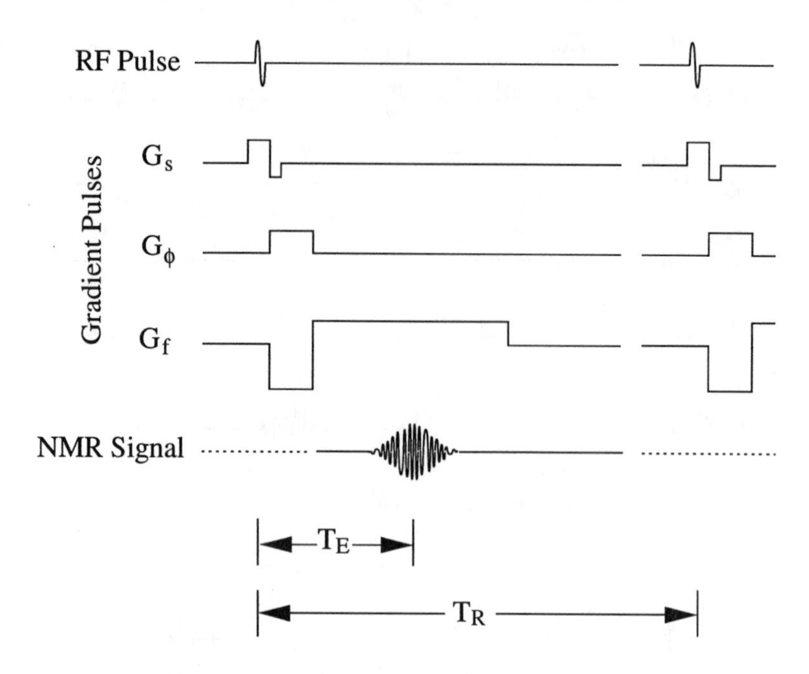


**Figure 1.22.** Gradient echo imaging sequence.

adjusting the experimental parameters, such as $T_E$, $T_I$, and $T_R$. For example, $T_1$ contrast can be achieved through $T_R$ and $T_I$, and $T_2$ contrast can be adjusted by $T_E$. This is a very attractive feature of MRI since biological tissues can be differentiated by their $T_1$, $T_2$, and spin density values.

## References


A. Abragam (1978), *The Principles of Nuclear Magnetism.* Oxford: Oxford University Press.

W. G. Bradley, T. H. Newton, and L. E. Crooks (1983), "Physical principles of nuclear magnetic resonance," *Modern Neuroradiology, Volume II: Advanced Imaging Techniques.* San Anselmo, CA: Clavadel Press.

D. Canet (1996), *Nuclear Magnetic Resonance: Concepts and Methods.* New York: John Wiley & Sons.

C. N. Chen and D. I. Hoult (1989), *Biomedical Magnetic Resonance Technology.* Bristol: Adam Hilger.

D. G. Gadian (1995), *NMR and its Applications to Living Systems* (2nd edition). Oxford: Oxford University Press.

J. P. Hornak (1996), *The Basics of MRI.* http://www.cis.rit.edu/htbooks/mri.

P. C. Lauterbur (1973), "Image formation by induced local interactions: examples employing nuclear magnetic resonance," *Nature,* vol. 242, pp. 190–191.

P. Mansfield and P. G. Morris (1982), *NMR Imaging in Biomedicine.* New York: Academic Press.

P. G. Morris (1986), *Nuclear Magnetic Resonance Imaging in Medicine and Biology.* Oxford: Oxford University Press.

W. H. Olendorf (1988), "A comparison of resistive, superconducting and permanent magnets," *Magnetic Resonance Imaging* (2nd edition). Philadelphia: W. B. Saunders Co.

A. M. Parikh (1991), *Magnetic Resonance Imaging Techniques.* New York: Elsevier.

R. R. Price, W. H. Stephens, and C. L. Partain (1988), "NMR physical principles," *Magnetic Resonance Imaging* (2nd edition). Philadelphia: W. B. Saunders Co.

P. Rinck (1993), *Magnetic Resonance in Medicine.* Oxford: Blackwell Scientific Publications.

R. Sigal (1988), *Magnetic Resonance Imaging: Basis for Interpretation.* New York: Springer-Verlag.

C. P. Slichter (1996), *Principles of Magnetic Resonance* (3rd edition). New York: Springer-Verlag.

D. Stark and W. G. Bradley (1992), *Magnetic Resonance Imaging.* St Louis, MO: Mosby Year Book.

M. T. Vlaardingerbroek and J. A. den Boer (1996), *Magnetic Resonance Imaging: Theory and Practice.* Berlin: Springer-Verlag.

S. W. Young (1984), *Nuclear Magnetic Resonance Imaging: Basic Principles.* New York: Raven Press.

# Chapter 2

# Basic Electromagnetic Theory

## 2.1 Introduction

To understand the basic principles of magnets, gradient coils, and radio-frequency (RF) resonators used in magnetic resonance imaging (MRI), we must first understand basic electromagnetic theory. In this chapter, we first review some basic concepts and formulae of vector analysis, and then review the basic theory of static magnetic fields and time-harmonic electromagnetic fields. Our emphasis is on the topics that are closely related to MRI. These include Helmholtz and Maxwell coils, inductance calculations, and the magnetic fields produced by some special cylindrical and spherical surface currents that form the foundation for birdcage coil and magnet designs. Some more advanced concepts will be introduced later. For a complete account of electromagnetic theory, the readers are referred to some of the many good textbooks, such as those by Cheng (1993), Elliot (1966), Hayt (1989), Jackson (1975), Johnk (1975), Kraus (1992), Miner (1996), Plonus (1978), and Rao (1994).

## 2.2 Brief Review of Vector Analysis

The most useful concepts in vector analysis are those of divergence, curl, and gradient. In this section, we present the definitions for these quantities and the related theorems.

Assume that **A** is a vector function whose magnitude and direction are functions of space. The divergence of vector function **A** is defined as

$$\nabla \cdot \mathbf{A} = \lim_{\Delta v \to 0} \frac{1}{\Delta v} \left[ \oiint_s \mathbf{A} \cdot d\mathbf{s} \right] \tag{2.1}$$

where $s$ is the surface enclosing volume $\Delta v$ and $\mathbf{ds}$ is normal to $s$ and points outward. The explicit expressions for the divergence in rectangular, cylindrical, and spherical coordinates are given in Appendix 2.A at the end of this chapter. From the definition of divergence, we can show that

$$\iiint_V \nabla \cdot \mathbf{A}\, dv = \oiint_S \mathbf{A} \cdot \mathbf{ds} \tag{2.2}$$

if vector $\mathbf{A}$ and its first derivative are continuous in volume $V$ as well as on its surface $S$. Equation (2.2) is known as the divergence theorem or Gauss's theorem.

The curl of vector function $\mathbf{A}$ is defined as

$$\nabla \times \mathbf{A} = \lim_{\Delta v \to 0} \frac{1}{\Delta v} \left[ \oiint_s \mathbf{ds} \times \mathbf{A} \right] \tag{2.3}$$

whose magnitude in the direction of $\hat{n}$ is given by

$$\hat{n} \cdot (\nabla \times \mathbf{A}) = \lim_{\Delta s \to 0} \frac{1}{\Delta s} \left[ \oint_c \mathbf{A} \cdot \mathbf{dl} \right] \tag{2.4}$$

where $c$ is the contour bounding surface $\Delta s$, and $\hat{n}$ denotes the unit vector normal to $\Delta s$. The directions of $\hat{n}$ and $\hat{l}$ are related by the right-hand rule. The explicit expressions for the curl in rectangular, cylindrical, and spherical coordinates are also given in Appendix 2.A. From the definition of curl, it can be shown that

$$\iint_S (\nabla \times \mathbf{A}) \cdot \mathbf{ds} = \oint_C \mathbf{A} \cdot \mathbf{dl} \tag{2.5}$$

if vector $\mathbf{A}$ and its first derivative are continuous on surface $S$ as well as along contour $C$ that bounds $S$. Equation (2.5) is known as the curl theorem or Stokes's theorem.

Assume that $F$ is a scalar function of space. The gradient of scalar function $F$ is defined as

$$\nabla F = \lim_{\Delta v \to 0} \frac{1}{\Delta v} \left[ \oiint_s F\, \mathbf{ds} \right] \tag{2.6}$$

whose magnitude in the direction of $\hat{n}$ is given by

$$\hat{n} \cdot \nabla F = \frac{dF}{dn}. \tag{2.7}$$

From the definition of gradient, we can show that

$$\iiint_V \nabla F\, dv = \oiint_S F\, \mathbf{ds} \tag{2.8}$$

if $F$ and its first derivative are continuous in volume $V$ as well as on its surface $S$. Equation (2.8) is known as the gradient theorem. The explicit expressions for the gradient in rectangular, cylindrical, and spherical coordinates are given in Appendix 2.A.

For the divergence, curl, and gradient, there are two very useful identities given by

$$\nabla \times (\nabla F) = 0 \tag{2.9}$$
$$\nabla \cdot (\nabla \times \mathbf{A}) = 0 \tag{2.10}$$

where $F$ and $\mathbf{A}$ are any functions that are continuous with a continuous first derivative. Both identities can be proven with the aid of the divergence and curl theorems and are easily verified in Cartesian coordinates. Another useful identity is

$$\nabla \times \nabla \times \mathbf{A} = \nabla\nabla \cdot \mathbf{A} - \nabla^2 \mathbf{A} \tag{2.11}$$

where $\nabla^2$ is known as the Laplacian, whose specific form in rectangular, cylindrical, and spherical coordinates is given in Appendix 2.A.

## 2.3 Magnetostatic Fields in Free Space

A steady electric current produces a static magnetic field. The flux density of the magnetic field, denoted by $\mathbf{B}$ and measured in webers per square meter (Wb/m$^2$) or Tesla (T), satisfies two equations given by

$$\oint\!\!\!\oint_S \mathbf{B} \cdot d\mathbf{s} = 0 \qquad \text{(Gauss's law—magnetic)} \tag{2.12}$$

$$\oint_C \mathbf{B} \cdot d\mathbf{l} = \mu_0 I \qquad \text{(Ampere's law).} \tag{2.13}$$

In Eq. (2.12), $S$ is an arbitrary closed surface and $d\mathbf{s} = \hat{n}ds$ with $\hat{n}$ denoting the outward unit vector normal to $S$. In Eq. (2.13), $C$ is an arbitrary closed contour and $d\mathbf{l} = \hat{l}dl$ with $\hat{l}$ denoting the unit vector tangential to $C$. Also, $\mu_0 = 4\pi \times 10^{-7}$ henrys per meter (H/m) is the permeability of free space, and $I$ is the total electric current passing through the surface bounded by $C$. Clearly, Eq. (2.12) indicates that there are no magnetic flow sources and, thus, the magnetic flux lines must close upon themselves.

Equations (2.12) and (2.13) are also known as the two fundamental postulates in integral form for magnetostatic fields. In many cases, it is useful to have their differential counterparts. Applying the divergence and curl theorems to Eqs. (2.12) and (2.13), respectively, we obtain their differential counterparts as

$$\nabla \cdot \mathbf{B} = 0 \qquad \text{(Gauss's law—magnetic)} \tag{2.14}$$

$$\nabla \times \mathbf{B} = \mu_0 \mathbf{J} \qquad \text{(Ampere's law)} \tag{2.15}$$

where $\mathbf{J}$ denotes the electric current density measured in amperes per square meter (A/m$^2$). Taking the divergence of Eq. (2.15) and invoking Eq. (2.10), we have

$$\nabla \cdot \mathbf{J} = 0 \qquad \text{(continuity equation)} \tag{2.16}$$

which indicates that the electric current must be conservative in the static case.

To solve Eqs. (2.14) and (2.15), we introduce a magnetic vector potential, denoted by $\mathbf{A}$, and let

$$\mathbf{B} = \nabla \times \mathbf{A}. \tag{2.17}$$

Because of the identity given in Eq. (2.10), Eq. (2.14) is satisfied automatically. To satisfy Eq. (2.15), we substitute into it Eq. (2.17) to find

$$\nabla \times \nabla \times \mathbf{A} = \mu_0 \mathbf{J} \tag{2.18}$$

which can also be written as

$$\nabla \nabla \cdot \mathbf{A} - \nabla^2 \mathbf{A} = \mu_0 \mathbf{J} \tag{2.19}$$

upon the application of Eq. (2.11). According to the Helmholtz theorem, a vector function is determined to within an additive constant if both its divergence and curl are specified. Therefore, in order to determine $\mathbf{A}$, we must specify its divergence and, with the intent of simplifying Eq. (2.19), we choose

$$\nabla \cdot \mathbf{A} = 0. \tag{2.20}$$

With this choice, Eq. (2.19) becomes

$$\nabla^2 \mathbf{A} = -\mu_0 \mathbf{J} \tag{2.21}$$

which is known as the vector Poisson's equation.

Equation (2.21) has a well-known physical solution given by

$$\mathbf{A}(\mathbf{r}) = \frac{\mu_0}{4\pi} \iiint_V \frac{\mathbf{J}(\mathbf{r}')}{R} \, dv' \tag{2.22}$$

where $R = |\mathbf{r} - \mathbf{r}'|$. In many applications in MRI, we are interested in finding the field produced by wires carrying a current. Assume that the path of a wire is $C$ and the current is $I$. Then, Eq. (2.22) becomes

$$\mathbf{A}(\mathbf{r}) = \frac{\mu_0 I}{4\pi} \int_C \frac{d\mathbf{l}'}{R}. \tag{2.23}$$

To find the magnetic field, we substitute this into Eq. (2.17) to find

$$\mathbf{B}(\mathbf{r}) = \nabla \times \mathbf{A}(\mathbf{r}) = \frac{\mu_0 I}{4\pi} \int_C \nabla \times \frac{d\mathbf{l}'}{R} \tag{2.24}$$

where we moved the del operator inside the integral because it operates on the observation point, whereas the integration is with respect to the source point. Employing the vector identity

$$\nabla \times (a\mathbf{b}) = a\nabla \times \mathbf{b} + \nabla a \times \mathbf{b} \tag{2.25}$$

we obtain

$$\nabla \times \frac{d\mathbf{l}'}{R} = \frac{1}{R}\nabla \times d\mathbf{l}' + \left(\nabla \frac{1}{R}\right) \times d\mathbf{l}' = \left(\nabla \frac{1}{R}\right) \times d\mathbf{l}'. \tag{2.26}$$

Further, realizing that

$$\nabla \frac{1}{R} = -\frac{\nabla R}{R^2} = -\frac{\mathbf{R}}{R^3} \tag{2.27}$$

where $\mathbf{R} = \mathbf{r} - \mathbf{r}'$, we can rewrite Eq. (2.24) as

$$\mathbf{B}(\mathbf{r}) = \frac{\mu_0 I}{4\pi} \int_C \frac{d\mathbf{l}' \times \mathbf{R}}{R^3} \qquad \text{(Biot-Savart's law)} \tag{2.28}$$

which provides a convenient formula to calculate the magnetic field from a line current. As noted, Eq. (2.28) is the well-known Biot-Savart's law.

To show the application of Biot-Savart's law, let us consider the following two examples. The results obtained for these two examples are useful because square and circular loops are basic building blocks for surface coils and coil arrays.

**Example 1.** A square loop of width $w$ carries electric current $I$. Find the magnetic flux density along the $z$-axis, which is perpendicular to the loop and passes through the center of the loop, as shown in Fig. 2.1.

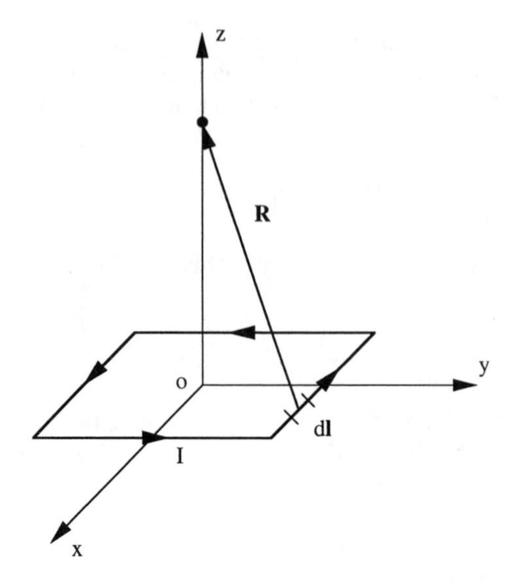


**Figure 2.1.** A square loop.

**Solution.** Let us consider first the magnetic field along the $z$-axis produced by the current segment located at $y = w/2$. For this, $d\mathbf{l}' = -\hat{x}dx'$, $\mathbf{R} = \hat{z}z - (\hat{x}x' + \hat{y}w/2)$. Hence, $d\mathbf{l}' \times \mathbf{R} = (\hat{y}z + \hat{z}w/2)dx'$ and

$$\begin{aligned}\mathbf{B}_1(z) &= \frac{\mu_0 I}{4\pi}\int_{-w/2}^{w/2}\frac{(\hat{y}z + \hat{z}w/2)\,dx'}{[z^2 + (w/2)^2 + x'^2]^{3/2}} \\ &= \frac{\mu_0 Iw(\hat{y}z + \hat{z}w/2)}{4\pi[z^2 + (w/2)^2]\sqrt{z^2 + 2(w/2)^2}}.\end{aligned} \tag{2.29}$$

Because of the symmetry, the current segment located at $y = -w/2$ will produce a magnetic field whose $z$-component is the same as that of $\mathbf{B}_1$, but whose $y$-component is the negative of the corresponding component in $\mathbf{B}_1$. With similar arguments for the current segments at $x = \pm w/2$, we conclude that the total magnetic field along the $z$-axis will have only a $z$-component, whose magnitude is given by

$$\mathbf{B}(z) = \hat{z}\frac{\mu_0 Iw^2}{2\pi[z^2 + (w/2)^2]\sqrt{z^2 + 2(w/2)^2}}. \tag{2.30}$$

Figure 2.2 plots $B_z$ as a function of $z$. As can be seen, the magnetic field decays rapidly as the observation point moves away from the loop.

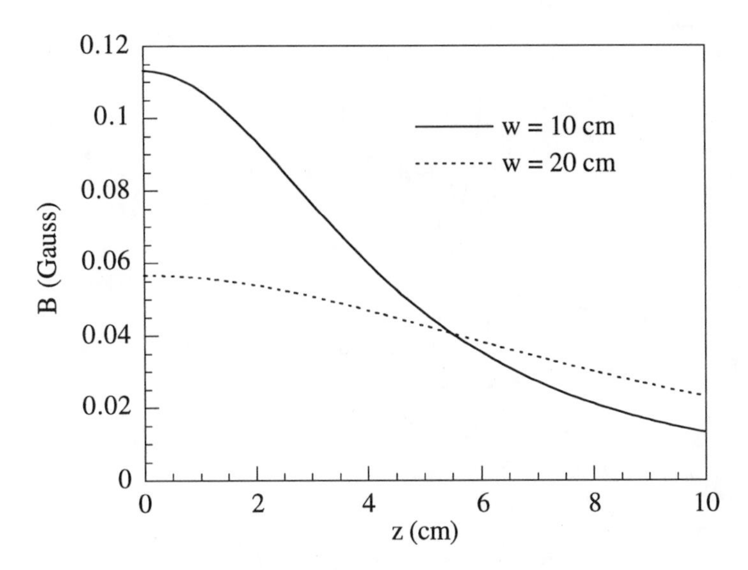


**Figure 2.2.** The magnetic field of a square loop along its axis ($I = 1$ A). Note: "Gauss" is another unit for magnetic flux density and is related to "Tesla" by 1 Gauss $= 10^{-4}$ Tesla.

Therefore, when this loop is used as an RF coil for MRI, its field of view is limited to within the region close to itself. Note that it is not difficult to calculate the field off the $z$-axis.

**Example 2.** A circular loop of radius $a$ carries an electric current $I$. Find the magnetic flux density along the $z$-axis, which is perpendicular to the loop and passes through the center of the loop, as shown in Fig. 2.3.

**Solution.** For this problem, $d\mathbf{l}' = \hat{\phi}' a\, d\phi'$, $\mathbf{R} = \hat{z} z - \hat{\rho}' a$, and $d\mathbf{l}' \times \mathbf{R} = \hat{\rho}' az\, d\phi' + \hat{z} a^2 d\phi'$. It is clear that the element $I\, d\mathbf{l}'$ produces both $z$- and $\rho'$-components for the magnetic field. However, because of the symmetry, the $\rho'$-component will be canceled by the element on the opposite side of the loop. Therefore, the total magnetic field along the $z$-axis will have only a $z$-component, which is given by

$$\mathbf{B}(z) = \frac{\mu_0 I}{4\pi} \int_0^{2\pi} \frac{\hat{z} a^2 d\phi'}{[z^2 + a^2]^{3/2}} = \hat{z} \frac{\mu_0 I a^2}{2[z^2 + a^2]^{3/2}}. \tag{2.31}$$

Figure 3.4 plots $B_z$ as a function of $z$. Again, the magnetic field decays rapidly as the observation point moves away from the loop.

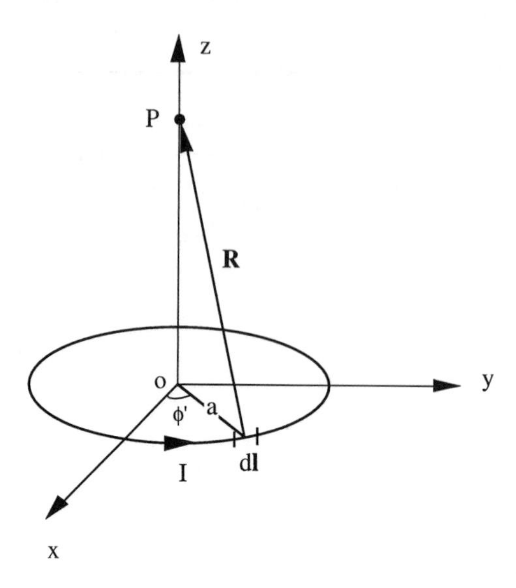


**Figure 2.3.** A circular loop.

The field off the $z$-axis has a more complicated expression and is given by

$$B_z = \frac{\mu_0 I k}{4\pi\sqrt{a\rho}}\left[K(k) + \frac{a^2 - \rho^2 - z^2}{(a-\rho)^2 + z^2}E(k)\right] \tag{2.32}$$

$$B_\rho = \frac{\mu_0 I k z}{4\pi\rho\sqrt{a\rho}}\left[-K(k) + \frac{a^2 + \rho^2 + z^2}{(a-\rho)^2 + z^2}E(k)\right] \tag{2.33}$$

where

$$k = \sqrt{\frac{4a\rho}{(a+\rho)^2 + z^2}} \tag{2.34}$$

and $K(k)$ and $E(k)$ are Legendre's complete elliptic integrals of the first and second kinds, defined as

$$K(k) = \int_0^{\pi/2} \frac{d\theta}{\sqrt{1 - k^2 \sin^2\theta}} \tag{2.35}$$

$$E(k) = \int_0^{\pi/2} \sqrt{1 - k^2 \sin^2\theta}\, d\theta \tag{2.36}$$

whose numerical evaluation is discussed by Zhang and Jin (1996).

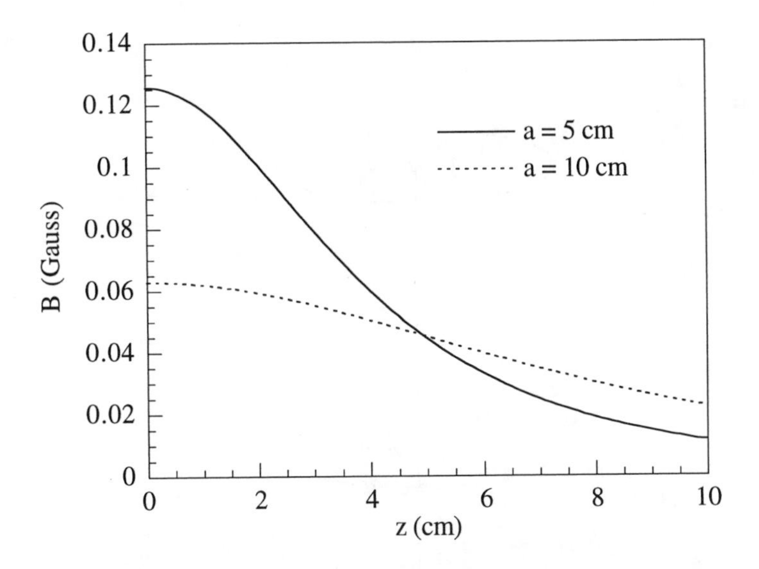


**Figure 2.4.** The magnetic field of a circular loop along its axis ($I = 1$ A).

The result obtained in Example 2 can be used to find the field inside a solenoid having $n$ turns per unit length. Assume that the center of the solenoid coincides with point $z = 0$ and the length of the solenoid is $L$. Then, the field along the $z$-axis is given by

$$\begin{aligned} \mathbf{B}(z) &= \hat{z} \int_{-L/2}^{L/2} \frac{\mu_0 n I a^2 \, dz'}{2[(z - z')^2 + a^2]^{3/2}} \\ &= \hat{z} \frac{\mu_0 n I}{2} \left[ \frac{L/2 - z}{\sqrt{(L/2 - z)^2 + a^2}} + \frac{L/2 + z}{\sqrt{(L/2 + z)^2 + a^2}} \right] \end{aligned} \tag{2.37}$$

which reduces to the well-known result for an infinitely long solenoid

$$\mathbf{B}(z) = \hat{z} \mu_0 n I \qquad \text{as } L \to \infty. \tag{2.38}$$

In fact, the result in Eq. (2.38) can be derived more easily from Eq. (2.13).

## 2.4 Helmholtz and Maxwell Coils

Consider two identical circular loops of radius $a$, separated by distance $d$, and carrying the same current in the same direction, as illustrated in Fig. 2.4. The magnetic field produced by these two loops is the sum of the

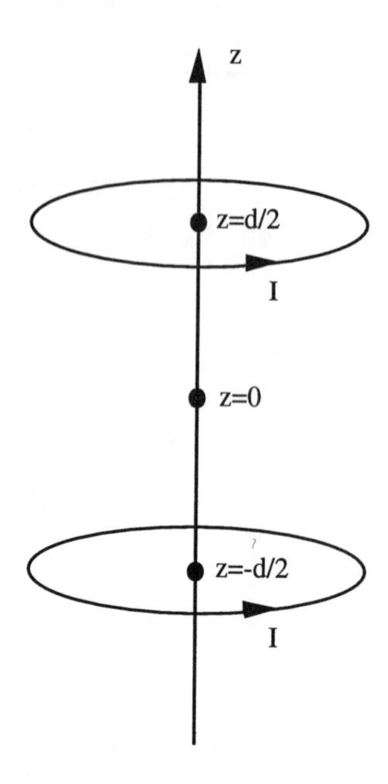


**Figure 2.5.** Helmholtz coil.

fields produced by the individual loops. Using the result obtained in the preceding section, we obtain the magnetic field along the $z$-axis as

$$B_z = \frac{\mu_0 I a^2}{2\left[(d/2-z)^2+a^2\right]^{3/2}} + \frac{\mu_0 I a^2}{2\left[(d/2+z)^2+a^2\right]^{3/2}}. \tag{2.39}$$

Now let us find the optimal distance so that the magnetic field is most uniform in the vicinity of their midpoint $z=0$. For this, we take the first derivative of Eq. (2.39) to find

$$\frac{dB_z}{dz} = \frac{3\mu_0 I a^2}{2}\left\{\frac{(d/2-z)}{\left[(d/2-z)^2+a^2\right]^{5/2}} - \frac{(d/2+z)}{\left[(d/2+z)^2+a^2\right]^{5/2}}\right\} \tag{2.40}$$

which vanishes at $z=0$ for any $d$. Next, we take the second derivative

$$\frac{d^2 B_z}{dz^2} = \frac{3\mu_0 I a^2}{2}\left\{\frac{4(d/2-z)^2-a^2}{\left[(d/2-z)^2+a^2\right]^{7/2}} + \frac{4(d/2+z)^2-a^2}{\left[(d/2+z)^2+a^2\right]^{7/2}}\right\} \tag{2.41}$$

which vanishes at $z=0$ for $d=a$. Since the third derivative, like all other odd derivatives, vanishes for any $d$, $B_z$ is uniform around $z=0$ through

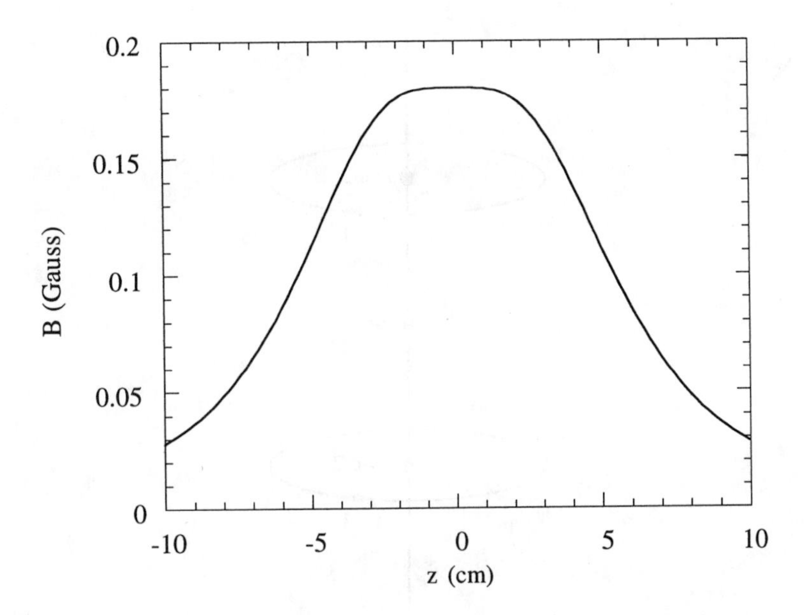


**Figure 2.6.** The magnetic field of the Helmholtz coil pair along the axis ($a = 5$ cm and $I = 1$ A).

the third power of $z$, that is,

$$B_z(z) = B_z(0) + O[(z/d)^4] \tag{2.42}$$

when the distance is chosen to be the same as the radius of the loops. Such a configuration is called the Helmholtz coil, which has found applications in MRI as RF coils because of its ability to generate a uniform field in the vicinity of their midpoint. (A more uniform field can be achieved using more coil pairs, see Problems 2.13 and 2.14.) Figure 2.6 shows $B_z$ for a Helmholtz coil pair.

If the currents in the two loops are in opposite directions, as illustrated in Fig. 2.7, the magnetic field along the $z$-axis is then

$$B_z = \frac{\mu_0 I a^2}{2\left[(d/2 - z)^2 + a^2\right]^{3/2}} - \frac{\mu_0 I a^2}{2\left[(d/2 + z)^2 + a^2\right]^{3/2}} \tag{2.43}$$

from which we find that $B_z$, as well as all the even derivatives, vanish at $z = 0$. Its third derivative is found as

$$\frac{d^3 B_z}{dz^3} = \frac{15\mu_0 I a^2}{2}$$

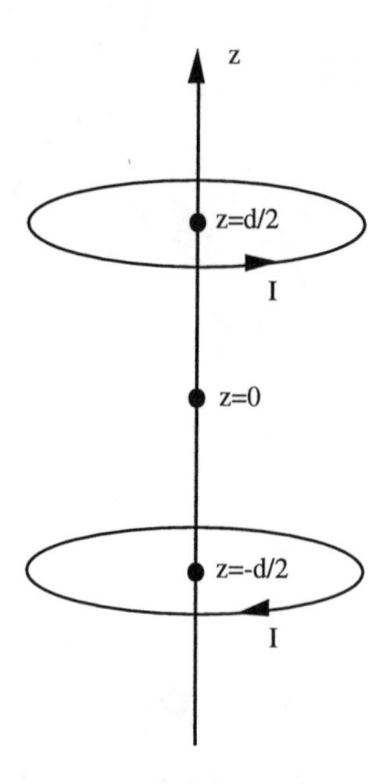


**Figure 2.7.** Maxwell coil.

$$\times \left\{ \frac{4(d/2-z)^3 - 3(d/2-z)a^2}{\left[(d/2-z)^2+a^2\right]^{9/2}} + \frac{4(d/2+z)^3 - 3(d/2+z)a^2}{\left[(d/2+z)^2+a^2\right]^{9/2}} \right\} \tag{2.44}$$

which vanishes at $z = 0$ for $d = \sqrt{3}a$. At this distance, the first derivative is nonzero; therefore, $B_z$ around $z = 0$ is linear along $z$ up through the fourth power of $z$, that is

$$B_z(z) = B_z'(0)\,z + O[(z/d)^5] \tag{2.45}$$

when the distance is chosen to be $\sqrt{3}$ times the radius of the loops. Such a configuration is called the Maxwell coil, which has found applications in MRI as a $z$-gradient coil. Figure 2.8 shows $B_z$ for a Maxwell coil pair.

## 2.5 Boundary Conditions for Magnetostatic Fields

In this section, instead of deriving boundary conditions for a general case, we derive the boundary conditions for magnetostatic fields across a current sheet in free space, which are useful in finding the magnetic fields produced by planar, cylindrical, and spherical surface currents.

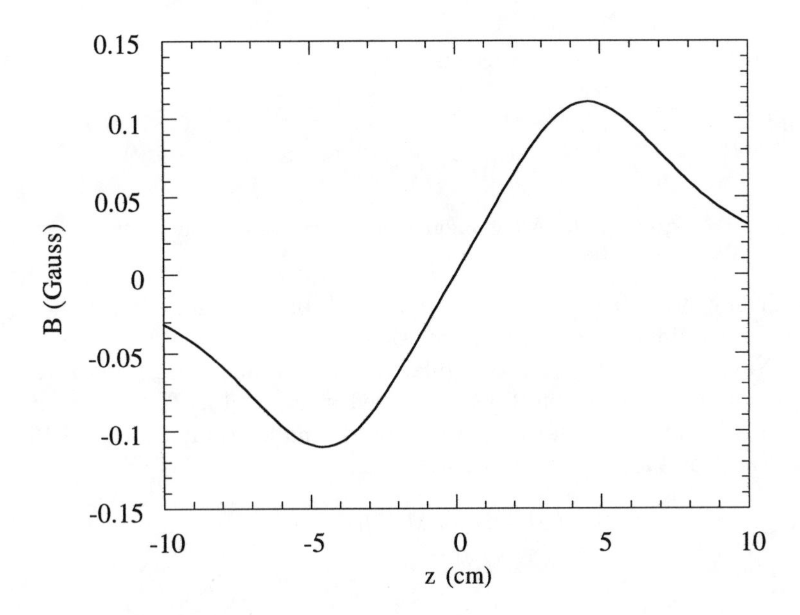


**Figure 2.8.** The magnetic field of the Maxwell coil pair along the axis ($a = 5$ cm and $I = 1$ A).

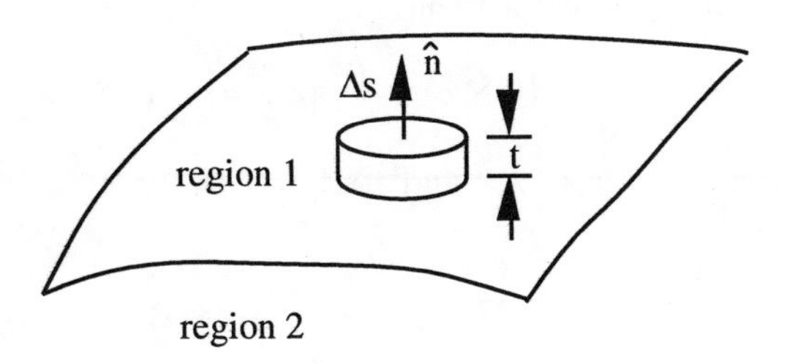


**Figure 2.9.** A pillbox across a current sheet.

Consider an infinitely thin current sheet carrying a surface current $\mathbf{J}_s$ measured in A/m. We construct a small pillbox with one of its faces in region 1 and the other in region 2, as illustrated in Fig. 2.9. Each face of the pillbox has an area $\Delta s$ and the thickness $t$ is vanishingly small. Applying Eq. (2.12) to this pillbox and letting $t \to 0$, we obtain

$$B_{1n}\Delta s - B_{2n}\Delta s = 0 \tag{2.46}$$

or

$$B_{1n} = B_{2n} \tag{2.47}$$

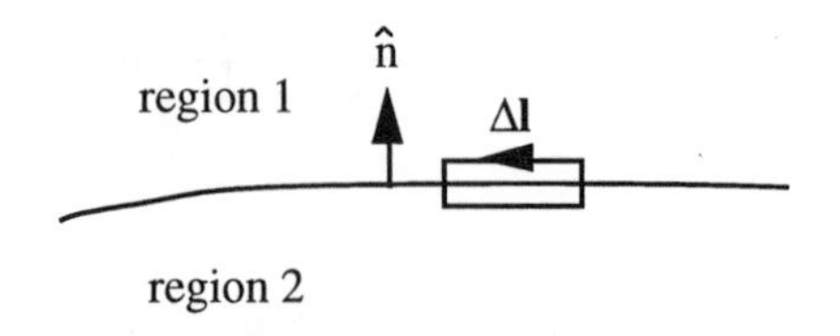


**Figure 2.10.** A rectangular path across a current sheet.

which indicates that the normal component of the magnetic flux density must be continuous across a current sheet.

Next, we construct a rectangular frame with one of its sides in region 1 and the other in region 2, as illustrated in Fig. 2.10. The length of the frame is $\Delta l$ and the width $t$ is vanishingly small. Applying Eq. (2.13) to this frame and letting $t \to 0$, we have

$$\mathbf{B}_1 \cdot \hat{l}\Delta l - \mathbf{B}_2 \cdot \hat{l}\Delta l = \mu_0 \mathbf{J}_s \cdot (\hat{n} \times \hat{l})\Delta l \tag{2.48}$$

or

$$\mathbf{B}_1 \cdot \hat{l} - \mathbf{B}_2 \cdot \hat{l} = \mu_0 (\mathbf{J}_s \times \hat{n}) \cdot \hat{l} \tag{2.49}$$

where we applied vector identity

$$\mathbf{a} \cdot (\mathbf{b} \times \mathbf{c}) = \mathbf{b} \cdot (\mathbf{c} \times \mathbf{a}) = \mathbf{c} \cdot (\mathbf{a} \times \mathbf{b}). \tag{2.50}$$

By rewriting $\hat{l} = \hat{n} \times \hat{l} \times \hat{n}$ and applying Eq. (2.50) again, Eq. (2.49) can be written as

$$(\hat{l} \times \hat{n}) \cdot (\hat{n} \times \mathbf{B}_1) - (\hat{l} \times \hat{n}) \cdot (\hat{n} \times \mathbf{B}_2) = \mu_0 \mathbf{J}_s \cdot (\hat{l} \times \hat{n}). \tag{2.51}$$

Since the orientation of $\hat{l}$ and, thus, $(\hat{l} \times \hat{n})$, is arbitrary, we have

$$\hat{n} \times (\mathbf{B}_1 - \mathbf{B}_2) = \mu_0 \mathbf{J}_s \tag{2.52}$$

which indicates that the tangential component of the magnetic flux density is discontinuous across a current sheet.

## 2.6 Magnetostatic Fields in Source-Free Regions

In this section, we derive the general solution of the magnetic field in source-free regions in cylindrical and spherical coordinates. These will be used later to determine the magnetic fields produced by cylindrical and spherical surface currents.

In a source-free region, Eqs. (2.14) and (2.15) become

$$\nabla \cdot \mathbf{B} = 0 \tag{2.53}$$

$$\nabla \times \mathbf{B} = 0. \tag{2.54}$$

To solve these two equations, we introduce a scalar magnetic potential, denoted as $\psi$, and defined by

$$\mathbf{B} = -\nabla\psi. \tag{2.55}$$

In light of the identity given in Eq. (2.9), Eq. (2.54) is satisfied automatically. To satisfy Eq. (2.53), we substitute into it Eq. (2.55) to find

$$\nabla \cdot (-\nabla\psi) = 0 \tag{2.56}$$

or

$$\nabla^2\psi = 0 \tag{2.57}$$

which is the well-known Laplace equation.

Equation (2.57) can be solved using the method of separation of variables. Assume that $\psi$ has no variation along the $z$-axis. The general solution of Eq. (2.57) in cylindrical coordinates is given by

$$\psi(\rho, \phi) = \sum_{m=-\infty}^{\infty} \rho^m (A_m \cos m\phi + B_m \sin m\phi) \tag{2.58}$$

where $A_m$ and $B_m$ are arbitrary constants to be determined by specific problems. From this, we obtain

$$\begin{aligned} \mathbf{B}(\rho, \phi) = &-\hat{\rho} \sum_{m=-\infty}^{\infty} m\rho^{m-1}(A_m \cos m\phi + B_m \sin m\phi) \\ &+ \hat{\phi} \sum_{m=-\infty}^{\infty} m\rho^{m-1}(A_m \sin m\phi - B_m \cos m\phi) \end{aligned} \tag{2.59}$$

which is a general expression for the magnetic field in cylindrical coordinates with the assumption that there is no variation along the $z$-axis.

In spherical coordinates, by neglecting the solution that is singular along the $z$-axis, the general solution of Eq. (2.57) is given by

$$\begin{aligned} \psi(r, \theta, \phi) = \sum_{n=0}^{\infty}\sum_{m=0}^{n} \Big\{ &r^n P_n^m(\cos\theta)(A_{nm} \cos m\phi + B_{nm} \sin m\phi) \\ &+ \frac{1}{r^{n+1}} P_n^m(\cos\theta)(C_{nm} \cos m\phi + D_{nm} \sin m\phi) \Big\} \end{aligned} \tag{2.60}$$

where $P_n^m(\cos\theta)$ denotes the associated Legendre polynomial and $A_{nm}$, $B_{nm}$, $C_{nm}$, and $D_{nm}$ are arbitrary constants to be determined by specific problems. The definition and some important properties of the associated Legendre polynomials are described in Appendix 2.B at the end of this chapter. From Eq. (2.55), we obtain

$$
\begin{aligned}
&\mathbf{B}(r,\theta,\phi) \\
&= -\hat{r}\sum_{n=0}^{\infty}\sum_{m=0}^{n}\left\{nr^{n-1}P_n^m(\cos\theta)(A_{nm}\cos m\phi + B_{nm}\sin m\phi)\right. \\
&\qquad\left. - \frac{n+1}{r^{n+2}}P_n^m(\cos\theta)(C_{nm}\cos m\phi + D_{nm}\sin m\phi)\right\} \\
&\quad + \hat{\theta}\sum_{n=0}^{\infty}\sum_{m=0}^{n}\sin\theta\left\{r^{n-1}P'^m_n(\cos\theta)(A_{nm}\cos m\phi + B_{nm}\sin m\phi)\right. \\
&\qquad\left. + \frac{1}{r^{n+2}}P'^m_n(\cos\theta)(C_{nm}\cos m\phi + D_{nm}\sin m\phi)\right\} \\
&\quad + \hat{\phi}\frac{1}{\sin\theta}\sum_{n=0}^{\infty}\sum_{m=0}^{n}m\left\{r^{n-1}P_n^m(\cos\theta)(A_{nm}\sin m\phi - B_{nm}\cos m\phi)\right. \\
&\qquad\left. + \frac{1}{r^{n+2}}P_n^m(\cos\theta)(C_{nm}\sin m\phi - D_{nm}\cos m\phi)\right\}.
\end{aligned}
\tag{2.61}
$$

## 2.7 Magnetostatic Fields Produced by Cylindrical and Spherical Surface Currents

With the boundary conditions and the general expressions for the fields in cylindrical and spherical coordinates, we can now find the magnetic fields produced by particular cylindrical and spherical surface currents.

Consider an infinitely long cylindrical surface carrying a $z$-directed surface current

$$\mathbf{J}_s = \hat{z}J_0\sin\phi \tag{2.62}$$

where $J_0$ is a constant. The radius of the cylinder is $a$. To find the magnetic field everywhere, we first have to find the general solution to the field inside and outside the cylinder. Consider first the field outside the cylinder. Since the field must decay as $\rho$ increases, from Eq. (2.59) we obtain

$$\mathbf{B}_1(\rho,\phi) = -\hat{\rho}\sum_{m=-\infty}^{-1}m\rho^{m-1}(A_m\cos m\phi + B_m\sin m\phi)$$

$$+\hat{\phi}\sum_{m=-\infty}^{-1} m\rho^{m-1}(A_m \sin m\phi - B_m \cos m\phi). \qquad (2.63)$$

Next, consider the field inside the cylinder. Since the field must remain finite at the center, we can have only the terms containing $\rho^{m-1}$ $(m \geq 1)$. Therefore, from Eq. (2.59) we have

$$\begin{aligned}\mathbf{B}_2(\rho,\phi) = &-\hat{\rho}\sum_{m=1}^{\infty} m\rho^{m-1}(A_m \cos m\phi + B_m \sin m\phi) \\ &+\hat{\phi}\sum_{m=1}^{\infty} m\rho^{m-1}(A_m \sin m\phi - B_m \cos m\phi). \qquad (2.64)\end{aligned}$$

Applying the boundary conditions across the cylindrical surface and solving for the constants, we obtain the only nonzero constants

$$A_1 = -\frac{\mu_0 J_0}{2}, \qquad A_{-1} = -\frac{\mu_0 J_0}{2}a^2. \qquad (2.65)$$

Substituting these into Eqs. (2.63) and (2.64), we have

$$\begin{aligned}\mathbf{B}_1(\rho,\phi) &= \hat{\rho}\left(\frac{a}{\rho}\right)^2 \frac{\mu_0 J_0}{2}\cos\phi + \hat{\phi}\left(\frac{a}{\rho}\right)^2 \frac{\mu_0 J_0}{2}\sin\phi \\ &= \left(\frac{a}{\rho}\right)^2 \frac{\mu_0 J_0}{2}(\hat{\rho}\cos\phi + \hat{\phi}\sin\phi) \qquad (2.66)\end{aligned}$$

and

$$\begin{aligned}\mathbf{B}_2(\rho,\phi) &= \hat{\rho}\frac{\mu_0 J_0}{2}\cos\phi - \hat{\phi}\frac{\mu_0 J_0}{2}\sin\phi \\ &= \frac{\mu_0 J_0}{2}(\hat{\rho}\cos\phi - \hat{\phi}\sin\phi) \\ &= \hat{x}\frac{\mu_0 J_0}{2}. \qquad (2.67)\end{aligned}$$

Note that the magnetic field inside the cylinder is $x$-directed and, more important, is a constant! Therefore, a $z$-directed surface current with $\sin\phi$ variation produces a uniform, or homogeneous, $x$-directed magnetic field inside the cylinder, as shown in Fig. 2.11. This fact provides the basis for the design of birdcage coils, as discussed in Chapter 4.

Now, consider a spherical surface having radius $a$ and carrying a surface current

$$\mathbf{J}_s = \hat{\phi}J_0 \sin\theta \qquad (2.68)$$

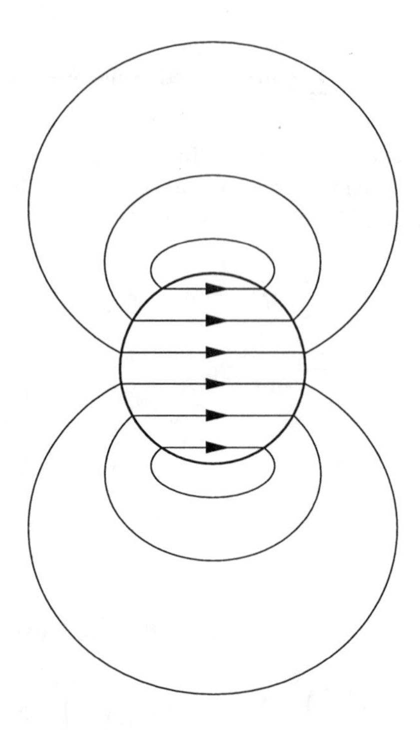

**Figure 2.11.** The magnetic flux lines inside and outside a cylindrical shell carrying a $z$-directed surface current with $\sin\phi$ variation.

where $J_0$ is a constant. (The solution to an arbitrary current is given in Appendix 2.C.) To find the magnetic field everywhere, we first note that the field outside the sphere must decay as $r \to \infty$ and the field inside the sphere must be finite at $r = 0$. Therefore, according to Eq. (2.61), the field outside the sphere can be represented by

$$\begin{aligned}\mathbf{B}_1(r,\theta,\phi) = \hat{r}\sum_{n=0}^{\infty}\sum_{m=0}^{n}\frac{n+1}{r^{n+2}}P_n^m(\cos\theta)(C_{nm}\cos m\phi + D_{nm}\sin m\phi) \\ + \hat{\theta}\sum_{n=0}^{\infty}\sum_{m=0}^{n}\frac{\sin\theta}{r^{n+2}}P'^m_n(\cos\theta)(C_{nm}\cos m\phi + D_{nm}\sin m\phi) \\ + \hat{\phi}\frac{1}{\sin\theta}\sum_{n=0}^{\infty}\sum_{m=0}^{n}\frac{m}{r^{n+2}}P_n^m(\cos\theta)(C_{nm}\sin m\phi - D_{nm}\cos m\phi)\end{aligned} \tag{2.69}$$

and the field inside the sphere can be represented by

$$\begin{aligned}\mathbf{B}_2(r,\theta,\phi) = &-\hat{r}\sum_{n=1}^{\infty}\sum_{m=0}^{n} nr^{n-1}P_n^m(\cos\theta)(A_{nm}\cos m\phi + B_{nm}\sin m\phi)\\ &+\hat{\theta}\sum_{n=1}^{\infty}\sum_{m=0}^{n} r^{n-1}\sin\theta P'^m_n(\cos\theta)(A_{nm}\cos m\phi + B_{nm}\sin m\phi)\\ &+\hat{\phi}\frac{1}{\sin\theta}\sum_{n=1}^{\infty}\sum_{m=0}^{n} mr^{n-1}P_n^m(\cos\theta)(A_{nm}\sin m\phi - B_{nm}\cos m\phi).\end{aligned} \tag{2.70}$$

Applying the boundary conditions across the spherical surface and solving for the constants, we obtain the only nonzero constants

$$A_{10} = -\frac{2}{3}\mu_0 J_0, \qquad C_{10} = \frac{1}{3}a^3\mu_0 J_0. \tag{2.71}$$

Substituting these into Eqs. (2.69) and (2.70), we obtain the field outside the sphere as

$$\begin{aligned}\mathbf{B}_1(r,\theta,\phi) &= \hat{r}\frac{2}{3}\left(\frac{a}{r}\right)^3\mu_0 J_0\cos\theta + \hat{\theta}\frac{1}{3}\left(\frac{a}{r}\right)^3\mu_0 J_0\sin\theta\\ &= \frac{\mu_0 J_0}{3}\left(\frac{a}{r}\right)^3(\hat{r}2\cos\theta + \hat{\theta}\sin\theta)\end{aligned} \tag{2.72}$$

and the field inside the sphere as

$$\begin{aligned}\mathbf{B}_2(r,\theta,\phi) &= \hat{r}\frac{2}{3}\mu_0 J_0\cos\theta - \hat{\theta}\frac{2}{3}\mu_0 J_0\sin\theta\\ &= \frac{2\mu_0 J_0}{3}(\hat{r}\cos\theta - \hat{\theta}\sin\theta)\\ &= \hat{z}\frac{2\mu_0 J_0}{3}.\end{aligned} \tag{2.73}$$

Note that the magnetic field inside the sphere is $z$-directed and, more important, is a constant! Therefore, a $\phi$-directed surface current with $\sin\theta$ variation produces a uniform, or homogeneous, $z$-directed magnetic field inside the sphere. This fact provides the basis for the design of the main magnet.

## 2.8 Inductance Calculation

For the analysis and design of gradient and RF coils, we often have to calculate the self-inductance of a conductor and the mutual inductance between two conductors.

Consider a conductor carrying a current density $\mathbf{J}$ in free space. The self-inductance $L$ is defined as the quantity related to its associated magnetic energy by

$$E_m = \frac{1}{2} L I^2 \tag{2.74}$$

where $I$ denotes the total current in the conductor. The magnetic energy is given by

$$E_m = \frac{1}{2} \iiint_V \mathbf{B} \cdot \mathbf{H} \, dv \tag{2.75}$$

where $\mathbf{B}$ and $\mathbf{H}$ are produced by $\mathbf{J}$. Since

$$\begin{aligned} \mathbf{B} \cdot \mathbf{H} &= (\nabla \times \mathbf{A}) \cdot \mathbf{H} = \mathbf{A} \cdot (\nabla \times \mathbf{H}) + \nabla \cdot (\mathbf{A} \times \mathbf{H}) \\ &= \mathbf{A} \cdot \mathbf{J} + \nabla \cdot (\mathbf{A} \times \mathbf{H}), \end{aligned} \tag{2.76}$$

Eq. (2.75) becomes

$$E_m = \frac{1}{2} \iiint_V \mathbf{A} \cdot \mathbf{J} \, dv + \frac{1}{2} \oiint_S (\mathbf{A} \times \mathbf{H}) \cdot d\mathbf{s} \tag{2.77}$$

where we applied the divergence theorem in Eq. (2.2). Since the field produced by $\mathbf{J}$ extends to infinity, $S$ in Eq. (2.77) is a spherical surface whose radius $r$ approaches infinity. However, when $r \to \infty$, $A \sim 1/r$ and $B \sim 1/r^2$. As a result, the surface integral in Eq. (2.77) vanishes and Eq. (2.77) becomes

$$E_m = \frac{1}{2} \iiint_V \mathbf{A} \cdot \mathbf{J} \, dv \tag{2.78}$$

where $V$ denotes the volume of the conductor and $\mathbf{A}$ is the magnetic vector potential generated by $\mathbf{J}$. From Eqs. (2.74) and (2.78), we obtain the expression of the self-inductance in terms of $\mathbf{A}$ and $\mathbf{J}$:

$$L = \frac{1}{I^2} \iiint_V \mathbf{A} \cdot \mathbf{J} \, dv. \tag{2.79}$$

Substituting Eq. (2.22) into Eq. (2.79) yields

$$L = \frac{\mu_0}{4\pi I^2} \iiint_V \iiint_V \frac{\mathbf{J}(\mathbf{r}) \cdot \mathbf{J}(\mathbf{r}')}{R} \, dv' \, dv \tag{2.80}$$

where $R = |\mathbf{r} - \mathbf{r}'|$.

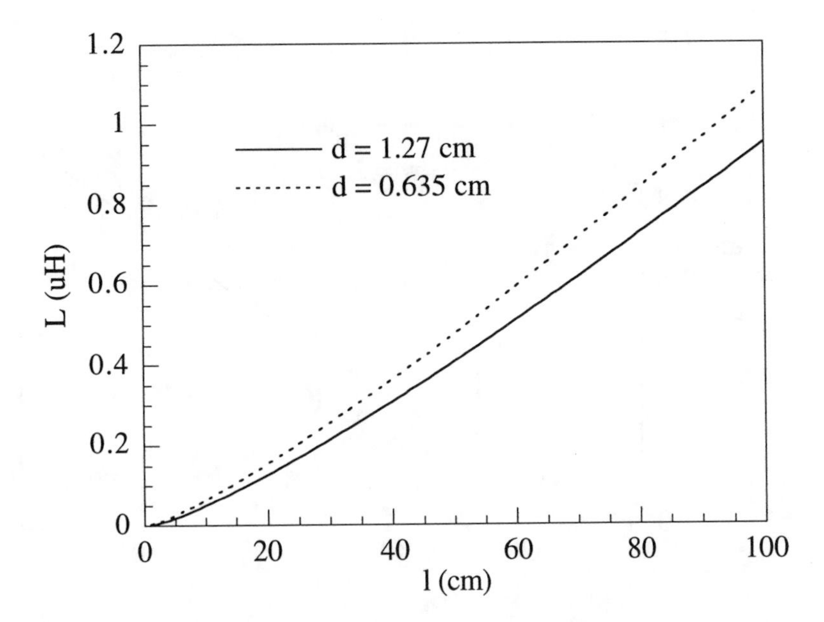


**Figure 2.12.** Self-inductance of a wire of diameter $d$.

To illustrate the use of Eq. (2.80), let us consider the evaluation of the self-inductance of a circular wire of radius $a$ and a strip of width $w$. For a straight circular wire of radius $a$ and length $l$, by assuming that the current is distributed uniformly over the surface of the wire, Eq. (2.80) can be written as

$$L = \frac{\mu_0}{4\pi(2\pi)^2} \int_0^{2\pi} \int_{-l/2}^{l/2} \int_0^{2\pi} \int_{-l/2}^{l/2} \frac{1}{R} dz' d\varphi' dz\, d\varphi \tag{2.81}$$

where $R = \sqrt{2a^2[1 - \cos(\varphi - \varphi')] + (z - z')^2}$. Apparently, the integrals are very complicated; however, with some approximations we can obtain (Grover 1962)

$$L = \frac{\mu_0 l}{2\pi} \left( \ln \frac{2l}{a} - 1 \right) \tag{2.82}$$

which is rather accurate when $l >> a$. Figure 2.12 plots the self-inductance of a wire.

For a strip of width $w$ and length $l$, Eq. (2.80) becomes

$$L = \frac{\mu_0}{4\pi w^2} \int_{-w/2}^{w/2} \int_{-l/2}^{l/2} \int_{-w/2}^{w/2} \int_{-l/2}^{l/2} \frac{1}{R} dz' dx' dz dx \tag{2.83}$$

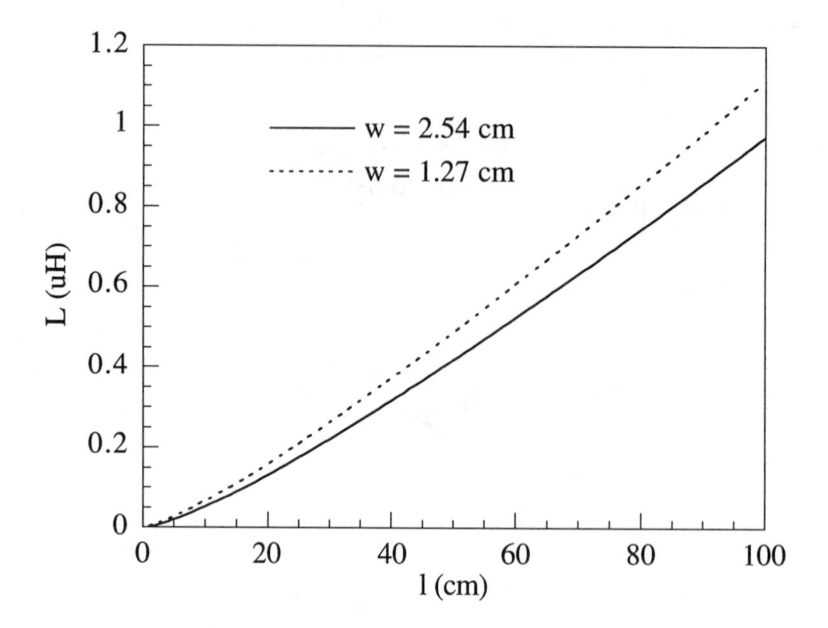


**Figure 2.13.** Self-inductance of a strip of width $w$.

where $R = \sqrt{(x-x')^2 + (z-z')^2}$. These integrals can be evaluated analytically, yielding

$$L = \frac{\mu_0}{4\pi w^2}\left[\frac{(x-x')(z-z')}{2}\{(x-x')\ln[(z-z')+R] + (z-z')\ln[(x-x')+R]\} - \frac{(x-x')(z-z')[(x-x')+(z-z')]}{4} - \frac{R^3}{6}\right]\Bigg|_{x'=-w/2}^{w/2}\Bigg|_{z'=-l/2}^{l/2}\Bigg|_{x=-w/2}^{w/2}\Bigg|_{z=-l/2}^{l/2}. \tag{2.84}$$

Although this expression is complicated, it can be easily implemented for numerical calculation. Equation (2.84) can also be approximated by a much simpler formula given by (Grover 1962)

$$L = \frac{\mu_0 l}{2\pi}\left(\ln\frac{2l}{w} + \frac{1}{2}\right) \tag{2.85}$$

whose accuracy improves when $l >> w$. Figure 2.13 gives the self-inductance of a strip.

To find the expression for calculating the mutual inductance, consider two conductors carrying currents $\mathbf{J}_1$ and $\mathbf{J}_2$ and occupying volumes $V_1$ and

$V_2$, respectively. The mutual inductances are defined as

$$M_{12} = \frac{1}{I_1 I_2} \iiint_{V_2} \mathbf{A}_1 \cdot \mathbf{J}_2 \, dv \tag{2.86}$$

and

$$M_{21} = \frac{1}{I_1 I_2} \iiint_{V_1} \mathbf{A}_2 \cdot \mathbf{J}_1 \, dv \tag{2.87}$$

where $I_1$ and $I_2$ denote the total currents in $V_1$ and $V_2$, respectively. Substituting Eq. (2.22) into Eqs. (2.86) and (2.87), we obtain

$$M_{12} = M_{21} = \frac{\mu_0}{4\pi I_1 I_2} \iiint_{V_1} \iiint_{V_2} \frac{\mathbf{J}_1(\mathbf{r}) \cdot \mathbf{J}_2(\mathbf{r}')}{R} \, dv' dv. \tag{2.88}$$

Apparently, for two wires perpendicular to each other, $M_{12} = M_{21} = 0$. For two parallel wires having the same length $l$ and distance $d$, the mutual inductance becomes

$$M_{12} = M_{21} = \frac{\mu_0}{4\pi} \int_{-l/2}^{l/2} \int_{-l/2}^{l/2} \frac{dz' dz}{\sqrt{d^2 + (z - z')^2}} \tag{2.89}$$

which can be evaluated analytically, yielding

$$M_{12} = M_{21} = \frac{\mu_0}{4\pi} \left[ R + z \ln(z' - z + R) + z \ln(z - z' + R) \right] \Big|_{z'=-l/2}^{l/2} \Big|_{z=-l/2}^{l/2} \tag{2.90}$$

where $R = \sqrt{d^2 + (z - z')^2}$. This result can be simplified as (Grover 1962)

$$M_{12} = M_{21} = \frac{\mu_0 l}{2\pi} \left[ \ln\left( \frac{l}{d} + \sqrt{1 + \frac{l^2}{d^2}} \right) - \sqrt{1 + \frac{d^2}{l^2}} + \frac{d}{l} \right] \tag{2.91}$$

which yields an almost identical result to that of Eq. (2.90). The calculation of the mutual inductance between two strips of different lengths is described in Appendix 2.D.

## 2.9 Time-Varying Electromagnetic Fields

As mentioned before, a steady electric current produces a static magnetic field. If the current varies with time, it not only produces a magnetic field, but also produces an electric field, both varying with time. The electric and magnetic fields must satisfy Maxwell's equations

$$\oint_C \mathbf{E} \cdot d\mathbf{l} = -\frac{d}{dt} \iint_S \mathbf{B} \cdot d\mathbf{s} \qquad \text{(Faraday's law)} \tag{2.92}$$

$$\oint_C \mathbf{H} \cdot d\mathbf{l} = \frac{d}{dt} \iint_S \mathbf{D} \cdot d\mathbf{s} + \iint_S \mathbf{J} \cdot d\mathbf{s} \qquad \text{(Maxwell-Ampere law)} \tag{2.93}$$

$$\oint\!\!\oint_S \mathbf{D} \cdot d\mathbf{s} = \iiint_V \rho_e \, dv \qquad \text{(Gauss's law)} \tag{2.94}$$

$$\oint\!\!\oint_S \mathbf{B} \cdot d\mathbf{s} = 0 \qquad \text{(Gauss's law—magnetic)} \tag{2.95}$$

where

$\mathbf{E}$ = electric field intensity (volts/meter)
$\mathbf{D}$ = electric flux density (coulombs/meter$^2$)
$\mathbf{H}$ = magnetic field intensity (amperes/meter)
$\mathbf{B}$ = magnetic flux density (webers/meter$^2$)
$\mathbf{J}$ = electric current density (amperes/meter$^2$)
$\rho_e$ = electric charge density (coulombs/meter$^3$).

Note that in Eqs. (2.92) and (2.93), $S$ is an open surface bounded by contour $C$, whereas in Eqs. (2.94) and (2.95), $S$ is a closed surface of volume $V$. Using the divergence and Stokes's theorems and vector identities, we can derive Maxwell's equations in differential form as

$$\nabla \times \mathbf{E} + \frac{\partial \mathbf{B}}{\partial t} = 0 \qquad \text{(Faraday's law)} \tag{2.96}$$

$$\nabla \times \mathbf{H} - \frac{\partial \mathbf{D}}{\partial t} = \mathbf{J} \qquad \text{(Maxwell-Ampere law)} \tag{2.97}$$

$$\nabla \cdot \mathbf{D} = \rho_e \qquad \text{(Gauss's law)} \tag{2.98}$$

$$\nabla \cdot \mathbf{B} = 0 \qquad \text{(Gauss's law—magnetic).} \tag{2.99}$$

Taking the divergence of Eq. (2.97) and employing Eqs. (2.10) and (2.98), we obtain

$$\nabla \cdot \mathbf{J} = -\frac{\partial \rho_e}{\partial t} \qquad \text{(equation of continuity).} \tag{2.100}$$

The quantities $\mathbf{E}$ and $\mathbf{D}$, $\mathbf{H}$ and $\mathbf{B}$, and $\mathbf{E}$ and $\mathbf{J}$ are related by the constitutive relations, which, for linear isotropic media, are given by

$$\mathbf{D} = \epsilon \mathbf{E} \tag{2.101}$$

$$\mathbf{B} = \mu \mathbf{H} \tag{2.102}$$

$$\mathbf{J} = \sigma \mathbf{E} \tag{2.103}$$

where

$$\epsilon = \text{permittivity (farads/meter)}$$
$$\mu = \text{permeability (henrys/meter)}$$
$$\sigma = \text{conductivity (siemens/meter)}.$$

Applying Eqs. (2.92)–(2.94) to the interface between two different media and using a similar approach as in the magnetostatic case, we obtain the boundary conditions across the interface as

$$D_{1n} - D_{2n} = \rho_s \tag{2.104}$$
$$E_{1t} = E_{2t} \tag{2.105}$$
$$B_{1n} = B_{2n} \tag{2.106}$$
$$\hat{n} \times (\mathbf{H}_1 - \mathbf{H}_2) = \mathbf{J}_s \tag{2.107}$$

where $\rho_s$ denotes the surface charge density, $\mathbf{J}_s$ denotes the surface current density on the interface and, again, $\hat{n}$ points from medium 2 to medium 1. Since a perfect conductor cannot sustain an electromagnetic field inside, the boundary conditions on a conducting surface become

$$D_n = \rho_s, \qquad E_t = 0 \tag{2.108}$$
$$B_n = 0, \qquad \hat{n} \times \mathbf{H} = \mathbf{J}_s. \tag{2.109}$$

## 2.10 Time-Harmonic Fields

When the fields are oscillating at a single frequency, each field quantity can be expressed as

$$\mathbf{A}(\mathbf{r}, t) = \text{Re}[\mathbf{A}(\mathbf{r})e^{-i\omega t}] \tag{2.110}$$

where $i = \sqrt{-1}$, $\omega$ is the angular frequency, and $\mathbf{A}(\mathbf{r})$ is a complex quantity called a phasor.[1] By expressing each quantity in the form of Eq. (2.110), Maxwell's equations can be reduced to

$$\nabla \times \mathbf{E} = i\omega\mathbf{B} \tag{2.111}$$
$$\nabla \times \mathbf{H} = -i\omega\mathbf{D} + \mathbf{J} \tag{2.112}$$
$$\nabla \cdot \mathbf{J} = i\omega\rho_e \tag{2.113}$$

[1] The time convention commonly adopted in electrical engineering is such that Eq. (2.110) becomes

$$\mathbf{A}(\mathbf{r}, t) = \text{Re}[\mathbf{A}(\mathbf{r})e^{j\omega t}]$$

where $j = \sqrt{-1}$. All the equations in this book can be converted to those with this time convention by replacing $i$ with $-j$.

and Eqs. (2.98) and (2.99) remain the same. Eliminating the magnetic field in Eqs. (2.111) and (2.112) with the aid of Eqs. (2.101) and (2.102), we obtain

$$\nabla \times \left( \frac{1}{\mu} \nabla \times \mathbf{E} \right) - \omega^2 \epsilon \mathbf{E} = i\omega \mathbf{J} \tag{2.114}$$

and, similarly, eliminating the electric field, we obtain

$$\nabla \times \left( \frac{1}{\epsilon} \nabla \times \mathbf{H} \right) - \omega^2 \mu \mathbf{H} = \nabla \times \left( \frac{1}{\epsilon} \mathbf{J} \right). \tag{2.115}$$

Equations (2.114) and (2.115) are the second-order uncoupled partial differential equations governing the electric and magnetic fields produced by the current **J**.

## 2.A Divergence, Curl, Gradient, and Laplacian Operations

1. In Rectangular (Cartesian) Coordinates

$$\nabla \cdot \mathbf{A} = \frac{\partial A_x}{\partial x} + \frac{\partial A_y}{\partial y} + \frac{\partial A_z}{\partial z} \tag{2.116}$$

$$\nabla \times \mathbf{A} = \hat{x} \left( \frac{\partial A_z}{\partial y} - \frac{\partial A_y}{\partial z} \right) + \hat{y} \left( \frac{\partial A_x}{\partial z} - \frac{\partial A_z}{\partial x} \right) + \hat{z} \left( \frac{\partial A_y}{\partial x} - \frac{\partial A_x}{\partial y} \right) \tag{2.117}$$

$$\nabla F = \hat{x} \frac{\partial F}{\partial x} + \hat{y} \frac{\partial F}{\partial y} + \hat{z} \frac{\partial F}{\partial z} \tag{2.118}$$

$$\nabla^2 F = \frac{\partial^2 F}{\partial x^2} + \frac{\partial^2 F}{\partial y^2} + \frac{\partial^2 F}{\partial z^2} \tag{2.119}$$

2. In Cylindrical Coordinates

$$\nabla \cdot \mathbf{A} = \frac{1}{\rho} \frac{\partial (\rho A_\rho)}{\partial \rho} + \frac{\partial A_\phi}{\rho \partial \phi} + \frac{\partial A_z}{\partial z} \tag{2.120}$$

$$\nabla \times \mathbf{A} = \hat{\rho} \left( \frac{\partial A_z}{\rho \partial \phi} - \frac{\partial A_\phi}{\partial z} \right) + \hat{\phi} \left( \frac{\partial A_\rho}{\partial z} - \frac{\partial A_z}{\partial \rho} \right) + \hat{z} \frac{1}{\rho} \left( \frac{\partial (\rho A_\phi)}{\partial \rho} - \frac{\partial A_\rho}{\partial \phi} \right) \tag{2.121}$$

$$\nabla F = \hat{\rho} \frac{\partial F}{\partial \rho} + \hat{\phi} \frac{\partial F}{\rho \partial \phi} + \hat{z} \frac{\partial F}{\partial z} \tag{2.122}$$

$$\nabla^2 F = \frac{1}{\rho} \frac{\partial}{\partial \rho} \left( \rho \frac{\partial F}{\partial \rho} \right) + \frac{1}{\rho^2} \frac{\partial^2 F}{\partial \phi^2} + \frac{\partial^2 F}{\partial z^2} \tag{2.123}$$

3. In Spherical Coordinates

$$\nabla \cdot \mathbf{A} = \frac{1}{r^2}\frac{\partial}{\partial r}(r^2 A_r) + \frac{1}{r \sin\theta}\frac{\partial}{\partial \theta}(A_\theta \sin\theta) + \frac{1}{r\sin\theta}\frac{\partial A_\phi}{\partial \phi} \tag{2.124}$$

$$\nabla \times \mathbf{A} = \hat{r}\frac{1}{r\sin\theta}\left[\frac{\partial}{\partial\theta}(A_\phi \sin\theta) - \frac{\partial A_\theta}{\partial \phi}\right] + \hat{\theta}\frac{1}{r}\left[\frac{1}{\sin\theta}\frac{\partial A_r}{\partial\phi} - \frac{\partial}{\partial r}(rA_\phi)\right] + \hat{\phi}\frac{1}{r}\left[\frac{\partial}{\partial r}(rA_\theta) - \frac{\partial A_r}{\partial\theta}\right] \tag{2.125}$$

$$\nabla F = \hat{r}\frac{\partial F}{\partial r} + \hat{\theta}\frac{\partial F}{r\partial\theta} + \hat{\phi}\frac{1}{r\sin\theta}\frac{\partial F}{\partial\phi} \tag{2.126}$$

$$\nabla^2 F = \frac{1}{r^2}\frac{\partial}{\partial r}\left(r^2\frac{\partial F}{\partial r}\right) + \frac{1}{r^2\sin\theta}\frac{\partial}{\partial\theta}\left(\sin\theta\frac{\partial F}{\partial\theta}\right) + \frac{1}{r^2\sin^2\theta}\frac{\partial^2 F}{\partial\phi^2} \tag{2.127}$$

## 2.B Associated Legendre Polynomials

The associated Legendre polynomial of the first kind, denoted by $P_n^m(\cos\theta)$, is one of the two linearly independent solutions of the associated Legendre differential equation

$$(1-x^2)\frac{d^2y}{dx^2} - 2x\frac{dy}{dx} + \left[n(n+1) - \frac{m^2}{1-x^2}\right]y(x) = 0 \tag{2.128}$$

where $x = \cos\theta$. The other solution, denoted by $Q_n^m(\cos\theta)$, is singular at $\theta = 0$ and $\pi$ and, therefore, not useful here. The $P_n^m(x)$ can be expressed as

$$P_n^m(x) = (-1)^m(1-x^2)^{m/2}\frac{d^m}{dx^m}P_n(x) \tag{2.129}$$

where $P_n(x)$ is the Legendre polynomial given by

$$P_n(x) = \frac{1}{2^n n!}\frac{d^n}{dx^n}(x^2-1)^n. \tag{2.130}$$

It is clear that the Legendre polynomial is related to the associated Legendre polynomial by $P_n(x) = P_n^0(x)$.

The first several associated Legendre polynomials $P_n^m(\cos\theta)$ are given by

$$\begin{aligned} P_0^0(\cos\theta) &= 1 \\ P_1^0(\cos\theta) &= \cos\theta \\ P_1^1(\cos\theta) &= -\sin\theta \end{aligned}$$

$$
\begin{aligned}
P_2^0(\cos\theta) &= \tfrac{1}{4}(3\cos 2\theta + 1) \\
P_2^1(\cos\theta) &= -3\sin\theta\cos\theta \\
P_2^2(\cos\theta) &= 3\sin^2\theta \\
P_3^0(\cos\theta) &= \tfrac{1}{8}(5\cos 3\theta + 3\cos\theta) \\
P_3^1(\cos\theta) &= -\tfrac{3}{8}(5\sin 3\theta + \sin\theta) \\
P_3^2(\cos\theta) &= \tfrac{15}{4}(\cos\theta - \cos 3\theta) \\
P_3^3(\cos\theta) &= -\tfrac{15}{4}(3\sin\theta - \sin 3\theta).
\end{aligned}
\tag{2.131}
$$

The associated Legendre polynomials have many important mathematical properties, which can be found in the book by Abramowitz and Stegun (1964). For example, at $x = 0$ and $x = \pm 1$ they have special values

$$
P_n^m(0) = \begin{cases} (-1)^{(m+n)/2}\dfrac{1\cdot 3\cdot 5\cdots(n+m-1)}{2\cdot 4\cdot 6\cdots(n-m)} & n+m = \text{even} \\ 0 & n+m = \text{odd} \end{cases} \tag{2.132}
$$

$$
P_n^m(\pm 1) = \begin{cases} (\pm 1)^n & m = 0 \\ 0 & m > 0. \end{cases} \tag{2.133}
$$

For negative orders and arguments, they have relations

$$
P_n^{-m}(x) = (-1)^m \frac{(n-m)!}{(n+m)!} P_n^m(x) \tag{2.134}
$$

$$
P_n^m(-x) = (-1)^{n-m} P_n^m(x). \tag{2.135}
$$

Some useful recurrence relations are given by

$$
P_n^m(x) = xP_{n-1}^m(x) - (n+m-1)\sqrt{1-x^2}\,P_{n-1}^{m-1}(x) \tag{2.136}
$$

$$
P_n^m(x) = -\frac{2(m-1)}{\sqrt{1-x^2}} xP_n^{m-1}(x) - (n+m-1)(n-m+2)P_n^{m-2}(x) \tag{2.137}
$$

$$
P_n^m(x) = \frac{1}{n-m}\left[(2n-1)xP_{n-1}^m(x) - (n+m-1)P_{n-2}^m(x)\right] \tag{2.138}
$$

from which other recurrence relations can be derived (Collin 1991). Their differentiation formulas are given by

$$
P'^m_n(x) = \frac{mx}{1-x^2}P_n^m(x) + \frac{(n+m)(n-m+1)}{\sqrt{1-x^2}}P_n^{m-1}(x) \tag{2.139}
$$

$$
P'^m_n(x) = \frac{1}{1-x^2}\left[(n+m)P_{n-1}^m(x) - nxP_n^m(x)\right]. \tag{2.140}
$$

The important orthogonal relations are

$$\int_{-1}^{1} P_n^m(x) P_{n'}^m(x)\, dx = \frac{2}{2n+1} \frac{(n+m)!}{(n-m)!} \delta_{nn'} \qquad (2.141)$$

$$\int_{-1}^{1} P_n^m(x) P_n^{m'}(x) (1-x^2)^{-1}\, dx = \frac{1}{m} \frac{(n+m)!}{(n-m)!} \delta_{mm'} \qquad (2.142)$$

where

$$\delta_{nn'} = \begin{cases} 1 & n' = n \\ 0 & n' \neq n \end{cases}, \qquad \delta_{mm'} = \begin{cases} 1 & m' = m \\ 0 & m' \neq m \end{cases} \qquad (2.143)$$

from which one can derive relations given in Eqs. (2.152) and (2.153) with the aid of Eq. (2.128).

The numerical evaluation of the associated Legendre polynomials is discussed by Zhang and Jin (1996). The following is a FORTRAN program for computing the value of $P_n^m(x)$ and its first derivative.

```
      SUBROUTINE LPMN(MM,M,N,X,PM,PD)
C
C     ======================================================
C     Purpose: Compute associated Legendre functions Pmn(x)
C              and their derivatives Pmn'(x)
C     Input :  x  --- Argument of Pmn(x)
C              m  --- Order of Pmn(x),  m = 0,1,2,..., n
C              n  --- Degree of Pmn(x), n = 0,1,2,..., N
C              mm --- Physical dimension of PM and PD
C     Output:  PM(m,n) --- Pmn(x)
C              PD(m,n) --- Pmn'(x)
C     ======================================================
C
      IMPLICIT DOUBLE PRECISION (P,X)
      DIMENSION PM(0:MM,0:N),PD(0:MM,0:N)
      DO 10 I=0,N
      DO 10 J=0,M
         PM(J,I)=0.0D0
10       PD(J,I)=0.0D0
      PM(0,0)=1.0D0
      IF (DABS(X).EQ.1.0D0) THEN
         DO 15 I=1,N
            PM(0,I)=X**I
15          PD(0,I)=0.5D0*I*(I+1.0D0)*X**(I+1)
         DO 20 J=1,N
         DO 20 I=1,M
```

```
                IF (I.EQ.1) THEN
                   PD(I,J)=1.0D+300
                ELSE IF (I.EQ.2) THEN
                   PD(I,J)=-0.25D0*(J+2)*(J+1)*J*(J-1)*X**(J+1)
                ENDIF
20          CONTINUE
            RETURN
         ENDIF
         XQ=DSQRT(1.0D0-X*X)
         XS=1.0D0-X*X
         DO 30 I=1,M
30          PM(I,I)=(1.0D0-2.0D0*I)*XQ*PM(I-1,I-1)
         DO 35 I=0,M
35          PM(I,I+1)=(2.0D0*I+1.0D0)*X*PM(I,I)
         DO 40 I=0,M
         DO 40 J=I+2,N
            PM(I,J)=((2.0D0*J-1.0D0)*X*PM(I,J-1)
     &              -(I+J-1.0D0)*PM(I,J-2))/(J-I)
40       CONTINUE
         PD(0,0)=0.0D0
         DO 45 J=1,N
45          PD(0,J)=J*(PM(0,J-1)-X*PM(0,J))/XS
         DO 50 I=1,M
         DO 50 J=I,N
            PD(I,J)=I*X*PM(I,J)/XS+(J+I)*(J-I+1.0D0)/XQ*PM(I-1,J)
50       CONTINUE
         RETURN
         END
```

## 2.C Magnetic Field Produced by a Spherical Surface Current

Consider an arbitrary surface current on a sphere of radius $r_0$. Based on the analysis presented in Section 2.7, the magnetic field inside the sphere can be expressed as Eq. (2.69) and that outside the sphere can be expressed as Eq. (2.70). Applying the boundary condition $B_{1r} = B_{2r}$ across the spherical surface, we obtain

$$-\sum_{n=0}^{\infty}\sum_{m=0}^{n} n r_0^{n-1} P_n^m(\cos\theta)(A_{nm}\cos m\phi + B_{nm}\sin m\phi)$$

$$= \sum_{n=0}^{\infty}\sum_{m=0}^{n} \frac{n+1}{r_0^{n+2}} P_n^m(\cos\theta)(C_{nm}\cos m\phi + D_{nm}\sin m\phi). \quad (2.144)$$

Using the orthogonal relations for the associated Legendre polynomials and trigonometric functions, we find

$$C_{nm} = -\frac{n}{n+1} r_0^{2n+1} A_{nm}, \qquad D_{nm} = -\frac{n}{n+1} r_0^{2n+1} B_{nm}. \quad (2.145)$$

Substituting these into the two equations obtained from the boundary condition $\hat{r} \times (\mathbf{B}_1 - \mathbf{B}_2) = \mu_0 \mathbf{J}_s$, we obtain

$$\sum_{n=0}^{\infty} \sum_{m=0}^{n} \frac{2n+1}{n+1} r_0^{n-1} \frac{\partial P_n^m(\cos\theta)}{\partial\theta} (A_{nm}\cos m\phi + B_{nm}\sin m\phi) = \mu_0 J_\phi \quad (2.146)$$

$$\sum_{n=0}^{\infty} \sum_{m=0}^{n} \frac{2n+1}{n+1} \frac{m}{\sin\theta} r_0^{n-1} P_n^m(\cos\theta)(A_{nm}\sin m\phi - B_{nm}\cos m\phi) = -\mu_0 J_\theta. \quad (2.147)$$

To determine $A_{nm}$ and $B_{nm}$, we first use the orthogonal relations for the trigonometric functions to find

$$\sum_{n=0}^{\infty} \frac{2n+1}{n+1} r_0^{n-1} \frac{\partial P_n^m(\cos\theta)}{\partial\theta} A_{nm} = \frac{\mu_0}{(1+\delta_{0m})\pi} \int_0^{2\pi} J_\phi \cos m\phi \, d\phi \quad (2.148)$$

$$\sum_{n=0}^{\infty} \frac{2n+1}{n+1} r_0^{n-1} \frac{\partial P_n^m(\cos\theta)}{\partial\theta} B_{nm} = \frac{\mu_0}{\pi} \int_0^{2\pi} J_\phi \sin m\phi \, d\phi \quad (2.149)$$

$$\sum_{n=0}^{\infty} \frac{2n+1}{n+1} \frac{m}{\sin\theta} r_0^{n-1} P_n^m(\cos\theta) A_{nm} = -\frac{\mu_0}{\pi} \int_0^{2\pi} J_\theta \sin m\phi \, d\phi \quad (2.150)$$

$$\sum_{n=0}^{\infty} \frac{2n+1}{n+1} \frac{m}{\sin\theta} r_0^{n-1} P_n^m(\cos\theta) B_{nm} = \frac{\mu_0}{(1+\delta_{0m})\pi} \int_0^{2\pi} J_\theta \cos m\phi \, d\phi \quad (2.151)$$

where $\delta_{0m} = 1$ for $m = 0$ and $\delta_{0m} = 0$ otherwise. We then use the orthogonal relations (Stratton 1941, Chew 1995)

$$\int_0^\pi \left[ \frac{\partial P_n^m(\cos\theta)}{\partial\theta} \frac{\partial P_{n'}^m(\cos\theta)}{\partial\theta} + \frac{m^2}{\sin^2\theta} P_n^m(\cos\theta) P_{n'}^m(\cos\theta) \right] \sin\theta d\theta = \delta_{nn'} \frac{2n(n+1)}{(2n+1)} \frac{(n+m)!}{(n-m)!} \quad (2.152)$$

$$\int_0^\pi \left[ \frac{\partial P_n^m(\cos\theta)}{\partial\theta} P_{n'}^m(\cos\theta) + P_n^m(\cos\theta) \frac{\partial P_{n'}^m(\cos\theta)}{\partial\theta} \right] d\theta = 0 \quad (2.153)$$

to finally obtain

$$A_{nm} = \alpha_{nm} \int_0^{\pi} \int_0^{2\pi} \left[ J_\phi \frac{\partial P_n^m(\cos\theta)}{\partial \theta} \cos m\phi - J_\theta \frac{m}{\sin\theta} P_n^m(\cos\theta) \sin m\phi \right] \times \sin\theta \, d\phi \, d\theta \tag{2.154}$$

$$B_{nm} = \alpha_{nm} \int_0^{\pi} \int_0^{2\pi} \left[ J_\theta \frac{m}{\sin\theta} P_n^m(\cos\theta) \cos m\phi + J_\phi \frac{\partial P_n^m(\cos\theta)}{\partial \theta} \sin m\phi \right] \times \sin\theta \, d\phi \, d\theta \tag{2.155}$$

where

$$\alpha_{nm} = \frac{1}{2n} \frac{(n-m)!}{(n+m)!} \frac{\mu_0}{(1+\delta_{0m})\pi} \frac{1}{r_0^{n-1}}. \tag{2.156}$$

In addition to these, we also obtain

$$\int_0^{\pi} \int_0^{2\pi} \left[ J_\phi \frac{m}{\sin\theta} P_n^m(\cos\theta) \cos m\phi - J_\theta \frac{\partial P_n^m(\cos\theta)}{\partial \theta} \sin m\phi \right] \sin\theta \, d\phi \, d\theta = 0 \tag{2.157}$$

$$\int_0^{\pi} \int_0^{2\pi} \left[ J_\phi \frac{m}{\sin\theta} P_n^m(\cos\theta) \sin m\phi + J_\theta \frac{\partial P_n^m(\cos\theta)}{\partial \theta} \cos m\phi \right] \sin\theta \, d\phi \, d\theta = 0. \tag{2.158}$$

Equations (2.157) and (2.158) can be considered as conditions that the current density must satisfy in order for the formulation described to be valid. It can be shown that if the current density satisfies the continuity condition stated in Eq. (2.16), these two are always satisfied. Therefore, they can be considered as an alternative form of the continuity equation.

With the expansion coefficients given in Eqs. (2.154) and (2.155), we can find the magnetic field both inside and outside the sphere. In particular, the $z$-component of the magnetic field inside the sphere is given by

$$\begin{aligned} B_z(r,\theta,\phi) &= \cos\theta \, B_r(r,\theta,\phi) - \sin\theta \, B_\theta(r,\theta,\phi) \\ &= -\sum_{n=0}^{\infty} \sum_{m=0}^{n} r^{n-1} \left[ n \cos\theta P_n^m(\cos\theta) - \sin\theta \frac{\partial P_n^m(\cos\theta)}{\partial\theta} \right] \\ &\quad \times (A_{nm} \cos m\phi + B_{nm} \sin m\phi) \\ &= -\sum_{n=0}^{\infty} \sum_{m=0}^{n} r^{n-1} (n+m) P_{n-1}^m(\cos\theta) \\ &\quad \times (A_{nm} \cos m\phi + B_{nm} \sin m\phi) \end{aligned} \tag{2.159}$$

which can be rewritten as

$$B_z(r,\theta,\phi) = -\sum_{n=0}^{\infty}\sum_{m=0}^{n} r^n(n+m+1)P_n^m(\cos\theta) \times (A_{n+1,m}\cos m\phi + B_{n+1,m}\sin m\phi). \quad (2.160)$$

As an example, a circular loop of radius $a$ placed at $z_0$ can be considered as a surface current placed on a sphere of radius $r_0 = \sqrt{a^2 + z_0^2}$, whose density is given by

$$J_\phi = I\frac{\delta(\theta - \theta_0)}{r_0}, \qquad J_\theta = 0 \quad (2.161)$$

where $\theta_0$ is determined by $\cos\theta_0 = z_0/r_0$ and $I$ is the current in the loop. Substituting this into Eqs. (2.154) and (2.155), we obtain the only nonzero coefficients as

$$A_{n0} = -\frac{\mu_0 I}{2r_0^n}\left[P_{n-1}(\cos\theta_0) - \cos\theta_0 P_n(\cos\theta_0)\right] \quad (2.162)$$

and then, from Eq. (2.160), we have

$$B_z(r,\theta,\phi) = \frac{\mu_0 I}{2r_0}\sum_{n=0}^{\infty}\left(\frac{r}{r_0}\right)^n (n+1)P_n(\cos\theta) \times \left[P_n(\cos\theta_0) - \cos\theta_0 P_{n+1}(\cos\theta_0)\right]. \quad (2.163)$$

Along the $z$-axis, this reduces to

$$B_z(r,0,\phi) = \frac{\mu_0 I}{2r_0}\sum_{n=0}^{\infty}\left(\frac{z}{r_0}\right)^n (n+1)\left[P_n(\cos\theta_0) - \cos\theta_0 P_{n+1}(\cos\theta_0)\right]. \quad (2.164)$$

## 2.D Computer Program for Inductance Calculation

Consider two parallel strips of different widths and different lengths in the same plane, as illustrated in Fig. 2.14. Without any loss of generality, we assume both strips are in the $xz$-plane and the lower-left corner of strip 1 is at the origin. The mutual inductance between the two strips is then given by

$$M = \frac{\mu_0}{4\pi w_1 w_2}\int_{x_1}^{x_2}\int_{z_1}^{z_2}\int_{x_1'}^{x_2'}\int_{z_1'}^{z_2'}\frac{1}{R}\,dz'dx'dzdx \quad (2.165)$$

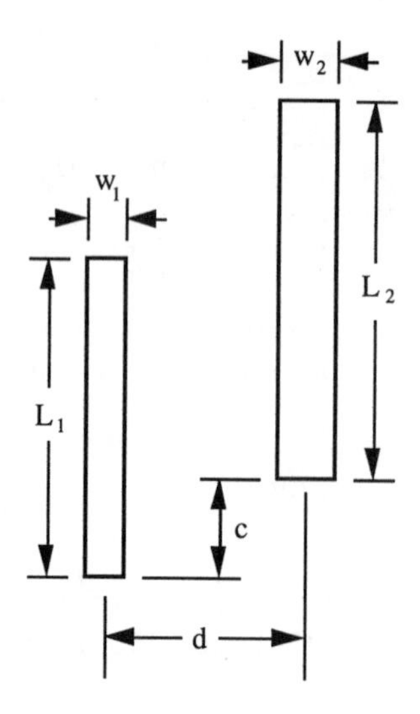


**Figure 2.14.** Two strips in the same plane.

where $x_1 = 0$, $x_2 = w_1$, $z_1 = 0$, $z_2 = L_1$, $x_1' = d + (w_1 - w_2)/2$, $x_2' = d + (w_1 + w_2)/2$, $z_1' = c$, and $z_2' = c + L_2$. These integrals can be evaluated analytically, yielding

$$M = \frac{\mu_0}{4\pi w_1 w_2}\left[\frac{(x-x')(z-z')}{2}\{(x-x')\ln[(z-z')+R] + (z-z')\ln[(x-x')+R]\} - \frac{(x-x')(z-z')[(x-x')+(z-z')]}{4} - \frac{R^3}{6}\right]\Bigg|_{x'=x_1'}^{x_2'}\Bigg|_{z'=z_1'}^{z_2'}\Bigg|_{x=x_1}^{x_2}\Bigg|_{z=z_1}^{z_2} \tag{2.166}$$

Apparently, when the two strips coincide with each other, Eq. (2.166) becomes the self-inductance given in Eq. (2.84). Equation (2.166) can be calculated using the FORTRAN computer program given below.

```
      REAL FUNCTION STRIPM(W1,W2,L1,L2,D,C)
C
C     ================================================================
C     Purpose: Compute the mutual inductance between two strips
C              or the self-inductance of a strip
C     Input:   W1 --- Width of strip 1 (in cm)
C              W2 --- Width of strip 2 (in cm)
C              L1 --- Length of strip 1 (in cm)
```

```
C              L2 --- Length of strip 2 (in cm)
C              D  --- Distance between two strips (in cm)
C              C  --- Longitudinal displacement (in cm)
C       Output STRIPM --- Mutual or self-inductance (in uH)
C       ============================================================
        REAL L1,L2
        XL=0.0
        XU=W1
        YL=0.0
        YU=L1
        XLP=D+0.5*W1-0.5*W2
        XUP=XLP+W2
        YLP=C
        YUP=YLP+L2
        A1=FINT(XUP,YUP,XU,YU)
        A2=FINT(XLP,YLP,XU,YU)
        A3=FINT(XLP,YUP,XU,YU)
        A4=FINT(XUP,YLP,XU,YU)
        A5=FINT(XUP,YUP,XL,YL)
        A6=FINT(XLP,YLP,XL,YL)
        A7=FINT(XLP,YUP,XL,YL)
        A8=FINT(XUP,YLP,XL,YL)
        A9=FINT(XUP,YUP,XL,YU)
        A10=FINT(XLP,YLP,XL,YU)
        A11=FINT(XLP,YUP,XL,YU)
        A12=FINT(XUP,YLP,XL,YU)
        A13=FINT(XUP,YUP,XU,YL)
        A14=FINT(XLP,YLP,XU,YL)
        A15=FINT(XLP,YUP,XU,YL)
        A16=FINT(XUP,YLP,XU,YL)
        G1=A1+A2-A3-A4+A5+A6-A7-A8-A9-A10+A11+A12-A13-A14+A15+A16
        STRIPM=0.001*G1/(W1*W2)
        RETURN
        END

        REAL FUNCTION FINT(XP,YP,X,Y)
        XX=X-XP
        YY=Y-YP
        R=SQRT(XX*XX+YY*YY)
        IF((ABS(XX).LE.0.0).OR.(ABS(YY).LE.0.0)) THEN
        SUM=-R*R*R/6.
        ELSE
        SUM=0.5*XX*YY*(XX*ALOG(YY+R)+YY*ALOG(XX+R))
       1    -0.25*XX*YY*(XX+YY)-R*R*R/6.
        END IF
```

```
FINT=SUM
RETURN
END
```

## Problems

2.1 Derive Gauss's theorem in Eq. (2.2) from the definition of the divergence in Eq. (2.1).

2.2 Derive the alternative definition of the curl in Eq. (2.4) from the definition given in Eq. (2.3). Derive Stokes's theorem in Eq. (2.5) from Eq. (2.4).

2.3 Derive the alternative definition of the gradient in Eq. (2.7) from the definition given in Eq. (2.6). Derive the gradient theorem in Eq. (2.8) from Eq. (2.6).

2.4 Verify the vector identities in Eqs. (2.9) and (2.10) in Cartesian coordinates.

2.5 Consider a triangular loop coil in the $xy$-plane, as sketched below, where the $z$-axis passes through the center of the triangle. The current in the loop is $I$. (1) Find the value of $\alpha$ so that the magnetic field along the $z$-axis has only a $z$-component. (2) Find the expression for this magnetic field along the $z$-axis.

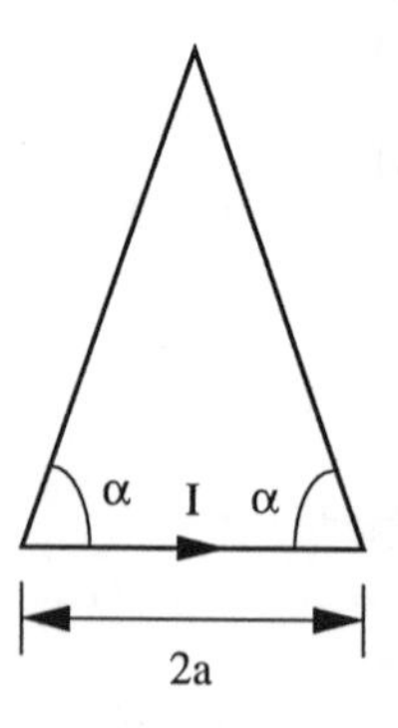


2.6 Derive the general expression for the magnetic field of a circular loop as given in Eqs. (2.32) and (2.33).

2.7 Using Eq. (2.61), find the magnetic fields of the Helmholtz and Maxwell coils in spherical coordinates.

2.8 A continuous, $z$-directed cylindrical surface current $\mathbf{J}_s = \hat{z} J_0 \sin\phi$ can be realized approximately by using $N$ equi-spaced line currents whose currents are given by

$$I_n = I_0 \sin[(n-1)\Delta\phi] \qquad (n = 1, 2, \ldots, N)$$

where $\Delta\phi = 2\pi/N$. Find the magnetic field inside the cylindrical surface and compare it with Eq. (2.67).

2.9 A continuous spherical surface current $\mathbf{J}_s = \hat{\phi} J_0 \sin\theta$ can be realized approximately by placing $N$ circular loops carrying the same current on the spherical surface. Find the location and radius of each loop for $N = 2$ and $N = 4$. Hint: The total current is given by

$$I = aJ_0 \int_0^\pi \sin\theta \, d\theta = 2aJ_0$$

where $a$ denotes the radius of the spherical surface. Hence, the current in each loop is $2aJ_0/N$, and the $n$th loop should be placed at $\theta_n$ which is specified by

$$\frac{2}{N}\left(n - \frac{1}{2}\right) = \int_0^{\theta_n} \sin\theta \, d\theta.$$

2.10 Given a square loop of length $l$ made of conducting strip of width $w$, find the self-inductance of the loop.

2.11 Show that the self-inductance of a circular loop of radius $a$, which is made of a circular wire of radius $b$, is given by

$$L = \mu_0 a \left(\ln \frac{8a}{b} - \frac{3}{2}\right)$$

when the current is distributed uniformly over the cross section of the wire and

$$L = \mu_0 a \left(\ln \frac{8a}{b} - 2\right)$$

when the current is distributed uniformly over the surface of the wire.

2.12 Consider two wires, whose lengths are denoted as $l_1$ and $l_2$, respectively, in the same axis, as illustrated below.

$l_1$ $l_2$

Using Eq. (2.82), find the mutual inductance between the two wires. Hint: Use the relation $L = L_1 + L_2 + 2M$, where $L$ denotes the self-inductance of a wire of length $l_1 + l_2$, $L_1$ and $L_2$ denote the self-inductances of the wires of length $l_1$ and $l_2$, respectively, and $M$ denotes the mutual inductance between the two wires. Note that the result also applies to strips because Eq. (2.85) has a similar form to Eq. (2.82).

2.13 Consider $N$ Helmholtz-type coil pairs, sketched below. Show that the expression for the derivative of $B_z$ is given by

$$\left.\frac{d^{2m}B_z}{dz^{2m}}\right|_{z=0} = \mu_0 \sum_{n=1}^{N} I_n \frac{(2m+1)!}{(z_n^2+a^2)^{m+1/2}} \left[P_{2m}(u_n) - u_n P_{2m+1}(u_n)\right]$$

where $u_n = z_n \Big/ \sqrt{z_n^2 + a^2}$ with $2z_n$ being the separation between the two loops of the $n$th pair, and $P_{2m}$ and $P_{2m+1}$ are the Legendre polynomials of degree $2m$ and $2m+1$, respectively. Hint: Use the result in Eq. (2.164).

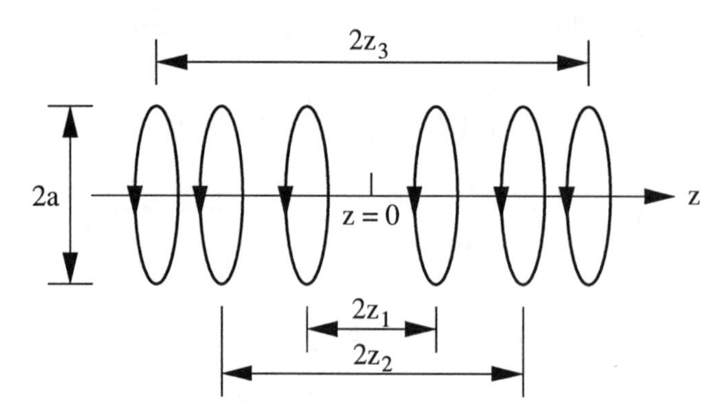


2.14 Using the expression in Problem 2.13, describe the procedure to design a magnet with three coil pairs (that is, $N = 3$) to produce a uniform magnetic field in the vicinity of the magnet's center. Show that it is possible to obtain a field that is uniform through the tenth power of $z$, that is,

$$B_z(z) = B_z(0) + O[(z/a)^{11}].$$

## References

M. Abramowitz and I. Stegun, Eds. (1964), *Handbook of Mathematical Functions.* Washington: National Bureau of Standards. Reprinted by New York: Dover Publications, 1968.

D. K. Cheng (1993), *Fundamentals of Engineering Electromagnetics.* Reading, MA: Addison-Wesley.

W. C. Chew (1995), *Waves and Fields in Inhomogeneous Media.* New York: IEEE Press, p. 187.

R. E. Collin (1991), *Field Theory of Guided Waves* (2nd edition). New York: IEEE Press, p. 837.

R. S. Elliot (1966), *Electromagnetics.* New York: McGraw-Hill.

F. W. Grover (1962), *Inductance Calculations: Working Formulas and Tables.* New York: Dover.

W. H. Hayt (1989), *Engineering Electromagnetics* (5th edition). New York: McGraw-Hill.

J. D. Jackson (1975), *Classical Electrodynamics* (2nd edition). New York: Wiley.

C. T. Johnk (1975), *Engineering Electromagnetic Fields and Waves.* New York: Wiley.

J. D. Kraus (1992), *Electromagnetics* (4th edition). New York: McGraw-Hill.

G. F. Miner (1996), *Lines and Electromagnetic Fields for Engineers.* New York: Oxford Univ. Press.

M. A. Plonus (1978), *Applied Electromagnetics.* New York: McGraw-Hill.

N. N. Rao (1994), *Elements of Engineering Electromagnetics* (4th edition). Englewood Cliffs, NJ: Prentice-Hall.

J. A. Stratton (1941), *Electromagnetic Theory.* New York: McGraw-Hill, p. 417.

S. Zhang and J. Jin (1996), *Computation of Special Functions.* New York: Wiley.

# Chapter 3

# Analysis and Design of Gradient Coils

## 3.1 Introduction

In a magnetic resonance imaging (MRI) scanner, the main magnet and a set of shim coils produce, along the $z$ direction, a very homogeneous static magnetic field—the $B_0$ field. To provide the spatial information of MR images, the magnetic field strength must be able to vary in space in a controllable manner. Such a variation is provided by a set of gradient coils, which produce magnetic fields whose $z$-component varies linearly along the $x$, $y$, and $z$ directions, respectively. The linearity of the gradient fields is measured by the constancy of the gradients, defined as

$$G_x = \frac{\partial B_z}{\partial x}, \qquad G_y = \frac{\partial B_z}{\partial y}, \qquad G_z = \frac{\partial B_z}{\partial z} \tag{3.1}$$

where $G_x$ and $G_y$ are called transverse gradients and $G_z$ is called the longitudinal gradient. For imaging purposes, the ideal gradient fields are such that $G_x$, $G_y$, and $G_z$ are constant within the volume of interest.

In this chapter, we discuss the basic principles for the analysis and design of gradient coils for MRI applications. We first examine the effect of the inductance of a gradient coil on its performance and the inductance compensation using a gradient driver. We then briefly describe the concept of the figure of merit to measure the quality of a gradient coil. After that, we discuss the design of gradient coils using discrete wires. This is followed by the description of the target field method for the design of gradient coils, including shielded coils, using distributed currents. Finally, we discuss the design of gradient coils with a minimum inductance or power dissipation using the Lagrange multiplier method. The chapter concludes with a description of the design of planar gradient coils.

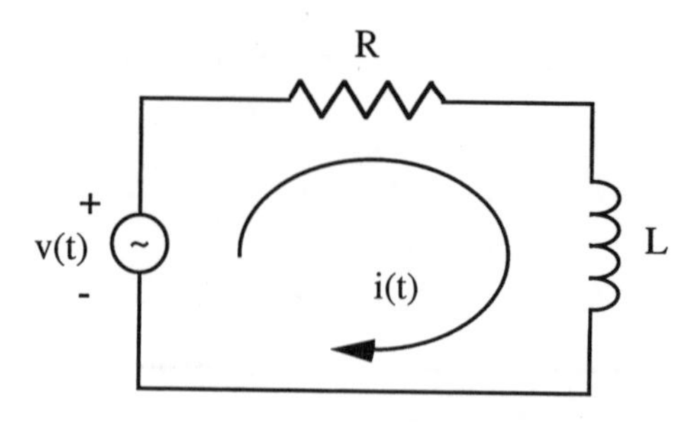


**Figure 3.1.** An *RL*-circuit.

## 3.2 Effect of Coil's Inductance

In the design of gradient coils for MRI applications, the inductance of a gradient coil is one of the major factors that measure the quality of the coil. A good gradient coil should have an inductance as small as possible so that the coil can be switched on and off quickly. A large inductance can reduce the switching speed. To illustrate this, let us consider the simple *RL*-circuit shown in Fig. 3.1. In accordance with Kirchhoff's voltage law, the current in the circuit is related to the voltage by

$$L\frac{di(t)}{dt} + Ri(t) = v(t). \tag{3.2}$$

Assume that the voltage turns on instantaneously at $t = 0$ and there is no current in the circuit before this moment. Solving Eq. (3.2), we obtain

$$i(t) = \frac{V}{R}\left[1 - e^{-(R/L)t}\right] \tag{3.3}$$

which is plotted in Fig. 3.2. It is clear that the current does not rise to its maximum instantaneously. Instead, it rises exponentially with a rise time directly proportional to the inductance. A time constant, defined as the time it takes for the current to rise 63% of its full value, is given by

$$\tau = L/R \tag{3.4}$$

which is proportional to the inductance. A similar phenomenon is observed when the voltage turns off at $t = 0$, as illustrated in Fig. 3.3.

It is evident from Eq. (3.4) that one method to reduce the rise time is to reduce the inductance ($R$ must be kept small to limit the power consumption). In addition to this, the rise time can also be reduced by

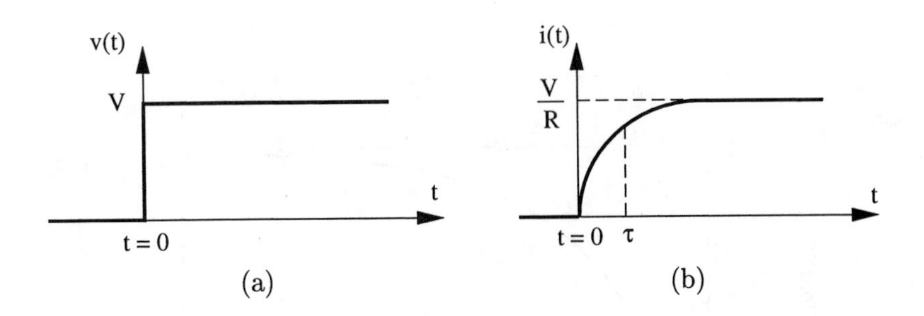


**Figure 3.2.** Response of an $RL$-circuit. (a) Input. (b) Output.

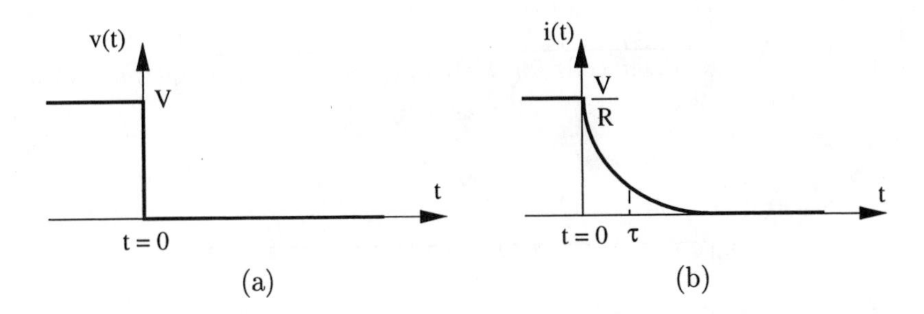


**Figure 3.3.** Response of an $RL$-circuit. (a) Input. (b) Output.

adjusting the gradient voltage at the cost of using a more powerful gradient driver. For example, if we wish to reduce the rise time by a factor of $q$, the desired current should have the form

$$i(t) = \frac{V}{R}\left[1 - e^{-q(R/L)t}\right]. \tag{3.5}$$

Substituting this into Eq. (3.2), we obtain the required voltage as

$$v(t) = V\left[1 + (q-1)e^{-q(R/L)t}\right] \tag{3.6}$$

from which it is apparent that the required gradient driver must be $q$ times more powerful. This is illustrated in Fig. 3.4 for the case of $\tau = 1$ and $q = 5$. The same technique can be applied to reduce the turn-off time illustrated in Fig. 3.3. This is left to the reader as an exercise.

Finally, we note that the inductance of most cylindrical coils is proportional to the fifth power of the radius. Therefore, it is important

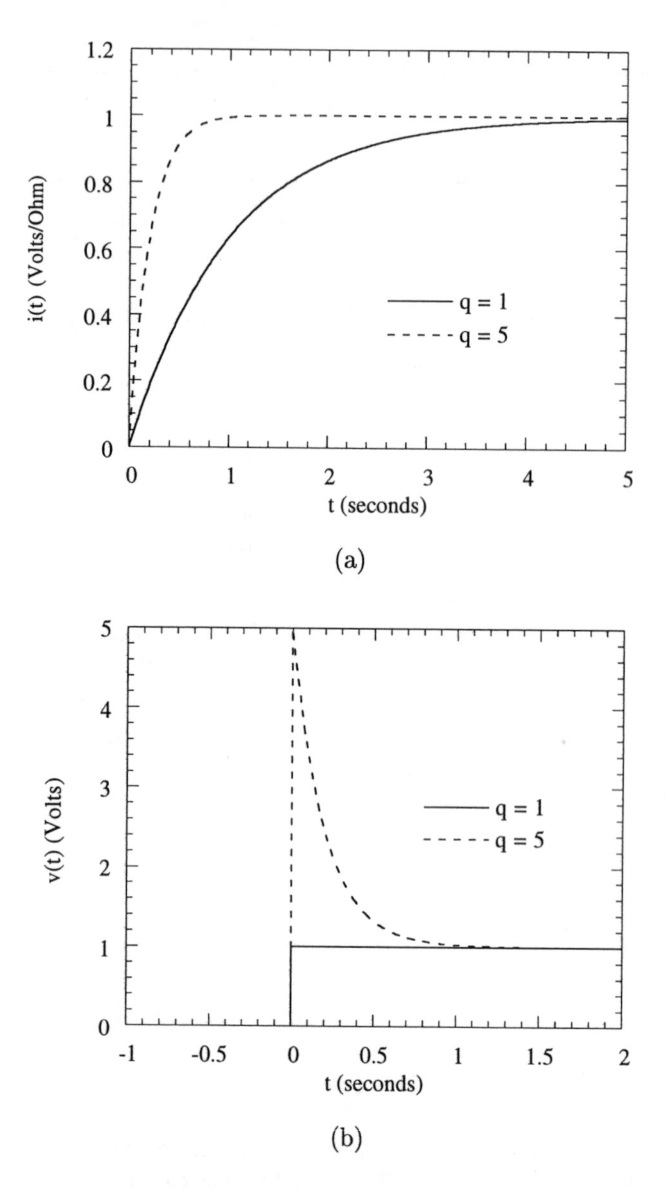


**Figure 3.4.** Compensation for the effect of inductance by adjusting the voltage waveform. (a) Desired current. (b) Required voltage.

to keep the coils as small as possible. Of course, this is necessary only for applications that require fast switching of the gradient fields.

## 3.3 Figure of Merit

For MRI applications, the quality of a gradient coil is measured primarily by three factors. The first factor is the coil efficiency, denoted by $\eta$, which is a measure of the field gradient at the center of the coil produced by a unit current. The second factor is the inductance, denoted by $L$. The third factor is the gradient homogeneity, which is the difference between the desired field and the field actually achieved over the volume of interest, that is,

$$\delta = \frac{1}{V} \iiint_V \left[ \frac{B_{\text{achieved}} - B_{\text{desired}}}{B_{\text{desired}}} \right]^2 dv. \tag{3.7}$$

A good gradient coil should have a coil efficiency as high as possible, an inductance as small as possible, and a very homogeneous gradient. To properly measure the quality of a gradient coil, Turner (1988, 1993) defined a figure of merit as

$$\beta = \frac{\eta^2}{L\sqrt{\delta}}. \tag{3.8}$$

Apparently, this figure is independent of the number of turns of coil; it depends only on the configuration and radius of the coil. For the purpose of comparison, the radius of a coil can be scaled to 1.0 m.

## 3.4 Gradient Coils Made of Discrete Wires

Gradient coils can be designed using either discrete or distributed currents. In this section, we discuss first the design using discrete currents.

### 3.4.1 Longitudinal Gradient

A simple and popular $z$-gradient coil is called the Maxwell coil pair, which consists of two circular loops having electric currents in opposite directions. As pointed out in Section 2.4, the Maxwell coil pair produces a magnetic field along its axis, designated as the $z$-axis, given by

$$B_z(z) = B_z'(0)\, z + O[(z/d)^5] \tag{3.9}$$

when the distance between the two loops is chosen to be $d = \sqrt{3}a$ with $a$ denoting the radius of the loops. The $z$-gradient then becomes

$$G_z(z) = \frac{dB_z(z)}{dz} = B'_z(0) + O[(z/d)^4] \tag{3.10}$$

which is a constant through the third order. A simple calculation shows that this gradient is uniform to 5% within a sphere of radius $0.5a$ and, at the center, the gradient efficiency is (Turner 1993)

$$\eta = \frac{8.058 \times 10^{-7}}{a^2} \mathrm{T} \cdot \mathrm{m}^{-1} \cdot \mathrm{A}^{-1}. \tag{3.11}$$

A straightforward approach to obtaining a better $z$-gradient field is to introduce more loops or a coil with multiple turns. Recalling that a pair of coils, carrying a current $I_n$ and placed at $z = z_n$ and $z = -z_n$, respectively, produces a magnetic field

$$B_z(z) = \frac{\mu_0 I_n a^2}{2\left[(z - z_n)^2 + a^2\right]^{3/2}} - \frac{\mu_0 I_n a^2}{2\left[(z + z_n)^2 + a^2\right]^{3/2}} \tag{3.12}$$

along the $z$-axis, the field produced by $N$ such pairs can then be written as

$$B_z(z) = \frac{\mu_0 a^2}{2} \sum_{n=1}^{N} I_n \left\{ \left[(z - z_n)^2 + a^2\right]^{-3/2} - \left[(z + z_n)^2 + a^2\right]^{-3/2} \right\}. \tag{3.13}$$

Because of the antisymmetric configuration, the field and all of its even derivatives vanish at $z = 0$. By properly selecting $z_n$ and $I_n$, we can systematically remove the third, fifth, and other higher-order odd derivatives, thus achieving a better $z$-gradient field. To do this, we have to find the expression for the derivative of Eq. (3.13), which is given by (Romeo and Hoult 1984)

$$\left. \frac{d^{2m+1} B_z}{dz^{2m+1}} \right|_{z=0} = \mu_0 \sum_{n=1}^{N} I_n \frac{(2m+2)!}{(z_n^2 + a^2)^{m+1}} \left[P_{2m+1}(u_n) - u_n P_{2m+2}(u_n)\right] \tag{3.14}$$

where $u_n = z_n \Big/ \sqrt{z_n^2 + a^2}$ and $P_{2m+1}$ and $P_{2m+2}$ are the Legendre polynomials (see Appendix 2.B). For example, for the case of two coil pairs ($N = 2$), we can select $z_1$, $z_2$, and the ratio $I_2/I_1$ to eliminate the third, fifth, and seventh derivatives. This results in a solution given by (Suits and Wilken 1989)

$$z_1 = 0.44a, \qquad z_2 = 1.19a, \qquad \frac{I_2}{I_1} = 7.47. \tag{3.15}$$

The resulting gradient is a constant through the seventh order and is uniform to 5% within a sphere of radius $0.8a$, compared to $0.5a$ for the case of one pair. The gradient efficiency is

$$\eta = \frac{2.809 \times 10^{-7}}{a^2}\ \mathrm{T \cdot m^{-1} \cdot A^{-1}} \tag{3.16}$$

which is lower than that of the Maxwell pair.

Another approach to finding the desired currents $I_n$ is to match their field at a number of discrete points $z_m$ with the desired field (Hoult 1973). Doing so, we obtain a set of linear equations

$$\sum_{n=1}^{N} A_{mn} I_n = B_z^{\text{desired}}(z_m) \tag{3.17}$$

where $B_z^{\text{desired}}(z_m)$ denotes the desired field at $z_m$ and

$$A_{mn} = \frac{\mu_0 a^2}{2}\left\{\left[(z_m - z_n)^2 + a^2\right]^{-3/2} - \left[(z_m + z_n)^2 + a^2\right]^{-3/2}\right\} \tag{3.18}$$

By choosing $N$ such discrete points within the volume of interest, we obtain a square-matrix equation

$$[A]\{I\} = \{B_z^{\text{desired}}\} \tag{3.19}$$

which can be solved for $I_n$ for a set of prefixed $z_n$. The drawback of this method, known as the point collocation method, is that the matrix $[A]$ is almost always singular and, therefore, Eq. (3.19) cannot be solved by direct matrix inversion methods such as Gaussian elimination and *LU* decomposition. Instead, it must be solved by an iterative method. The solution obtained often requires large variations in current from one turn to another and sometimes even current reversal. One approach to reduce the large variation is to deliberately set a high tolerance in the iterative method to allow a slight yet permissible deviation of the actual field from the desired field. In addition to the point collocation method, one can also solve for $I_n$ using the least squares method, which minimizes an error defined by

$$\varepsilon = \int_{-L}^{L} \left[B_z(z) - B_z^{\text{desired}}(z)\right]^2 dz \tag{3.20}$$

where $(-L, L)$ denotes the region of interest along the $z$-axis. Substituting Eq. (3.13) into Eq. (3.20) and setting the partial derivative of $\varepsilon$ with respect to $I_n$ to zero

$$\frac{\partial \varepsilon}{\partial I_n} = 0 \qquad (n = 1, 2, \ldots, N) \tag{3.21}$$

we obtain a set of linear equations, which can be solved for $I_n$ for a set of prefixed $z_n$. This method also suffers from the drawback discussed above. Also note that any deviation from the predicted currents and positions, which is inevitable in practice, can introduce some degree of gradient inhomogeneity and, in addition, the linearity of the field off the $z$-axis cannot be guaranteed. The second drawback, however, can be alleviated by replacing the line integral in Eq. (3.20) with an integral over the volume of interest.

Obtaining $I_n$ for a set of prefixed $z_n$, as described above, may not be the best way to design gradient coils since in practice one cannot achieve an arbitrary current at a fixed point. If the coil is made of a wire carrying a current $i_0$, the achievable current can only be $k \cdot i_0$ where $k$ denotes the number of turns at that point. Also, physically piling up many turns at one position can make it difficult to maintain the accuracy of positioning. An alternative, or preferred, approach is to fix $I_n$ and search for $z_n$ so that Eq. (3.20) is minimized. Because $z_n$ is involved in a complicated function, we cannot derive a set of linear equations to solve for $z_n$. Instead, we have to employ a minimization or optimization technique to search for $z_n$. Techniques such as the conjugate gradient method (Wong *et al.* 1991), the simulated annealing (SA) method (Crozier and Doddrell 1993), and the genetic algorithm (GA) can be used for this purpose. The potential advantage of the latter two (SA and GA) over traditional optimization methods is their ability to find the global optima, which may be hidden among many local optima. The simulated annealing is a multivariate or combinatorial optimization technique, which mimics the way that a metal slowly cools and anneals to a stable state of minimum energy. The reader is referred to Press *et al.* (1992) for an easy-to-understand discussion of the method. The genetic algorithm is an iterative search procedure that starts with a selected population of potential solutions that gradually evolve toward better solutions through the application of genetic operators. These genetic operators are modeled after processes of procreation observed in nature. Their repetitive application to a population of potential solutions results in an optimization process that resembles natural evolution. For a detailed discussion of the genetic algorithm, the reader is referred to Goldberg (1989). Finally, we note that when using the optimization methods, not only can one minimize the gradient inhomogeneity, but one can also minimize the inductance and power dissipation and maximize the efficiency simultaneously by properly defining an error as the weighted combination of these factors (Wong *et al.* 1991, Crozier and Doddrell 1993). To avoid a large $z_n$, one can also impose a constraint on the optimization.

### 3.4.2 Transverse Gradients

To understand how to design a transverse gradient coil, we consider a negative $x$-directed straight current placed at $y = b$, as shown in Fig. 3.5(a). This current will produce a $z$-directed field along the $y$-axis, whose $y$-gradient can be expressed as

$$G_y(y) = \frac{dB_z(y)}{dy} = B_z'(0) + O(y/b). \tag{3.22}$$

To double the gradient strength, we can place another straight current at $y = -b$ flowing in the negative $x$ direction, as shown in Fig. 3.5(b). Because of the antisymmetry of the $B_z$ along the $y$-axis, the even derivatives of $B_z$ with respect to $y$ vanish. Hence, the $y$-gradient can be expressed as

$$G_y(y) = \frac{dB_z(y)}{dy} = B_z'(0) + O[(y/b)^2] \tag{3.23}$$

where $B_z'(0)$ has twice the value of that in Eq. (3.22). The gradient field so obtained has poor gradient uniformity off the $y$-axis. To achieve better uniformity, we can employ two such pairs placed at $z = \pm d$, respectively, as shown in Fig. 3.5(c). A proper choice of $d$ can remove the third derivative of $B_z$ with respect to $y$; hence, the $y$-gradient can be expressed as

$$G_y(y) = \frac{\partial B_z(y)}{\partial y} = G_y(0) + O[(y/b)^4] \tag{3.24}$$

which is uniform through the third order.

To find the specific values for $b$ and $d$, we have to consider the specific expression of the field produced by the configuration in Fig. 3.5(c). The $B_z$ produced by the current at $y = b$ and $z = d$ can be written as

$$B_z(y,z) = \frac{\mu_0 I}{2\pi}\frac{b-y}{(b-y)^2+(d-z)^2} \tag{3.25}$$

which can be written as the real part of a simple complex function (Zupancic 1962, Zupancic and Pirs 1976)

$$\begin{aligned} B_z(y,z) &= \frac{\mu_0 I}{2\pi}\mathrm{Re}[(b+id)-(y+iz)]^{-1} \\ &= \frac{\mu_0 I}{2\pi}\mathrm{Re}[\rho e^{i\varphi}-\xi]^{-1} \end{aligned} \tag{3.26}$$

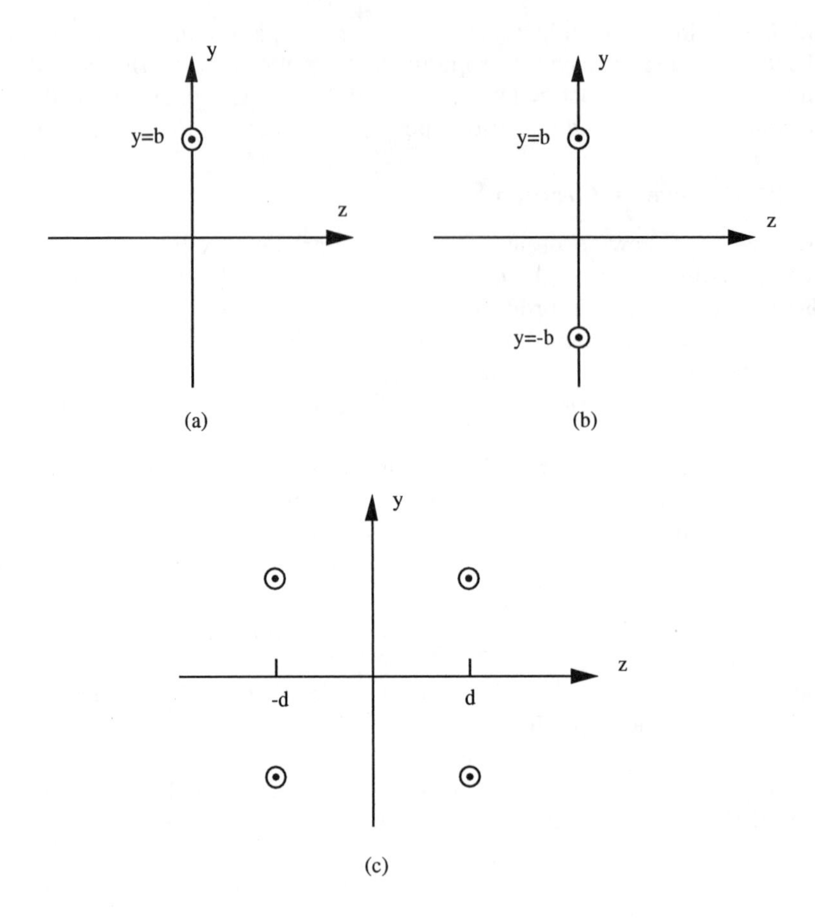


**Figure 3.5.** Evolution of a four-wire $y$-gradient coil.

where $\rho e^{i\varphi} = b + id$ and $\xi = y + iz$. Expanding Eq. (3.26) into a Taylor series, we obtain

$$B_z(\xi) = \frac{\mu_0 I}{2\pi\rho}\mathrm{Re}\sum_{n=0}^{\infty}\left(\frac{\xi}{\rho}\right)^n e^{-i(n+1)\varphi} \qquad (|\xi| < \rho). \tag{3.27}$$

Therefore, the total $B_z$ produced by the four currents is

$$B_z(\xi) = \frac{\mu_0 I}{2\pi\rho}\mathrm{Re}\sum_{n=0}^{\infty}\left(\frac{\xi}{\rho}\right)^n \times\left[e^{-i(n+1)\varphi} + e^{i(n+1)\varphi} + e^{-i(n+1)(\pi-\varphi)} + e^{i(n+1)(\pi-\varphi)}\right]$$

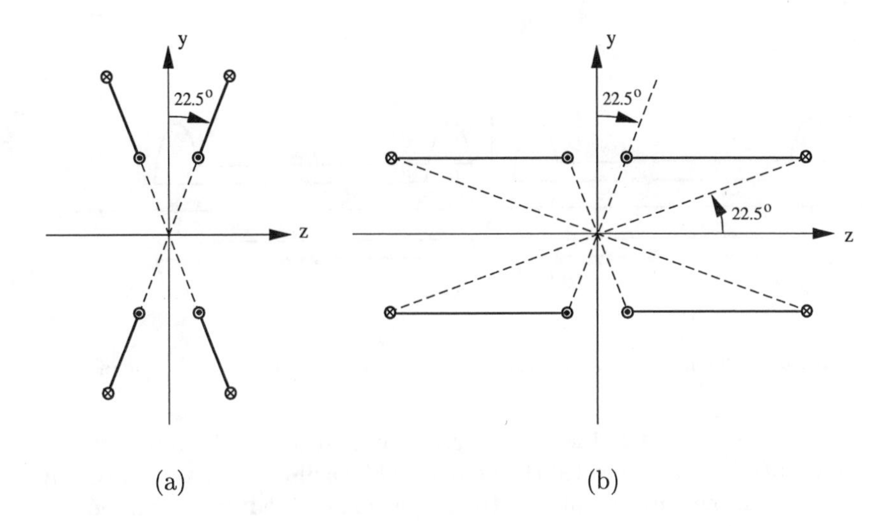


**Figure 3.6.** Arrangement of a four-wire $y$-gradient coil with return paths.

$$= \frac{\mu_0 I}{\pi\rho} \sum_{n=0}^{\infty} \frac{\mathrm{Re}(\xi^n)}{\rho^n} \left[1 + (-1)^{n+1}\right] \cos(n+1)\varphi \qquad (|\xi| < \rho). \tag{3.28}$$

Apparently, all even-order terms vanish in Eq. (3.28) and $B_z$ is therefore an odd function of $\xi$. To be more specific, Eq. (3.28) can be written as

$$B_z(\xi) = \frac{2\mu_0 I}{\pi\rho} \left[\frac{y}{\rho}\cos 2\varphi + \frac{\mathrm{Re}(\xi^3)}{\rho^3}\cos 4\varphi + \frac{\mathrm{Re}(\xi^5)}{\rho^5}\cos 6\varphi + \cdots\right] \qquad (|\xi| < \rho). \tag{3.29}$$

The first term provides the $y$-gradient. The next term is the third-order term, which can be made zero by setting $\cos 4\varphi = 0$, from which we obtain $\varphi = \pi/8 = 22.5°$ and $\varphi = 3\pi/8 = 67.5°$. Therefore, if $d$ is chosen such that $d/b = \cos(\pi/8) = 0.924$ or $d/b = \cos(3\pi/8) = 0.383$, the $y$-gradient is uniform through the third order. Two practical configurations containing return paths are depicted in Fig. 3.6 (Mansfield and Morris 1982, Thomas *et al.* 1988). The configuration in Fig. 3.6(a) forms the basis for the design of the trapezoidal gradient coil (Bangert and Mansfield 1982), which has a relatively low inductance.

In most MRI scanners, the gradient coils are made of wires wound on a cylindrical surface. Doing so, the four wires in Fig. 3.5(c) then become the four inner arcs shown in Fig. 3.7. In Fig. 3.7, eight additional wires

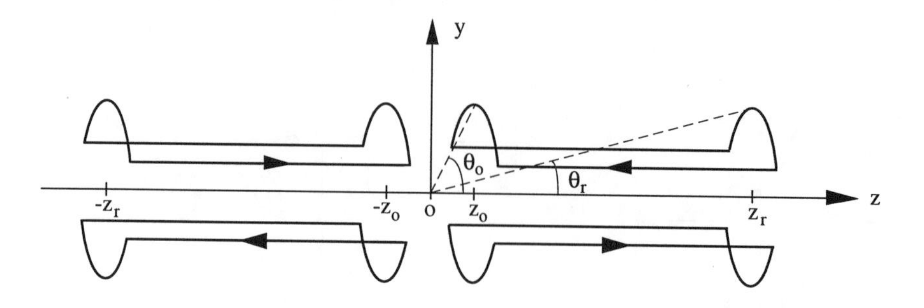


**Figure 3.7.** "Golay" transverse gradient coil. The arcs subtend an angle of 120°.

parallel to the $z$-axis and four outer arcs are used to provide return paths. The resulting design is called the double-saddle coil or "Golay" coil (Golay 1957). Since the wires parallel to the $z$-axis do not produce a $z$-component of magnetic field, they do not affect the gradient field. To determine the length and position of the inner and outer arcs, we consider first the $z$-component of the magnetic field produced by an arc on a cylinder of radius $a$. Since $B_z$ satisfies the Laplace equation $\nabla^2 B_z = 0$, it can be expanded in the vicinity of the origin as (Romeo and Hoult 1984, Carlson 1987)

$$B_z(r,\theta,\phi) = \sum_{n=0}^{\infty} \sum_{m=0}^{n} r^n P_n^m(\cos\theta)(A_{nm}\cos m\phi + B_{nm}\sin m\phi) \quad (3.30)$$

where $P_n^m(\cos\theta)$ denotes the associated Legendre polynomial and $A_{nm}$ and $B_{nm}$ are the expansion coefficients. For an arc that extends from $\phi_1$ to $\phi_2$ and is placed at $z_0$, $A_{nm}$ and $B_{nm}$ are given by

$$A_{nm} = \frac{\mu_0 I}{4(1+\delta_{0m})\pi} \int_{\phi_1}^{\phi_2} \frac{a}{r_0^{n+2}} f_{nm}(\theta_0) \cos m\phi \, d\phi \quad (3.31)$$

$$B_{nm} = \frac{\mu_0 I}{4\pi} \int_{\phi_1}^{\phi_2} \frac{a}{r_0^{n+2}} f_{nm}(\theta_0) \sin m\phi \, d\phi \quad (3.32)$$

where $\delta_{0m} = 1$ for $m = 0$, $\delta_{0m} = 0$ otherwise, $r_0^2 = a^2 + z_0^2$, and

$$f_{nm}(\theta_0) = \frac{(n-m)!}{(n+m)!} \{2(n+1)\sin\theta_0 P_n^m(\cos\theta_0) - \cos\theta_0 \left[P_n^{m+1}(\cos\theta_0) - (n+m)(n-m+1)P_n^{m-1}(\cos\theta_0)\right]\} \quad (3.33)$$

in which $\sin\theta_0 = a/r_0$ and $\cos\theta_0 = z_0/r_0$. The explicit expressions for the first several $f_{nm}$ are given by

$$\begin{aligned}
f_{00}(\theta_0) &= 2\sin\theta_0 \\
f_{10}(\theta_0) &= 6\sin\theta_0\cos\theta_0 \\
f_{11}(\theta_0) &= \cos^2\theta_0 - 2\sin^2\theta_0 \\
f_{20}(\theta_0) &= 3(4\sin\theta_0\cos^2\theta_0 - \sin^3\theta_0) \\
f_{21}(\theta_0) &= \cos^3\theta_0 - 4\sin^2\theta_0\cos\theta_0 \\
f_{22}(\theta_0) &= \tfrac{1}{4}(3\sin^3\theta_0 - 2\sin\theta_0\cos^2\theta_0) \\
f_{30}(\theta_0) &= 5(4\sin\theta_0\cos^3\theta_0 - 3\sin^3\theta_0\cos\theta_0) \\
f_{31}(\theta_0) &= \tfrac{1}{4}(4\sin^4\theta_0 - 27\sin^2\theta_0\cos^2\theta_0 + 4\cos^4\theta_0) \\
f_{32}(\theta_0) &= \tfrac{1}{4}(5\sin^3\theta_0\cos\theta_0 - 2\sin\theta_0\cos^3\theta_0) \\
f_{33}(\theta_0) &= \tfrac{1}{24}(3\sin^2\theta_0\cos^2\theta_0 - 4\sin^4\theta_0).
\end{aligned} \tag{3.34}$$

Now, consider the magnetic field produced by the four inner arcs in Fig. 3.7, two placed at $z = z_0$ and another two placed at $z = -z_0$, and assume that the angle subtended by each arc is $\psi$. For this case, we find that $A_{nm} = 0$ for all $m$ and $B_{nm} = 0$ when $n$ or $m$ is even. When both $n$ and $m$ are odd, we obtain the only nonzero coefficients as

$$B_{nm} = \frac{2\mu_0 I}{m\pi}\frac{a}{r_0^{n+2}} f_{nm}(\theta_0)(-1)^{(m-1)/2}\sin\frac{m\psi}{2}. \tag{3.35}$$

Therefore, among the first ten $B_{nm}$, only $B_{11}$, $B_{31}$, and $B_{33}$ are nonzero, and the expression for $B_z$ becomes

$$\begin{aligned}
B_z(r,\theta,\phi) = &-B_{11}r\sin\theta\sin\phi + B_{31}r^3P_3^1(\cos\theta)\sin\phi \\
&+ B_{33}r^3P_3^3(\cos\theta)\sin 3\phi + \cdots .
\end{aligned} \tag{3.36}$$

Apparently, the first term is a linear function of $y$ because $y = r\sin\theta\sin\phi$. The $B_{33}$ term can be made zero by choosing $\psi$ such that $\sin(3\psi/2) = 0$ from which we find $\psi = 2\pi/3 = 120°$. The $B_{31}$ term can be made zero by choosing $\theta_0$ such that $f_{31}(\theta_0) = 0$, that is,

$$4\sin^4\theta_0 - 27\sin^2\theta_0\cos^2\theta_0 + 4\cos^4\theta_0 = 0 \tag{3.37}$$

from which we find two solutions: $\theta_0 = 21.27°$ ($z_0 = 2.57a$) and $68.73°$ ($z_0 = 0.39a$). As expected, these two solutions are very close to those ($22.5°$ and $67.5°$) with straight wires. Under such arrangements, the expression for $B_z$ becomes

$$B_z(r,\theta,\phi) = -B_{11}y + O(r^5) \tag{3.38}$$

and the $y$-gradient is uniform through the third order.

A practical design based on the analysis described above is shown in Fig. 3.7 with four inner arcs placed at $\theta_0 = 68.73°$ ($z_0 = 0.39a$) and four outer arcs placed at $\theta_0 = 21.27°$ ($z_0 = 2.57a$). The gradient is uniform to 5% within a sphere of radius $0.4a$. A simple calculation gives the efficiency as (Turner 1993)

$$\eta = \frac{9.18 \times 10^{-7}}{a^2} \mathrm{T} \cdot \mathrm{m}^{-1} \cdot \mathrm{A}^{-1}. \tag{3.39}$$

In some cases, the gradient coil in Fig. 3.7 may be too long. By considering the effect of the inner arcs at $\theta_0$ and outer arcs at $\theta_r$ together, the $B_{31}$ can still be made zero by choosing $\theta_0$ and $\theta_r$ such that (Suits and Wilken 1989)

$$f_{31}(\theta_0) - f_{31}(\theta_r) = 0. \tag{3.40}$$

In addition to the solution obtained earlier ($\theta_0 = 68.73°$ and $\theta_r = 21.27°$), one finds another solution given by $\theta_0 = 68.2°$ ($z_0 = 0.40a$) and $\theta_r = 31.37°$ ($z_r = 1.64a$). The second solution reduces the overall length significantly.

As can be seen, the gradient uniformity of the Golay coil is rather poor. A possible improvement is to employ more arcs with different arc lengths placed at different positions to eliminate more higher-order terms in Eq. (3.36). Some examples are given in Frenkiel *et al.* (1988), Suits and Wilken (1989), and Siebold (1990). These can be classified into three designs. The first one splits the inner arcs into two sets with the same arc length ($\psi = 120°$). One set is placed at $z_1$ and $-z_1$ and carries current $I_1$. The other set is placed at $z_2$ and $-z_2$ and carries current $I_2$. Therefore, one can eliminate $B_{31}$, $B_{51}$, and $B_{71}$ by setting

$$I_1 f_{n1}(\theta_1) + I_2 f_{n1}(\theta_2) - (I_1 + I_2) f_{n1}(\theta_r) = 0 \qquad (n = 3, 5, 7). \tag{3.41}$$

By letting $z_r = 2.0a$, Suits and Wilken (1989) calculated one solution: $z_1 = 0.22a$, $z_2 = 0.80a$, and $I_1/I_2 = 1.81$. The second design uses two sets of saddle coils at the same position, but with different arc lengths. Assume that one set subtends an angle $\psi_1$ and carries current $I_1$ and the other set subtends an angle $\psi_2$ and carries current $I_2$. Apparently, one can eliminate $B_{nm}$ ($m = 3, 5, 7$) by setting

$$I_1 \sin\frac{m\psi_1}{2} + I_2 \sin\frac{m\psi_2}{2} = 0 \qquad (m = 3, 5, 7). \tag{3.42}$$

A useful solution is $\psi_1 = 72°$, $\psi_1 = 144°$, and $I_1/I_2 = -0.618$ (Suits and Wilken 1989). As can be expected, naturally, the third design is a combination of the first two. It uses two sets of split-arc saddle coils with different arc lengths. By using the positions of the split coil and the arc lengths calculated above, one eliminates $B_{nm}$ with $n = 3, 5, 7$ and $m = 3, 5, 7$, leaving the highest contaminating term as $B_{91}$. The gradient so obtained is uniform to 5% within a sphere of radius of $0.6a$.

Finally, we note that the $x$-gradient can be obtained simply by rotating the $y$-gradient coil 90°.

## 3.5 Magnetic Field Produced by a Cylindrical Surface Current

To design gradient coils using distributed currents on a cylindrical surface, we first have to find the magnetic field produced by a cylindrical surface current. As discussed in Sections 2.6 and 2.7, this amounts to solving the Laplace equation given in Eq. (2.57) in cylindrical coordinates. In Section 2.6, we found such a solution for the case when the current and field have no variation along the $z$-axis. Here we consider the general case without this restriction.

In cylindrical coordinates, Eq. (2.57) can be written as

$$\frac{1}{\rho}\frac{\partial}{\partial \rho}\left(\rho\frac{\partial \psi}{\partial \rho}\right) + \frac{1}{\rho^2}\frac{\partial^2 \psi}{\partial \phi^2} + \frac{\partial^2 \psi}{\partial z^2} = 0 \tag{3.43}$$

which can be solved using the method of separation of variables. To do this, we let

$$\psi(\rho, \phi, z) = R(\rho)\Phi(\phi)Z(z) \tag{3.44}$$

and substitute it into Eq. (3.43) to find

$$\frac{d^2 Z(z)}{dz^2} + k^2 Z(z) = 0 \tag{3.45}$$

$$\frac{d^2 \Phi(\phi)}{d\phi^2} + m^2 \Phi(\phi) = 0 \tag{3.46}$$

$$\rho^2 \frac{d^2 R(\rho)}{d\rho^2} + \rho\frac{dR(\rho)}{d\rho} - (m^2 + k^2\rho^2)R(\rho) = 0 \tag{3.47}$$

where $k$ and $m$ are separation constants. In particular, $k$ is an arbitrary constant, but $m$ should be an integer to ensure a single-valued, periodic $\Phi(\phi)$. Equations (3.45) and (3.46) have well-known solutions given by

$$Z(z) = e^{\pm ikz} \quad \text{and} \quad \Phi(\phi) = e^{\pm im\phi} \tag{3.48}$$

respectively. Equation (3.47) is recognized as the modified Bessel's equation whose two independent solutions are given by

$$R_1(\rho) = I_m(|k|\,\rho) \quad \text{and} \quad R_2(\rho) = K_m(|k|\,\rho) \tag{3.49}$$

where $I_m(|k|\,\rho)$ and $K_m(|k|\,\rho)$ are the modified Bessel functions of the first and second kinds, respectively. Some basic properties of the modified Bessel functions are discussed in Appendix 3.A at the end of this chapter. Here we only need to point out that

$$I_m(|k|\,\rho) \to \infty \qquad \text{as } \rho \to \infty \tag{3.50}$$

and

$$K_m(|k|\,\rho) \to \infty \qquad \text{as } \rho \to 0. \tag{3.51}$$

For our problem, the potential $\psi$ must be finite both at the origin and infinity. Hence, the general solution of Eq. (3.47) is

$$\psi(\rho,\phi,z) = \int_{-\infty}^{\infty} \sum_{m=-\infty}^{\infty} e^{im\phi} e^{ikz} \left\{ \begin{array}{c} A_m(k) I_m(|k|\,\rho) \\ B_m(k) K_m(|k|\,\rho) \end{array} \right\} dk \quad \begin{array}{l} \text{for } \rho \le a \\ \text{for } \rho \ge a \end{array} \tag{3.52}$$

where $a$ denotes the radius of the cylindrical surface and $A_m(k)$ and $B_m(k)$ are constants to be determined. Substituting Eq. (3.52) into Eq. (2.55), we find the expression for the magnetic field to be

$$\begin{aligned} \mathbf{B}(\rho,\phi,z) = & -\hat{\rho} \int_{-\infty}^{\infty} \sum_{m=-\infty}^{\infty} e^{im\phi} e^{ikz} \left\{ \begin{array}{c} A_m(k) I'_m(|k|\,\rho) \\ B_m(k) K'_m(|k|\,\rho) \end{array} \right\} |k|\; dk \\ & -\hat{\phi}\frac{1}{\rho} \int_{-\infty}^{\infty} \sum_{m=-\infty}^{\infty} (im) e^{im\phi} e^{ikz} \left\{ \begin{array}{c} A_m(k) I_m(|k|\,\rho) \\ B_m(k) K_m(|k|\,\rho) \end{array} \right\} dk \\ & -\hat{z} \int_{-\infty}^{\infty} \sum_{m=-\infty}^{\infty} (ik) e^{im\phi} e^{ikz} \left\{ \begin{array}{c} A_m(k) I_m(|k|\,\rho) \\ B_m(k) K_m(|k|\,\rho) \end{array} \right\} dk \\ & \qquad \begin{array}{l} \text{for } \rho \le a \\ \text{for } \rho \ge a. \end{array} \end{aligned} \tag{3.53}$$

To determine $A_m(k)$ and $B_m(k)$, we apply the boundary conditions given in Eqs. (2.47) and (2.52) across the cylindrical surface current. First, from the continuity of the normal component (that is, $B_\rho$), we obtain

$$\begin{aligned} & \int_{-\infty}^{\infty} \sum_{m=-\infty}^{\infty} e^{im\phi} e^{ikz} A_m(k) I'_m(|k|\,a)\,|k|\; dk \\ & \qquad = \int_{-\infty}^{\infty} \sum_{m=-\infty}^{\infty} e^{im\phi} e^{ikz} B_m(k) K'_m(|k|\,a)\,|k|\; dk. \end{aligned} \tag{3.54}$$

Multiplying both sides by $e^{-im'\phi}$ and $e^{-ik'z}$ and then integrating it from $-\pi$ to $\pi$ with respect to $\phi$ and from $-\infty$ to $\infty$ with respect to $z$, we obtain

$$A_m(k)I'_m(|k|\,a) = B_m(k)K'_m(|k|\,a). \tag{3.55}$$

In arriving at this result, we employed the following well-known relations

$$\int_{-\pi}^{\pi} e^{i(m-m')\phi}d\phi = \begin{cases} 2\pi & m = m' \\ 0 & m \neq m' \end{cases} \tag{3.56}$$

$$\int_{-\infty}^{\infty}\int_{-\infty}^{\infty} e^{i(k-k')z} f(k)\,dk\,dz = 2\pi \int_{-\infty}^{\infty} \delta(k-k')f(k)\,dk = 2\pi f(k') \tag{3.57}$$

where $f(k)$ is an arbitrary function. Second, we apply the condition to the tangential component [that is, $\hat{n} \times (\mathbf{B}_1 - \mathbf{B}_2) = \mathbf{J}_s$ where $\mathbf{J}_s$ denotes the surface current density] to find

$$\int_{-\infty}^{\infty} \sum_{m=-\infty}^{\infty} (im)e^{im\phi}e^{ikz}B_m(k)K_m(|k|\,a)\,dk - \int_{-\infty}^{\infty} \sum_{m=-\infty}^{\infty} (im)e^{im\phi}e^{ikz}A_m(k)I_m(|k|\,a)\,dk = -\mu_0 a J_z(\phi, z) \tag{3.58}$$

$$\int_{-\infty}^{\infty} \sum_{m=-\infty}^{\infty} (ik)e^{im\phi}e^{ikz}B_m(k)K_m(|k|\,a)\,dk - \int_{-\infty}^{\infty} \sum_{m=-\infty}^{\infty} (ik)e^{im\phi}e^{ikz}A_m(k)I_m(|k|\,a)\,dk = \mu_0 J_\phi(\phi, z) \tag{3.59}$$

where $J_z(\phi, z)$ and $J_\phi(\phi, z)$ are the $z$- and $\phi$-components of $\mathbf{J}_s$. Among these two equations, it is sufficient to consider one of them because they are not independent. This becomes obvious if we multiply both sides of Eqs. (3.58) and (3.59) by $e^{-im'\phi}$ and $e^{-ik'z}$ and then integrate them from $-\pi$ to $\pi$ with respect to $\phi$ and from $-\infty$ to $\infty$ with respect to $z$. Using Eqs. (3.56) and (3.57), we obtain

$$imB_m(k)K_m(|k|\,a) - imA_m(k)I_m(|k|\,a) = -\frac{\mu_0 a}{2\pi} j_z^{(m)}(k) \tag{3.60}$$

$$ikB_m(k)K_m(|k|\,a) - ikA_m(k)I_m(|k|\,a) = \frac{\mu_0}{2\pi} j_\phi^{(m)}(k) \tag{3.61}$$

where

$$j_z^{(m)}(k) = \frac{1}{2\pi}\int_{-\infty}^{\infty}\int_{-\pi}^{\pi} e^{-im\phi}e^{-ikz}J_z(\phi, z)\,d\phi\,dz \tag{3.62}$$

$$j_\phi^{(m)}(k) = \frac{1}{2\pi}\int_{-\infty}^{\infty}\int_{-\pi}^{\pi} e^{-im\phi}e^{-ikz} J_\phi(\phi, z)\, d\phi\, dz. \tag{3.63}$$

From Eqs. (3.60) and (3.61), we have

$$m\, j_\phi^{(m)}(k) + ka\, j_z^{(m)}(k) = 0 \tag{3.64}$$

which, as will be shown later, is the current continuity equation in terms of $j_z^{(m)}(k)$ and $j_\phi^{(m)}(k)$. Solving Eqs. (3.55) and one of Eqs. (3.60) and (3.61), we obtain

$$A_m(k) = \frac{\mu_0 a}{i2\pi k}\, |k|\, j_\phi^{(m)}(k) K_m'(|k|\, a). \tag{3.65}$$

Substituting this into Eq. (3.53), we obtain the $z$-component of the magnetic field inside the cylindrical surface as

$$B_z(\rho, \phi, z) = -\frac{\mu_0 a}{2\pi}\int_{-\infty}^{\infty}\sum_{m=-\infty}^{\infty} e^{im\phi}e^{ikz}\, |k|\; j_\phi^{(m)}(k) I_m(|k|\,\rho) K_m'(|k|\, a)\, dk \qquad (\rho \le a) \tag{3.66}$$

which is the result we intended to derive. Before proceeding, we note that Eqs. (3.62) and (3.64) are the well-known Fourier transforms of $J_z(\phi, z)$ and $J_\phi(\phi, z)$. Their inverse transforms are given by

$$J_z(\phi, z) = \int_{-\infty}^{\infty}\sum_{m=-\infty}^{\infty} e^{im\phi}e^{ikz} j_z^{(m)}(k)\, dk \tag{3.67}$$

$$J_\phi(\phi, z) = \int_{-\infty}^{\infty}\sum_{m=-\infty}^{\infty} e^{im\phi}e^{ikz} j_\phi^{(m)}(k)\, dk. \tag{3.68}$$

Substituting these two expressions into the current continuity equation

$$\nabla_s \cdot \mathbf{J}_s = \frac{\partial J_\phi}{a\partial\phi} + \frac{\partial J_z}{\partial z} = 0 \tag{3.69}$$

we obtain

$$m\, j_\phi^{(m)}(k) + ka\, j_z^{(m)}(k) = 0 \tag{3.70}$$

which is the same as Eq. (3.64). Finally, we note that Eq. (3.66) can also be derived using a vector potential, which is left to the reader as an exercise (see Appendix 3.B).

To illustrate the use of Eq. (3.66), let us revisit the design of the Maxwell and Golay coils considered in the preceding section.

**Example 1.** Design a Maxwell coil pair to produce a longitudinal gradient. We first consider the $B_z$ produced by a pair of coils depicted in Fig. 2.7. From Eq. (3.63), we find

$$j_\phi^{(m)}(k) = \begin{cases} -2iI\sin(kd/2) & m = 0 \\ 0 & m \neq 0. \end{cases} \tag{3.71}$$

Substituting this into Eq. (3.66) yields

$$B_z(\rho, \phi, z) = \frac{2\mu_0 I a}{\pi} \int_0^\infty \sin kz \, \sin(kd/2) \, k \, I_0(k\rho) K_1(ka) \, dk \tag{3.72}$$

which is an odd function of $z$. Therefore, its value and those of the even derivatives with respect to $z$ are zero at $z = 0$. The first derivative provides the $z$ gradient and its optimization can be achieved by choosing a value for $d$ such that the third derivative of $B_z$ is eliminated. This requires

$$\int_0^\infty \sin(kd/2) \, k^4 \, K_1(ka) \, dk = 0 \tag{3.73}$$

which can be solved using a numerical method such as the secant method to find that $d = \sqrt{3}a$.

For a gradient coil consisting of two Maxwell pairs, $B_z$ is given by

$$B_z(\rho, \phi, z) = \frac{2\mu_0 a}{\pi} \int_0^\infty \sin kz \, [I_1 \sin(kd_1/2) + I_2 \sin(kd_2/2)] \times k \, I_0(k\rho) K_1(ka) \, dk \tag{3.74}$$

where $I_1$ and $d_1$ denote the current and length of the first pair and $I_2$ and $d_2$ denote the current and length of the second pair. In this case, one can select $d_1$, $d_2$, and the ratio $I_2/I_1$ to eliminate the third, fifth, and seventh derivatives of $B_z$ with respect to $z$. This requires

$$I_1 Q_n(d_1) + I_2 Q_n(d_2) = 0 \qquad (n = 4, 6, 8) \tag{3.75}$$

where $Q_n$ is defined as

$$Q_n = \int_0^\infty \sin(kd/2) \, k^n \, K_1(ka) \, dk. \tag{3.76}$$

**Example 2.** Design a "Golay" or double-saddle coil to produce a transverse gradient. Consider the configuration depicted in Fig. 3.7. From Eq. (3.63), we find

$$j_\phi^{(m)}(k) = \frac{4I}{im\pi} [\cos kz_0 - \cos kz_r] \sin \frac{m\psi}{2} \sin \frac{m\pi}{2}. \tag{3.77}$$

Apparently, $j_\phi^{(m)}(k) = 0$ for all even $m$. Furthermore, if $\psi = 120°$, $\sin(m\psi/2) = 0$ for $m = 3, 6, 9, \ldots$. Therefore,

$$B_z(\rho, \phi, z) = \frac{4\mu_0 I a}{\pi^2} \int_{-\infty}^{\infty} \sum_{m=1,5,7,\ldots}^{\infty} \frac{\sin m\phi}{m} e^{ikz} |k| \\ \times [\cos kz_r - \cos kz_0] \, I_m(|k| \rho) K'_m(|k| a) \, dk. \quad (3.78)$$

Since

$$I_m(k\rho) = \sum_{n=0}^{\infty} \frac{(k\rho/2)^{2n+m}}{n! \, (n+m)!} \quad (3.79)$$

it is clear that the term $m = 1$ is of the first order in $y$, which provides the desired $y$-gradient, and also of the third and higher orders in $x$, $y$, and $z$, whereas the term $m = 5$ is of the fifth and higher orders in $x$, $y$, and $z$. Therefore, one should choose $z_0$ and $z_r$ to eliminate the third order terms. This requires

$$\int_0^{\infty} k^4 \, [\cos kz_r - \cos kz_0] \, K'_1(ka) \, dk = 0 \quad (3.80)$$

from which we can solve for $z_0$ and $z_r$ in terms of $a$. In passing, we note that the same approach can be employed for the design of the split and double-set saddle coils. The procedure is however more tedious than that described in the preceding section.

## 3.6 Target Field Method

With the formulas derived in the preceding section, we are now ready to describe the target field method, a powerful method developed by Turner (1986) for the design of gradient coils. The general principle of this method is first to specify a desired field—the target field—over a cylindrical surface whose radius $c$ is less than the radius of the cylindrical surface carrying the current. Let us denote this field as $B_z(c, \phi, z)$ and substitute it into Eq. (3.66). After taking the Fourier transform of the resultant equation, we obtain

$$b_z^{(m)}(c, k) = -\mu_0 a \, |k| \, j_\phi^{(m)}(k) I_m(|k| \, c) K'_m(|k| \, a) \qquad (c \leq a) \quad (3.81)$$

where

$$b_z^{(m)}(c, k) = \frac{1}{2\pi} \int_{-\infty}^{\infty} \int_{-\pi}^{\pi} e^{-im\phi} e^{-ikz} B_z(c, \phi, z) \, d\phi \, dz. \quad (3.82)$$

From Eq. (3.81), we obtain

$$j_\phi^{(m)}(k) = -\frac{b_z^{(m)}(c,k)}{\mu_0 a\,|k|\,I_m(|k|\,c)K_m'(|k|\,a)} \qquad (c \le a) \tag{3.83}$$

and from Eq. (3.70), we have

$$j_z^{(m)}(k) = -\frac{m}{ka} j_\phi^{(m)}(k). \tag{3.84}$$

Once we obtain $j_z^{(m)}(k)$ and $j_\phi^{(m)}(k)$, we can perform the inverse Fourier transform, Eqs. (3.67) and (3.68), to find the desired current density $J_z(\phi, z)$ and $J_\phi(\phi, z)$ that generate the desired field $B_z(c, \phi, z)$. Although Eqs. (3.67) and (3.68) contain both an infinite integral and infinite summation, for gradient coils the infinite summation has only one or two nonzero terms.

As can be seen, the target field method finds the current to generate the desired field specified over a cylindrical surface ($\rho = c < a$). However, our interest is in the volume rather than on this cylindrical surface. Now, we show that the field at other points varies in a way very similar to the target field $B_z(c, \phi, z)$. To show this, we first substitute Eq. (3.83) into Eq. (3.66) to find the field at other points as

$$B_z(\rho, \phi, z) = \frac{1}{2\pi} \int_{-\infty}^{\infty} \sum_{m=-\infty}^{\infty} e^{im\phi} e^{ikz} \frac{I_m(|k|\,\rho)}{I_m(|k|\,c)}\, b_z^{(m)}(c,k)\, dk \qquad (\rho \le a). \tag{3.85}$$

Second, we note that for the inverse Fourier transform of $j_\phi^{(m)}(k)$ to exist, the right-hand side of Eq. (3.83) must tend to zero as $k \to \infty$. Since

$$kK_m'(ka)I_m(kc) \to e^{-k(a-c)} \qquad \text{as } k \to \infty \tag{3.86}$$

$b_z^{(m)}(c,k)$ must tend to zero faster than $e^{-k(a-c)}$. This implies that the only significant contribution to the integral in Eq. (3.85) comes from small $k$. However, for small $k$,

$$I_m(k\rho) \sim \left(\frac{k\rho}{2}\right)^{|m|} \tag{3.87}$$

and, therefore (Turner 1986),

$$B_z(\rho, \phi, z) \approx \frac{1}{2\pi} \sum_{m=-\infty}^{\infty} \left(\frac{\rho}{c}\right)^{|m|} e^{im\phi} \int_{-\infty}^{\infty} e^{ikz}\, b_z^{(m)}(c,k)\, dk \qquad (\rho \le a) \tag{3.88}$$

or

$$B_z(\rho, \phi, z) \approx \frac{1}{2\pi} \sum_{m=-\infty}^{\infty} \left(\frac{\rho}{c}\right)^{|m|} e^{im\phi} B_z^{(m)}(c, z) \qquad (\rho \leq a) \quad (3.89)$$

where

$$B_z^{(m)}(c, z) = \int_{-\infty}^{\infty} e^{ikz}\, b_z^{(m)}(c, k)\, dk. \quad (3.90)$$

Now, let us consider two examples. First, if the target field $B_z(c, \phi, z)$ is independent of $\phi$ such as the case for a $z$-gradient field, then, $m = 0$ and $B_z(\rho, \phi, z) = B_z(c, \phi, z)$ as desired. Second, if the target field is an $x$-gradient field, that is,

$$\begin{aligned} B_z(c, \phi, z) &= G_x x\, g(z) \\ &= G_x c \cos\phi\, g(z) \\ &= G_x \frac{c}{2} \left(e^{i\phi} + e^{-i\phi}\right) g(z) \end{aligned} \quad (3.91)$$

where $G_x$ is a constant and $g(z)$ specifies the variation with $z$, then $m = \pm 1$ and

$$\begin{aligned} B_z(\rho, \phi, z) &\approx \frac{\rho}{c} \left(e^{i\phi} + e^{-i\phi}\right) G_x \frac{c}{2} g(z) \\ &= G_x \rho \cos\phi\, g(z) \\ &= G_x x\, g(z) \end{aligned} \quad (3.92)$$

which is the desired field. The same is true for the $y$-gradient field. As pointed out by Turner (1986), in general, the azimuthal variation of $B_z(\rho, \phi, z)$ will be the same as that of the target field $B_z(c, \phi, z)$ and the variations in $\rho$ and $z$ will be similar.

Similar to the matrix inversion method, the target field method may also yield a solution with rapid current variation, which is difficult to fabricate, because the method requires the current to produce a field that matches exactly the target field. This problem can be overcome by multiplying Eqs. (3.83) and (3.84) by a Gaussian function to remove or reduce their high spectral components before they are Fourier-transformed back into $J_z(\phi, z)$ and $J_\phi(\phi, z)$. Turner (1988) suggested use of the Gaussian function

$$t(k) = e^{-2k^2h^2} \quad (3.93)$$

where $h$ is large enough to ensure that $j_\phi^{(m)}(k)t(k)$ tends to zero as $k \to \infty$, so that its inverse Fourier transform exists. Turner called this procedure apodization and $h$ the apodization length.

Let us now proceed step by step to illustrate the design process using the target field approach. To design a $z$-gradient coil, we can choose $B_z(c, \phi, z)$ as

$$B_z(c, \phi, z) = G_z z g(z) \tag{3.94}$$

where $G_z$ is a constant and $g(z)$ specifies the variation with $z$, which can have the form (Turner 1986)

$$g(z) = \left[1 + \left(\frac{z}{d}\right)^6\right]^{-1} \tag{3.95}$$

in which we can choose $d = 1.7a$ such that $g(z) \approx 1$ for a small $z$. The field specified by Eq. (3.94) is shown in Fig. 3.8 as the solid line. Then, from Eq. (3.82) we have

$$b_z^{(m)}(c, k) = \delta_{0m} \, G_z \, \tilde{g}(k) \tag{3.96}$$

where $\delta_{0m} = 1$ when $m = 0$ and $\delta_{0m} = 0$ otherwise, and

$$\tilde{g}(k) = \int_{-\infty}^{\infty} z \, g(z) e^{-ikz} dz. \tag{3.97}$$

Therefore, from Eqs. (3.83) and (3.84) we obtain

$$j_\phi^{(m)}(k) = -\frac{\delta_{0m} \, G_z \, \tilde{g}(k)}{\mu_0 a \, |k| \, I_0(|k| \, c) K_0'(|k| \, a)} \tag{3.98}$$

$$j_z^{(m)}(k) = 0 \tag{3.99}$$

which is plotted in Fig. 3.9 as the solid line. As can be seen, $j_\phi^{(m)}(k) \to \infty$ as $k \to \infty$ and, therefore, its inverse Fourier transform does not exist. This difficulty can be alleviated by apodization, that is, multiplying Eq. (3.98) by Eq. (3.93). This new function is plotted in Fig. 3.9 as the dashed line for $h = 0.1$ and it is obvious that $j_\phi^{(m)}(k)t(k) \to 0$ as $k \to \infty$. Taking the inverse Fourier transform, we obtain the current

$$J_\phi(\phi, z) = -2\frac{iG_z}{\mu_0 a} \int_0^{\infty} \frac{\tilde{g}(k) \sin kz}{kI_0(kc)K_0'(ka)} t(k) \, dk \tag{3.100}$$

$$J_z(\phi, z) = 0 \tag{3.101}$$

which is plotted in Fig. 3.10. The integrated current can be calculated as

$$I(z) = \int_0^z J_\phi(z') \, dz' \tag{3.102}$$

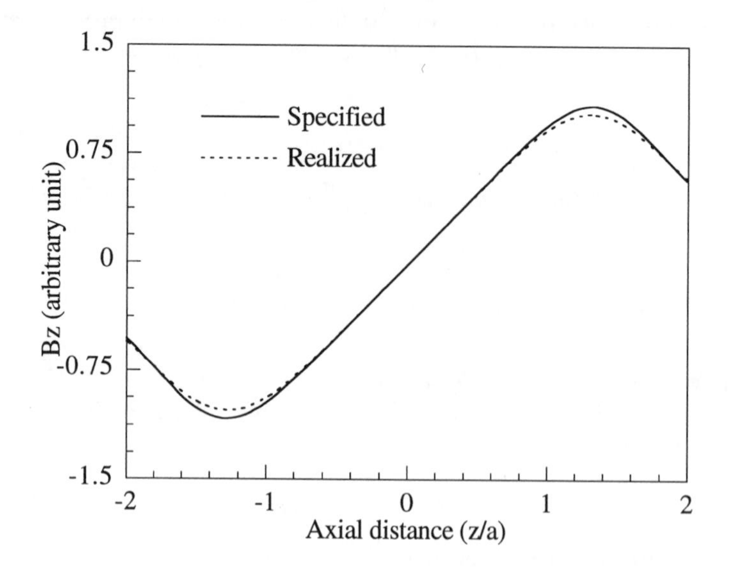


**Figure 3.8.** Specified and realized $z$-gradient field.

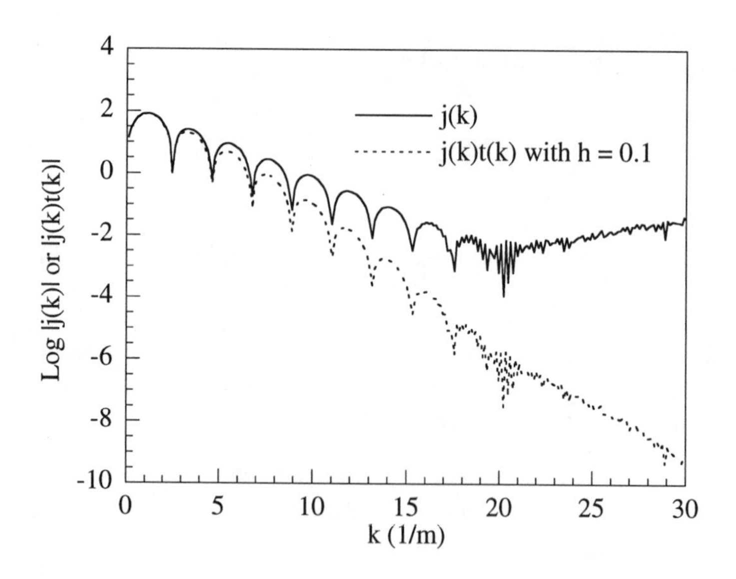


**Figure 3.9.** Plots of $j_\phi^{(m)}(k)$ and $j_\phi^{(m)}(k)t(k)$.

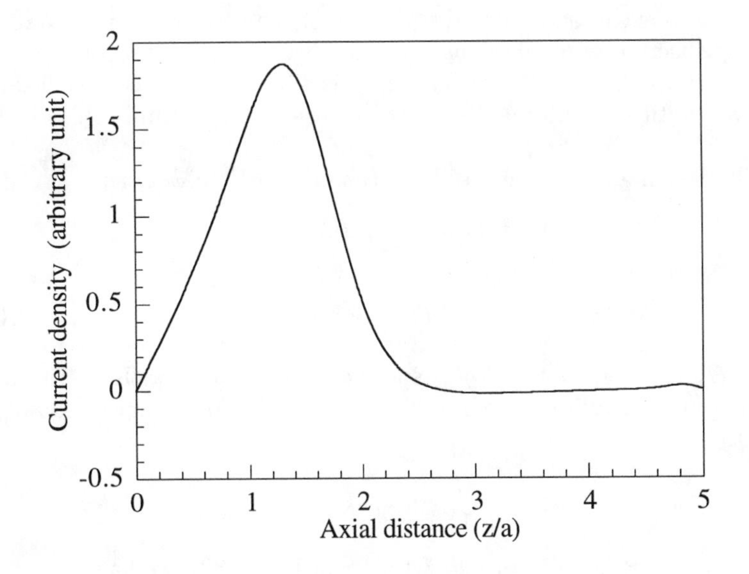


**Figure 3.10.** The current distribution $J_\phi(z)$ for a $z$-gradient coil.

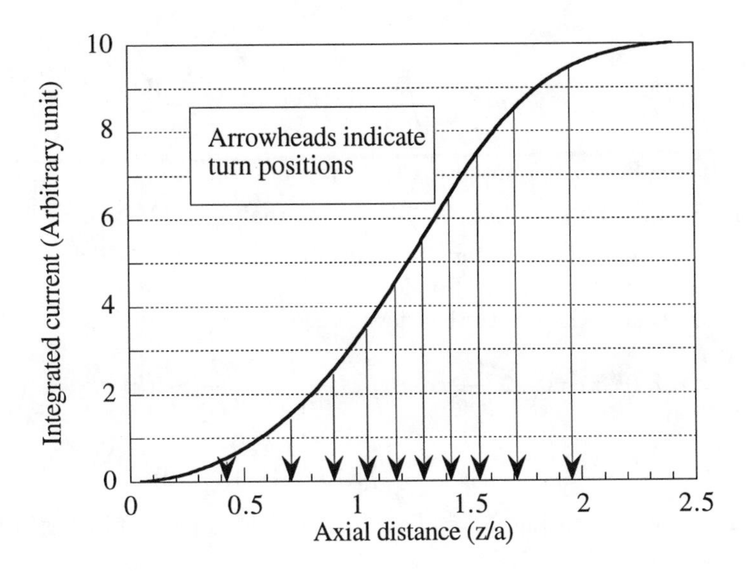


**Figure 3.11.** The integrated current and turn positions for a $z$-gradient coil.

from which we can determine the position of the turns if we wish to realize it using discrete wires, as illustrated in Fig. 3.11. As can be expected, because of apodization, the realized field is different from the specified one; however, with $h = 0.1$ the difference is very small, as can be seen in Fig. 3.8.

To design an $x$-gradient coil, we can choose $B_z(c, \phi, z)$ as

$$\begin{aligned} B_z(c, \phi, z) &= G_x x\, g(z) \\ &= G_x c \cos\phi\, g(z) \\ &= G_x \frac{c}{2} \left(e^{i\phi} + e^{-i\phi}\right) g(z) \end{aligned} \tag{3.103}$$

where $G_x$ is a constant and $g(z)$ specifies the variation with $z$. To satisfy the continuity condition given in Eq. (3.69) or (3.70), we must choose $g(z)$ such that

$$\int_{-\infty}^{\infty} g(z)\, dz = 0. \tag{3.104}$$

One such choice is given in Fig. 3.12. From Eq. (3.82), we have

$$b_z^{(m)}(c, k) = G_x \frac{c}{2}(\delta_{-1m} + \delta_{1m}) g(k) \tag{3.105}$$

where

$$g(k) = \int_{-\infty}^{\infty} g(z) e^{-ikz} dz. \tag{3.106}$$

Substituting Eq. (3.105) into Eq. (3.83), we obtain $j_\phi^{(m)}(k)$ , which is plotted in Fig. 3.13 as the solid line. Again, we see that $j_\phi^{(m)}(k) \to \infty$ as $k \to \infty$, and, therefore, it is necessary to multiply $j_\phi^{(m)}(k)$ by $t(k)$ given in Eq. (3.93). The new function is also plotted in Fig. 3.13 as the dashed line with $h = 0.13$. Taking the inverse Fourier transform, we obtain

$$J_\phi(\phi, z) = -2\frac{cG_x}{\mu_0 a} \cos\phi \int_0^{\infty} \frac{g(k) \cos kz}{kI_1(kc)K_1'(ka)} t(k)\, dk \tag{3.107}$$

$$J_z(\phi, z) = -2\frac{cG_x}{\mu_0 a^2} \sin\phi \int_0^{\infty} \frac{g(k) \sin kz}{k^2 I_1(kc)K_1'(ka)} t(k)\, dk \tag{3.108}$$

which are plotted in Fig. 3.14. The realized field is plotted in Fig. 3.12 as the dashed line.

Apparently, there are many possible choices for $g(z)$ which satisfy Eq. (3.104). Figure 3.15 shows another choice. The corresponding Fourier transform of the current is given in Fig. 3.16 and the current distribution is displayed in Fig. 3.17.

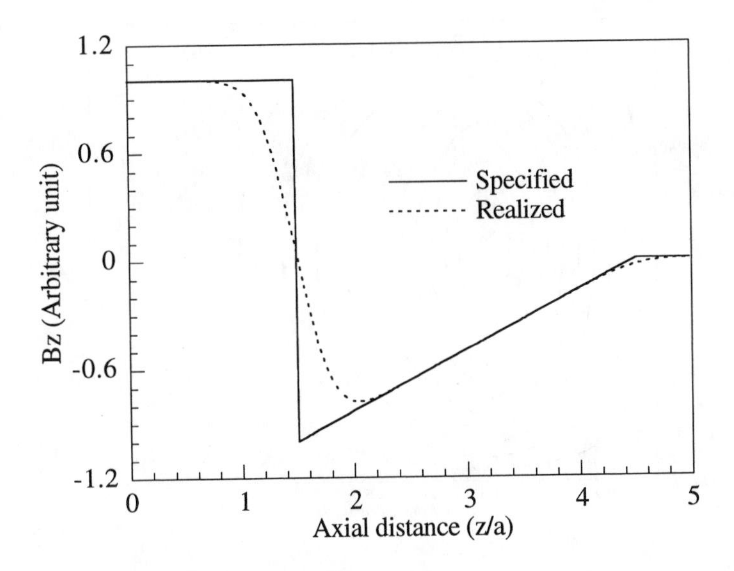


**Figure 3.12.** Specified and realized $x$-gradient field.

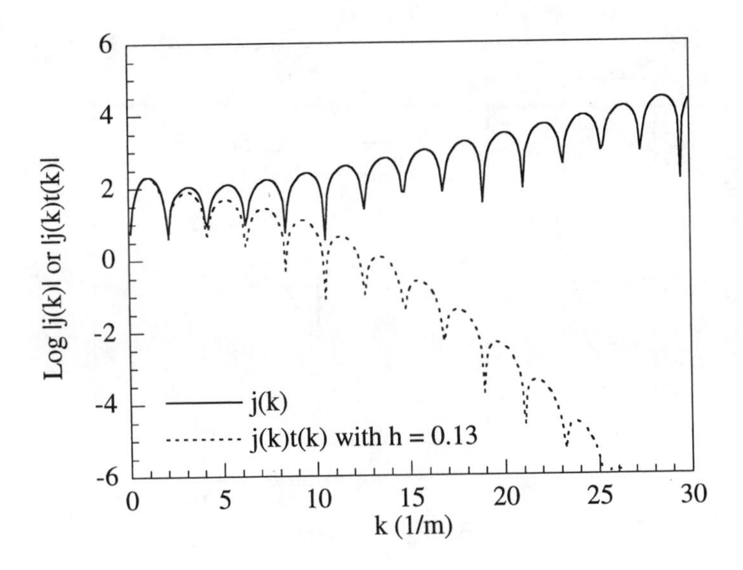


**Figure 3.13.** Plots of $j_\phi^{(m)}(k)$ and $j_\phi^{(m)}(k)t(k)$.

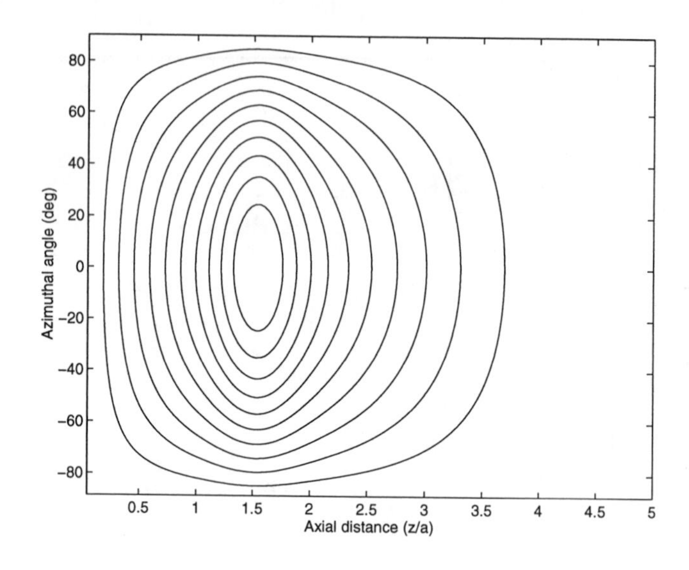


**Figure 3.14.** The current distribution for a transverse gradient coil. Only one octant is shown and the complete set forms a double saddle-type arrangement.

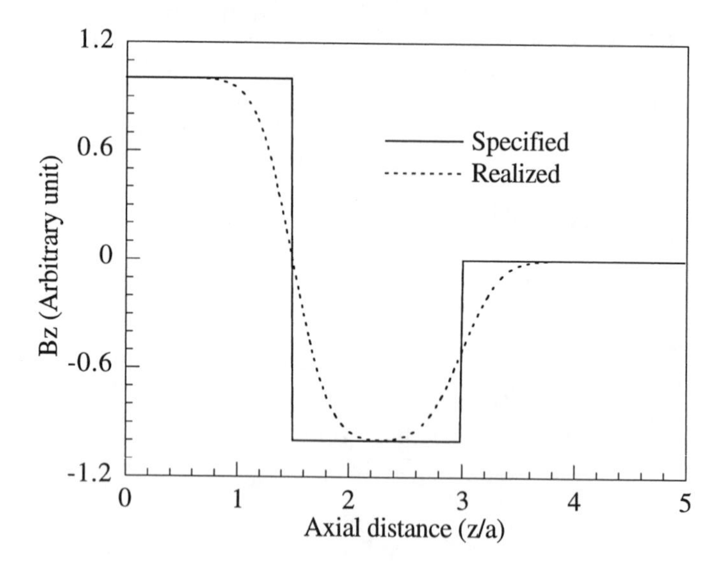


**Figure 3.15.** Specified and realized $x$-gradient field.

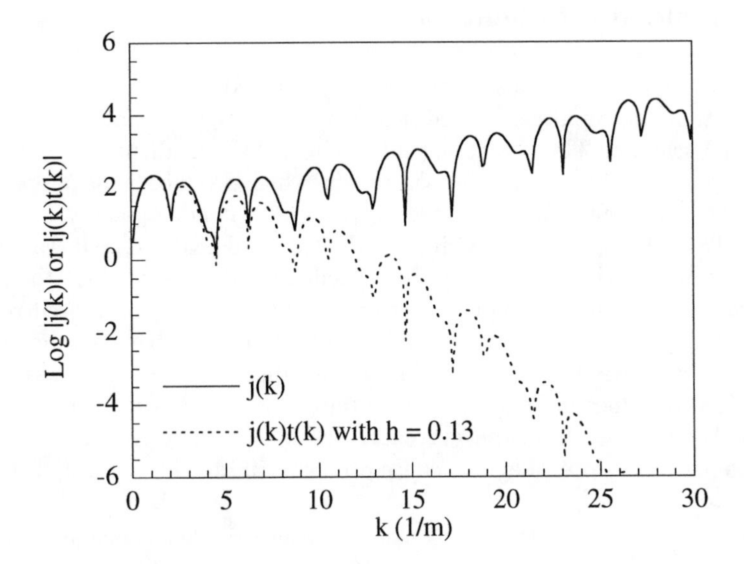


**Figure 3.16.** Plots of $j_{\phi}^{(m)}(k)$ and $j_{\phi}^{(m)}(k)t(k)$.

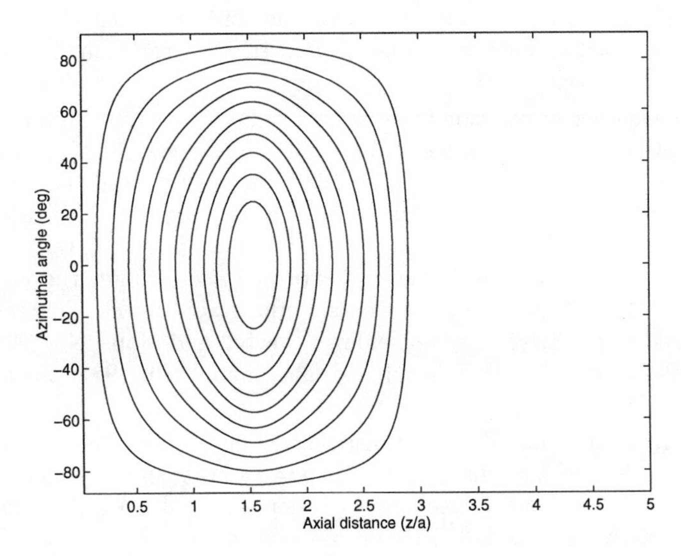


**Figure 3.17.** The current distribution for a transverse gradient coil. Only one octant is shown and the complete set forms a double saddle-type arrangement.

## 3.7 Shielded Gradient Coils

One of the major problems in the use of switched gradient coils is the interaction of the rapidly switched fields with other conducting structures in an MRI scanner. The magnetic field produced by a gradient coil induces eddy currents in other conducting structures, which produce fields opposing that of the gradient coil. As a result, the gradient homogeneity can be degraded and the rise and decay times of the switched field can be increased. One solution (Morich *et al.* 1988, Van Vaals and Bergman 1990) to this problem is to adjust the voltage waveform to produce the desired current and thus the field, in a manner similar to that discussed in Section 3.2. However, the eddy currents induced in other structures still exist and their rise and decay times are determined by the inductances of the structures. The fields produced by these currents vary in the same manner as the currents and, therefore, they can cause problems in imaging resolution and speed.

Another solution is to place a shield between gradient coils and their surrounding structures so that the gradient field is reduced to zero outside the shield. For the shield to be effective, its thickness must be much greater than the skin depth. Under this condition, the time dependence of the field produced by the eddy current in the shield will be the same as that of the gradient coil and one needs to consider only the spatial variation of the gradient field. This technique is often referred to as passive shielding (Turner and Bowley 1986).

An even better solution is to design gradient coils that do not produce a magnetic field outside the coils and thus do not induce eddy currents in other conducting structures. Such coils must consist of at least two coils of different sizes. The inner coil is often referred to as the primary coil and the outer coil is referred to as the shield coil. Basically, the shield coil produces a field that cancels that of the primary coil outside the shield coil. As a result, the total field is zero outside the gradient coil. This technique is referred to as active or self shielding (Bowtell and Mansfield 1990, 1991; Mansfield *et al.* 1985; Mansfield and Chapman 1986, 1987; Roemer and Hickey 1986).

To find the required current distribution on the shield coil, we consider two cylindrical surface currents, one at $\rho = a$ whose current is denoted as $\mathbf{J}$ and the other at $\rho = b$ whose current is denoted as $\mathbf{J}^s$. The field produced by these currents outside the shield coil is then

$$B_\rho(\rho, \phi, z) = -\frac{\mu_0 a}{2\pi i} \int_{-\infty}^{\infty} \sum_{m=-\infty}^{\infty} e^{im\phi} e^{ikz} \frac{|k|^2}{k} j_\phi^{(m)}(k) I'_m(|k|\, a) K'_m(|k|\, \rho)\, dk$$

$$
- \frac{\mu_0 b}{2\pi i} \int_{-\infty}^{\infty} \sum_{m=-\infty}^{\infty} e^{im\phi} e^{ikz} \frac{|k|^2}{k} j_\phi^{s(m)}(k) I'_m(|k|\,b) K'_m(|k|\,\rho)\, dk \tag{3.109}
$$

$$
B_\phi(\rho,\phi,z) = -\frac{\mu_0 a}{2\pi\rho} \int_{-\infty}^{\infty} \sum_{m=-\infty}^{\infty} e^{im\phi} e^{ikz} m \frac{|k|}{k} j_\phi^{(m)}(k) I'_m(|k|\,a) K_m(|k|\,\rho)\, dk - \frac{\mu_0 b}{2\pi} \int_{-\infty}^{\infty} \sum_{m=-\infty}^{\infty} e^{im\phi} e^{ikz} m \frac{|k|}{k} j_\phi^{s(m)}(k) I'_m(|k|\,b) K_m(|k|\,\rho)\, dk \tag{3.110}
$$

$$
B_z(\rho,\phi,z) = -\frac{\mu_0 a}{2\pi} \int_{-\infty}^{\infty} \sum_{m=-\infty}^{\infty} e^{im\phi} e^{ikz} |k|\, j_\phi^{(m)}(k) I'_m(|k|\,a) K_m(|k|\,\rho)\, dk - \frac{\mu_0 b}{2\pi} \int_{-\infty}^{\infty} \sum_{m=-\infty}^{\infty} e^{im\phi} e^{ikz} |k|\, j_\phi^{s(m)}(k) I'_m(|k|\,b) K_m(|k|\,\rho)\, dk \tag{3.111}
$$

where $j_\phi^{(m)}$ and $j_\phi^{s(m)}$ are the Fourier transforms of the $\phi$-component of $\mathbf{J}$ and $\mathbf{J}^s$, respectively. Apparently, all these field components would vanish if $j_\phi^{s(m)}$ is chosen to satisfy

$$
a\, j_\phi^{(m)}(k) I'_m(|k|\,a) + b\, j_\phi^{s(m)}(k) I'_m(|k|\,b) = 0 \tag{3.112}
$$

or

$$
j_\phi^{s(m)}(k) = -\frac{a\, I'_m(|k|\,a)}{b\, I'_m(|k|\,b)} j_\phi^{(m)}(k). \tag{3.113}
$$

The $j_\phi^{(m)}$ can then be determined using the target field method. The magnetic field inside the primary coil is given by

$$
B_z(\rho,\phi,z) = \frac{\mu_0 a}{2\pi} \int_{-\infty}^{\infty} \sum_{m=-\infty}^{\infty} e^{im\phi} e^{ikz} |k|\, j_\phi^{(m)}(k) \times \left[ \frac{I'_m(|k|\,a)}{I'_m(|k|\,b)} K'_m(|k|\,b) - K'_m(|k|\,a) \right] I_m(|k|\,\rho)\, dk \qquad (\rho \leq a). \tag{3.114}
$$

Its Fourier transform is

$$
b_z^{(m)}(\rho,k) = \mu_0 a\, |k|\, j_\phi^{(m)}(k) \left[ \frac{I'_m(|k|\,a)}{I'_m(|k|\,b)} K'_m(|k|\,b) - K'_m(|k|\,a) \right] I_m(|k|\,\rho) \qquad (\rho \leq a). \tag{3.115}
$$

Specifying the desired field on the target surface at $\rho = c$, we find the required current

$$j_\phi^{(m)}(k) = \frac{b_z^{(m)}(c,k)}{\mu_0 a\,|k|\,I_m(|k|\,c)} \left[\frac{I'_m(|k|\,a)}{I'_m(|k|\,b)} K'_m(|k|\,b) - K'_m(|k|\,a)\right]^{-1} \tag{3.116}$$

whose inverse transform gives the current in the primary coil. The current in the shield coil can be found using Eq. (3.113).

**Example 1.** Design a self-shielded Maxwell coil pair. The Fourier transform of the current in the primary Maxwell coils is given by Eq. (3.71). The Fourier transform of the current in the shield is then

$$j_\phi^{s(m)}(k) = \begin{cases} 2iI\dfrac{aI_1(|k|\,a)}{bI_1(|k|\,b)}\sin\dfrac{kd}{2} & m = 0 \\ 0 & m \neq 0 \end{cases} \tag{3.117}$$

and the $B_z$ is

$$B_z(\rho,\phi,z) = \frac{2\mu_0 I a}{\pi} \int_0^\infty \sin kz \sin\frac{kd}{2}\, k\, I_0(k\rho) \times \left[K_1(ka) - \frac{I_1(ka)}{I_1(kb)} K_1(kb)\right] dk. \tag{3.118}$$

To eliminate the third-order derivative of $B_z$, we set

$$\int_0^\infty k^4 \sin\frac{kd}{2} \left[K_1(ka) - \frac{I_1(ka)}{I_1(kb)} K_1(kb)\right] dk = 0 \tag{3.119}$$

from which we can find the desired $d$ for given $a$ and $b$. A design curve is given by Turner and Bowley (1986), showing the value of $d$ as a function of $b/a$. Figure 3.18 shows the current distribution on the shield of a Maxwell coil pair for two different radii. The design procedure for a shielded gradient coil consisting of four circular loops is similar.

**Example 2.** Design a self-shielded double-saddle coil. The Fourier transform of the current in the primary coil is given in Eq. (3.77). The Fourier transform of the current in the shield is then

$$j_\phi^{s(m)}(k) = \frac{4iI}{m\pi}\left[\cos kz_0 - \cos kz_r\right] \sin\frac{m\psi}{2} \sin\frac{m\pi}{2} \frac{aI'_m(ka)}{bI'_m(kb)} \tag{3.120}$$

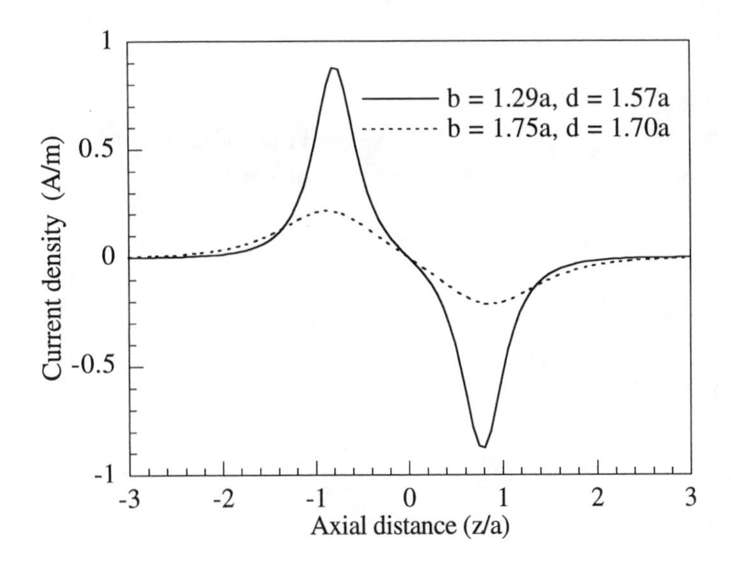


**Figure 3.18.** Current distribution on the shield of a Maxwell coil pair.

and the $B_z$ for $\psi = 120°$ becomes

$$B_z(\rho,\phi,z) = \frac{4\mu_0 I a}{\pi^2} \int_{-\infty}^{\infty} \sum_{m=1,5,7,\ldots}^{\infty} \frac{\sin m\phi}{m} \cos\frac{m\pi}{6}\, e^{ikz}\left[\cos kz_r - \cos kz_0\right] \times |k|\; I_m(|k|\,\rho)\left[K'_m(|k|\,a) - \frac{I'_m(|k|\,a)}{I'_m(|k|\,b)} K'_m(|k|\,b)\right] dk. \tag{3.121}$$

For the same reason as discussed in Section 3.5, to achieve a uniform $y$-gradient, one should choose $z_0$ and $z_r$ by solving

$$\int_0^{\infty} k^4 \left[\cos kz_r - \cos kz_0\right]\left[K'_1(ka) - \frac{I'_1(ka)}{I'_1(kb)} K'_1(kb)\right] dk = 0. \tag{3.122}$$

Turner and Bowley (1986) gave one set of solutions by solving

$$\int_0^{\infty} k^4 \cos kz_{0,r}\left[K'_1(ka) - \frac{I'_1(ka)}{I'_1(kb)} K'_1(kb)\right] dk = 0. \tag{3.123}$$

Another set of solutions can be obtained by solving Eq. (3.122) directly. The latter solution results in a significant reduction in the coil length.

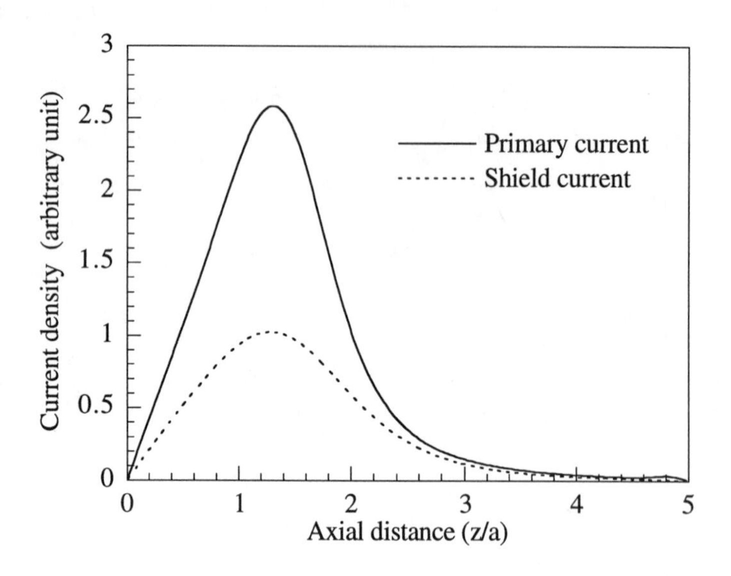


**Figure 3.19.** The current distribution on the primary and shield coils for a shielded $z$-gradient coil ($b = 1.4a$).

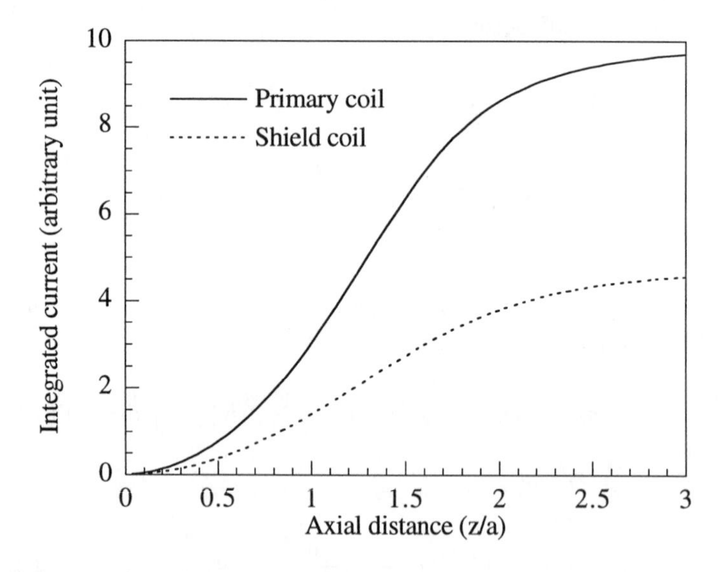


**Figure 3.20.** The integrated current on the primary and shield coils for a shielded $z$-gradient coil ($b = 1.4a$).

The design procedure using the target field method is similar to that described in the preceding section. Figure 3.19 shows the current distribution on the primary and shield coils of a shielded $z$-gradient coil. The integrated currents are given in Fig. 3.20, from which the position of the turns can be determined. The corresponding curves for the nonshielded coil are given in Figs. 3.10 and 3.11.

Finally, Fig. 3.21 displays the current distribution on the primary and shield coils of a shielded transverse gradient coil, corresponding to the nonshielded one shown in Fig. 3.14. The one corresponding to Fig. 3.17 is shown in Fig. 3.22.

## 3.8 Minimization of Inductance and Power Dissipation

To minimize the inductance of gradient coils, we first have to calculate the value of the inductance. From Eq. (2.77), we have

$$L = \frac{\mu_0}{4\pi I^2} \iiint_V \iiint_V \frac{\mathbf{J}(\mathbf{r}) \cdot \mathbf{J}(\mathbf{r}')}{R} dv' dv. \tag{3.124}$$

For a current confined to a cylindrical surface of radius $a$, there is no radial component and the current density can be written as

$$\mathbf{J}(\mathbf{r}') = [\hat{\phi}' J_\phi(\phi', z') + \hat{z} J_z(\phi', z')]\delta(\rho' - a) \tag{3.125}$$

from which we obtain

$$L = \frac{\mu_0 a^2}{4\pi I^2} \int_{-\infty}^{\infty} \int_0^{2\pi} \int_{-\infty}^{\infty} \int_0^{2\pi} \frac{1}{R} [J_z(\phi, z) J_{z'}(\phi', z') + \cos(\phi - \phi') J_\phi(\phi, z) J_{\phi'}(\phi', z')] \, d\phi' dz' d\phi dz \tag{3.126}$$

where $R = |\mathbf{r} - \mathbf{r}'|$ with both $\mathbf{r}$ and $\mathbf{r}'$ on the cylindrical surface. Substituting into the above the well-known expansion

$$\frac{1}{R} = \frac{1}{\pi} \int_{-\infty}^{\infty} \sum_{m=-\infty}^{\infty} e^{im(\phi-\phi')} e^{ik(z-z')} I_m(|k|\, a) K_m(|k|\, a) dk \tag{3.127}$$

we obtain

$$L = \frac{\mu_0 a^2}{2I^2} \int_{-\infty}^{\infty} \sum_{m=-\infty}^{\infty} \Big[ 2 j_z^{(m)}(k) j_z^{(-m)}(-k) + j_\phi^{(m+1)}(k) j_\phi^{(-m-1)}(-k) + j_\phi^{(m-1)}(k) j_\phi^{(-m+1)}(-k) \Big] I_m(|k|\, a) K_m(|k|\, a) \, dk \tag{3.128}$$

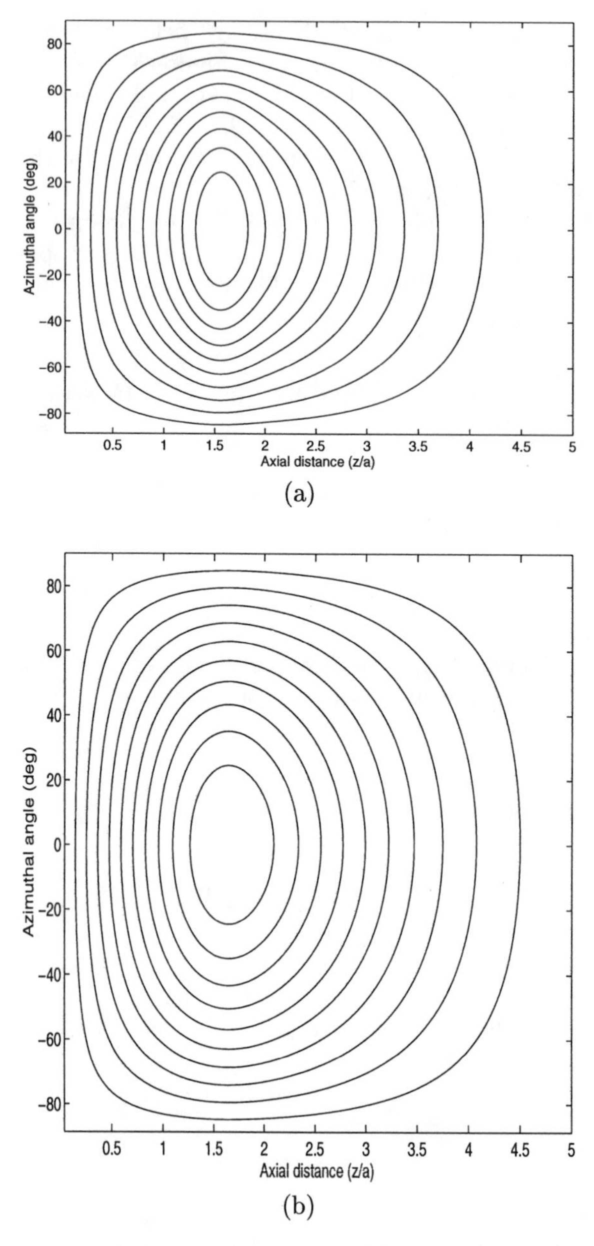


**Figure 3.21.** The current distribution for a shielded transverse gradient coil ($b = 1.4a$). Only one octant is shown and the complete set forms a double saddle-type arrangement. (a) Current on the primary coil. (b) Current on the shield coil.

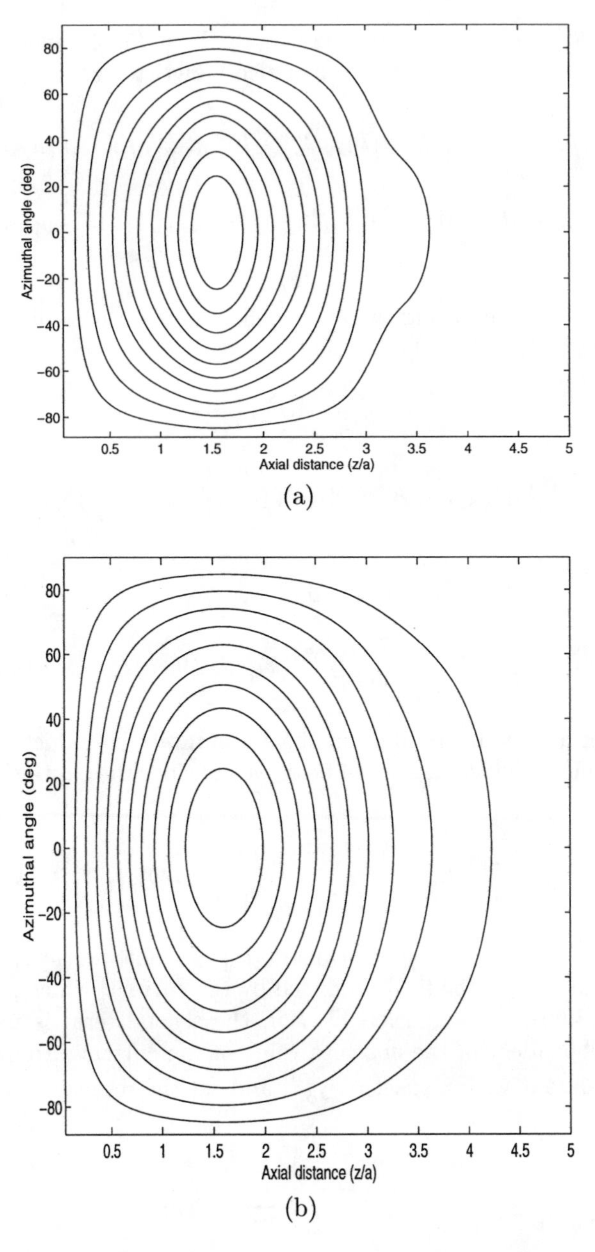


**Figure 3.22.** The current distribution for a shielded transverse gradient coil ($b = 1.4a$). Only one octant is shown and the complete set forms a double saddle-type arrangement. (a) Current on the primary coil. (b) Current on the shield coil.

where $j_z^{(m)}(k)$ and $j_\phi^{(m)}(k)$ are defined by Eqs. (3.62) and (3.63). By rearranging the index, Eq. (3.128) can also be written as

$$L = \frac{\mu_0 a^2}{2I^2} \int_{-\infty}^{\infty} \sum_{m=-\infty}^{\infty} \Big\{ 2 j_z^{(m)}(k) j_z^{(-m)}(-k) I_m(|k|\,a) K_m(|k|\,a) + j_\phi^{(m)}(k) \cdot j_\phi^{(-m)}(-k) [I_{m-1}(|k|\,a) K_{m-1}(|k|\,a) + I_{m+1}(|k|\,a) K_{m+1}(|k|\,a)] \Big\}\, dk. \tag{3.129}$$

This can be simplified using the recurrence and Wronskian formulas given in Eqs. (3.192)–(3.196), resulting in

$$L = \frac{\mu_0 a^2}{I^2} \int_{-\infty}^{\infty} \sum_{m=-\infty}^{\infty} \Big\{ j_z^{(m)}(k) j_z^{(-m)}(-k) I_m(|k|\,a) K_m(|k|\,a) - j_\phi^{(m)}(k) \cdot j_\phi^{(-m)}(-k) [I'_m(|k|\,a) K'_m(|k|\,a) + (m/ka)^2 I_m(|k|\,a) K_m(|k|\,a)] \Big\}\, dk. \tag{3.130}$$

Applying Eq. (3.64), we finally obtain

$$L = -\frac{\mu_0 a^2}{I^2} \int_{-\infty}^{\infty} \sum_{m=-\infty}^{\infty} \left| j_\phi^{(m)}(k) \right|^2 I'_m(|k|\,a) K'_m(|k|\,a)\, dk. \tag{3.131}$$

To seek a current distribution that minimizes the inductance and, at the same time, produces a desired field, we consider the expression (Turner 1988)

$$U = L[j_\phi^{(m)}(k)] + \frac{1}{I} \sum_{n=1}^{N} \lambda_n \left\{ B_n^{\text{desired}} - B_n[j_\phi^{(m)}(k)] \right\} \tag{3.132}$$

where $\lambda_n$ are called Lagrange multipliers, $B_n^{\text{desired}}$ denotes the specified field at point $n$, and $B_n$ is the field produced by the current, which is calculated using Eq. (3.66). The division by $I$ in the second term is necessary to make it independent of the absolute value of the current. To minimize $U$, we differentiate it with respect to $j_\phi^{(m)}$ and set the resultant expression to zero:

$$\frac{\partial U}{\partial j_\phi^{(m)}} = \frac{\partial L}{\partial j_\phi^{(m)}} - \frac{1}{I} \sum_{n=1}^{N} \lambda_n \frac{\partial B_n}{\partial j_\phi^{(m)}} = 0 \tag{3.133}$$

where

$$\frac{\partial L}{\partial j_\phi^{(m)}} = -\frac{2\mu_0 a^2}{I^2} \int_{-\infty}^{\infty} j_\phi^{(m)}(k) I'_m(|k|\,a) K'_m(|k|\,a) dk. \tag{3.134}$$

Using Eq. (3.66), we also find

$$\frac{\partial B_n}{\partial j_\phi^{(m)}} = -\frac{\mu_0 a}{2\pi}\int_{-\infty}^{\infty} e^{im\phi_n} e^{ikz_n}\,|k|\, I_m(|k|\,\rho_n) K_m'(|k|\,a)\,dk. \quad (3.135)$$

Substituting these into Eq. (3.133), we obtain

$$j_\phi^{(m)} = \frac{I\,|k|}{4\pi a I_m'(|k|\,a)}\sum_{n=1}^{N} \lambda_n e^{im\phi_n} e^{ikz_n} I_m(|k|\,\rho_n) \quad (3.136)$$

which provides a constraint on the current density for the minimization of inductance. Equation (3.136) contains the Lagrange multipliers $\lambda_n$. To determine $\lambda_n$, we can substitute it into Eq. (3.66). Doing so, we obtain

$$\begin{aligned} B_z(\rho,\phi,z) = &-\frac{\mu_0 I}{8\pi^2}\sum_{n=1}^{N}\lambda_n\int_{-\infty}^{\infty}\sum_{m=-\infty}^{\infty} k^2\frac{K_m'(|k|\,a)}{I_m'(|k|\,a)} \\ &\times e^{im(\phi+\phi_n)} e^{ik(z+z_n)} I_m(|k|\,\rho_n) I_m(|k|\,\rho)\,dk. \end{aligned} \quad (3.137)$$

Applying this at the specified points, we obtain a matrix equation given by

$$[A]\{\lambda\} = \{b\} \quad (3.138)$$

where $\{\lambda\} = [\lambda_1, \lambda_2, \ldots, \lambda_n]^T$, $\{b\} = [B_1^{\text{desired}}, B_2^{\text{desired}}, \ldots, B_N^{\text{desired}}]^T$, and

$$\begin{aligned} A_{n',n} = &-\frac{\mu_0 I}{8\pi^2}\int_{-\infty}^{\infty}\sum_{m=-\infty}^{\infty} k^2\frac{K_m'(|k|\,a)}{I_m'(|k|\,a)} \\ &\times e^{im(\phi_{n'}+\phi_n)} e^{ik(z_{n'}+z_n)} I_m(|k|\,\rho_n) I_m(|k|\,\rho_{n'})\,dk. \end{aligned} \quad (3.139)$$

Obviously, $[A]$ is a symmetric matrix. Solving Eq. (3.138), we obtain the values for $\lambda_n$, which can be substituted into Eq. (3.136) to calculate $j_\phi^{(m)}$. The desired current distribution can then be obtained via an inverse transform from Eqs. (3.67) and (3.68) with the aid of Eq. (3.64). Several examples can be found in Turner (1988).

The same method can be employed to minimize the power dissipation in the design of a gradient coil. The power dissipated in a gradient coil can be expressed as

$$P_d = \frac{\rho_r a}{t}\int_{-\infty}^{\infty}\int_0^{2\pi}\left[|J_z(\phi,z)|^2 + |J_\phi(\phi,z)|^2\right] d\phi\,dz \quad (3.140)$$

where $\rho_r$ denotes the resistivity and $t$ denotes the thickness of the conductor. Substituting Eqs. (3.67) and (3.68) into the above and performing the integration with respect to $\phi$ and $z$, we obtain

$$P_d = \frac{\rho_r a}{t}(4\pi)^2 \int_{-\infty}^{\infty} \sum_{m=-\infty}^{\infty} \left[ \left| j_z^{(m)}(k) \right|^2 + \left| j_\phi^{(m)}(k) \right|^2 \right] dk \quad (3.141)$$

where we have employed the relations in Eqs. (3.56) and (3.57). Applying Eq. (3.64), we obtain

$$P_d = \frac{\rho_r a}{t}(4\pi)^2 \int_{-\infty}^{\infty} \sum_{m=-\infty}^{\infty} \left| j_\phi^{(m)}(k) \right|^2 \left( 1 + \frac{m^2}{k^2 a^2} \right) dk. \quad (3.142)$$

By repeating the procedure of the inductance minimization with $L$ replaced by $P_d/I^2$, we can find the desired current distribution that minimizes power dissipation. One can also minimize both inductance and power dissipation by defining a properly weighted quantity of the two.

Figure 3.23 depicts the primary coil's wire layout of a shielded transverse gradient coil obtained by minimizing the inductance and power dissipation (Turner 1993). The primary coil has a radius 0.1 m, the shield has a radius 0.15 m, and the coil efficiency is 0.5 $\mathrm{mT \cdot m^{-1} \cdot A^{-1}}$. The target cylinder radii are 0.01 m and 0.07 m, the axial spacing of target points is 0.5 mm, and the number of target points per cylinder is 8.

## 3.9 Planar Gradient Coils

The principle of the design of planar gradient coils is very similar to that for the design of cylindrical gradient coils (Yoda 1990, Martens *et al.* 1991). In fact, the mathematics involved is much simpler.

### 3.9.1 Magnetic Field Produced by a Planar Surface Current

Let us start with the formulation of the static magnetic field generated by a surface current located in the plane of $y = y_0$. We consider first the solution of the Laplace equation in the Cartesian or rectangular coordinate system

$$\nabla^2 \psi = 0 \quad \text{or} \quad \frac{\partial^2 \psi}{\partial x^2} + \frac{\partial^2 \psi}{\partial y^2} + \frac{\partial^2 \psi}{\partial z^2} = 0. \quad (3.143)$$

Using the method of separation of variables, we find the general solution given by

$$\psi(x, y, z) = \int_{-\infty}^{\infty} \int_{-\infty}^{\infty} A^{(\pm)}(k_x, k_z) e^{i(k_x x + k_z z) \mp k_y y} dk_x dk_z \qquad \text{for } y \gtrless y_0 \quad (3.144)$$

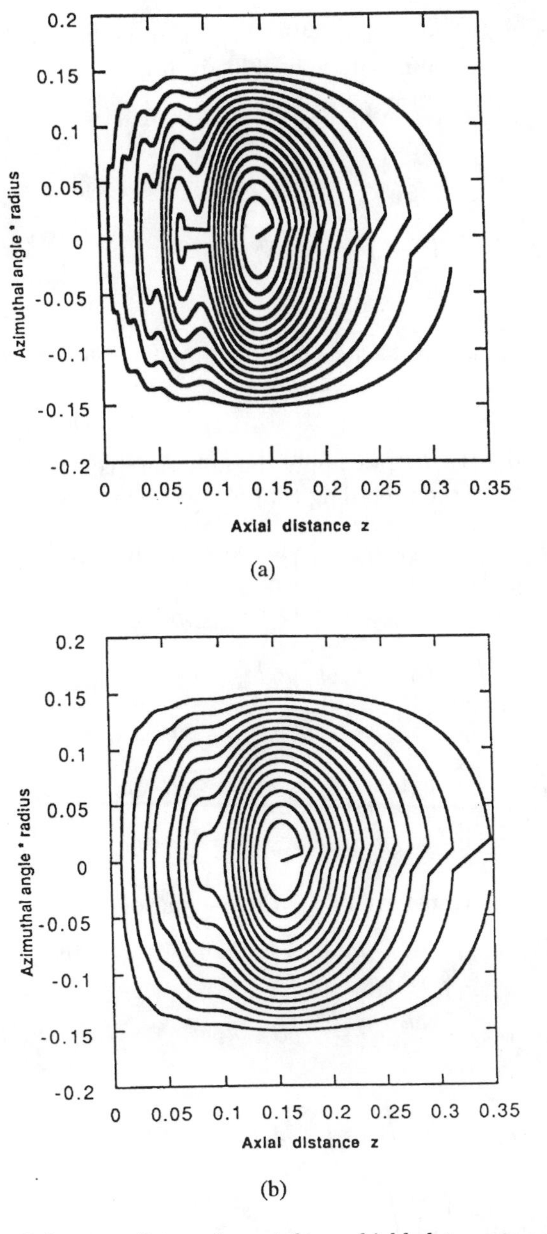


**Figure 3.23.** Primary coil turn layout for a shielded transverse gradient coil. (a) Obtained with inductance minimization. (b) Obtained with power dissipation minimization. Reproduced from Turner (1993) with permission from Elsevier Science.

where $k_y = \sqrt{k_x^2 + k_z^2}$ and $A^{(\pm)}(k_x, k_z)$ are the coefficients to be determined. Hence, the magnetic field is given by

$$B_x(x,y,z) = -i\int_{-\infty}^{\infty}\int_{-\infty}^{\infty} A^{(\pm)}(k_x,k_z)e^{i(k_x x+k_z z)\mp k_y y}k_x dk_x dk_z \quad \text{for } y \gtrless y_0 \tag{3.145}$$

$$B_y(x,y,z) = \pm\int_{-\infty}^{\infty}\int_{-\infty}^{\infty} A^{(\pm)}(k_x,k_z)e^{i(k_x x+k_z z)\mp k_y y}k_y dk_x dk_z \quad \text{for } y \gtrless y_0 \tag{3.146}$$

$$B_z(x,y,z) = -i\int_{-\infty}^{\infty}\int_{-\infty}^{\infty} A^{(\pm)}(k_x,k_z)e^{i(k_x x+k_z z)\mp k_y y}k_z dk_x dk_z \quad \text{for } y \gtrless y_0. \tag{3.147}$$

To determine $A^{(\pm)}(k_x, k_z)$, we apply the boundary conditions given in Eqs. (2.47) and (2.52) of the preceding chapter, yielding

$$\int_{-\infty}^{\infty}\int_{-\infty}^{\infty}\left[A^{(+)}(k_x,k_z)e^{-k_y y_0} - A^{(-)}(k_x,k_z)e^{k_y y_0}\right] \times e^{i(k_x x+k_z z)}k_x dk_x dk_z = -i\mu_0 J_z(x,z) \tag{3.148}$$

$$\int_{-\infty}^{\infty}\int_{-\infty}^{\infty}\left[A^{(+)}(k_x,k_z)e^{-k_y y_0} + A^{(-)}(k_x,k_z)e^{k_y y_0}\right] \times e^{i(k_x x+k_z z)}k_y dk_x dk_z = 0 \tag{3.149}$$

$$\int_{-\infty}^{\infty}\int_{-\infty}^{\infty}\left[A^{(+)}(k_x,k_z)e^{-k_y y_0} - A^{(-)}(k_x,k_z)e^{k_y y_0}\right] \times e^{i(k_x x+k_z z)}k_z dk_x dk_z = i\mu_0 J_x(x,z). \tag{3.150}$$

Taking the Fourier transform of the three equations above, we obtain

$$k_x A^{(+)}(k_x,k_z)e^{-k_y y_0} - k_x A^{(-)}(k_x,k_z)e^{k_y y_0} = -i\mu_0 j_z(k_x,k_z) \tag{3.151}$$

$$A^{(+)}(k_x,k_z)e^{-k_y y_0} + A^{(-)}(k_x,k_z)e^{k_y y_0} = 0 \tag{3.152}$$

$$k_z A^{(+)}(k_x,k_z)e^{-k_y y_0} - k_z A^{(-)}(k_x,k_z)e^{k_y y_0} = i\mu_0 j_x(k_x,k_z) \tag{3.153}$$

where

$$j_x(k_x,k_z) = \int_{-\infty}^{\infty}\int_{-\infty}^{\infty} J_x(x,z)\,e^{-i(k_x x+k_z z)}dx\,dz \tag{3.154}$$

$$j_z(k_x,k_z) = \int_{-\infty}^{\infty}\int_{-\infty}^{\infty} J_z(x,z)\,e^{-i(k_x x+k_z z)}dx\,dz. \tag{3.155}$$

From Eqs. (3.151)–(3.153), we obtain

$$A^{(\pm)}(k_x,k_z) = \pm\frac{i\mu_0}{2k_z}j_x(k_x,k_z)e^{\pm k_y y_0} \tag{3.156}$$

and

$$k_x j_x(k_x, k_z) + k_z j_z(k_x, k_z) = 0. \tag{3.157}$$

Substituting Eq. (3.156) into Eqs. (3.145)–(3.147), we obtain the field produced by a planar surface current placed at $y = y_0$.

Finally, we note that the inverse transforms of Eqs. (3.154) and (3.155) are given by

$$J_x(x, z) = \frac{1}{(2\pi)^2} \int_{-\infty}^{\infty} \int_{-\infty}^{\infty} j_x(k_x, k_z) e^{i(k_x x + k_z z)} dk_x dk_z \tag{3.158}$$

$$J_z(x, z) = \frac{1}{(2\pi)^2} \int_{-\infty}^{\infty} \int_{-\infty}^{\infty} j_z(k_x, k_z) e^{i(k_x x + k_z z)} dk_x dk_z. \tag{3.159}$$

Substituting these into the current continuity equation

$$\nabla \cdot \mathbf{J} = \frac{\partial J_x}{\partial x} + \frac{\partial J_z}{\partial z} = 0 \tag{3.160}$$

we obtain Eq. (3.157). Thus, Eq. (3.157) is simply the Fourier transform of the continuity equation of current.

### 3.9.2 Target Field Method

To illustrate the application of the target field method, we consider the design of bi-planar gradient coils; the design of single planar coils can be treated as a special case. We assume that one plane is placed at $y = b$ carrying a surface current $\mathbf{J}^{(1)}(x, z)$, and the other plane is placed at $y = -b$ carrying a surface current $\mathbf{J}^{(2)}(x, z)$. The $z$-component of the magnetic field between the two planes is then given by

$$B_z(x, y, z) = -\frac{\mu_0}{2} \int_{-\infty}^{\infty} \int_{-\infty}^{\infty} \left[ j_x^{(1)}(k_x, k_z) e^{k_y(y-b)} - j_x^{(2)}(k_x, k_z) e^{-k_y(y+b)} \right] \times e^{i(k_x x + k_z z)} dk_x dk_z. \tag{3.161}$$

We then specify the desired fields on two planes, one at $y = c$ and the other at $y = -c$, where $c < b$. Denote the desired fields as $B_z(x, c, z)$ and $B_z(x, -c, z)$, respectively, and substitute them into Eq. (3.161). Taking the Fourier transform, we obtain

$$j_x^{(1)}(k_x, k_z) e^{-k_y(b-c)} - j_x^{(2)}(k_x, k_z) e^{-k_y(b+c)} = -2b_z(k_x, k_z, c)/\mu_0 \tag{3.162}$$

$$j_x^{(1)}(k_x, k_z) e^{-k_y(b+c)} - j_x^{(2)}(k_x, k_z) e^{-k_y(b-c)} = -2b_z(k_x, k_z, -c)/\mu_0 \tag{3.163}$$

where $b_z(k_x, k_z, c)$ and $b_z(k_x, k_z, -c)$ are the Fourier transforms of $B_z(x, c, z)$ and $B_z(x, -c, z)$, respectively. From Eqs. (3.162) and (3.163), we find

$$j_x^{(1)}(k_x, k_z) = -e^{k_y b}\text{csch}(2k_y c)\left[b_z(k_x, k_z, c)e^{k_y c} - b_z(k_x, k_z, -c)e^{-k_y c}\right]/\mu_0 \tag{3.164}$$

$$j_x^{(2)}(k_x, k_z) = -e^{k_y b}\text{csch}(2k_y c)\left[b_z(k_x, k_z, c)e^{-k_y c} - b_z(k_x, k_z, -c)e^{k_y c}\right]/\mu_0. \tag{3.165}$$

Substituting these into Eqs. (3.158) and (3.159), we obtain the physical currents to generate the desired field.

### 3.9.3 Shielded Planar Coils

To design a shielded coil, we place two additional surface currents, one on the plane of $y = d$ whose current is denoted as $\mathbf{J}^{(s1)}$ and the other on the plane of $y = -d$ whose current is denoted as $\mathbf{J}^{(s2)}$. The $z$-component of the magnetic field for $y > d$ is then given by

$$\begin{aligned} B_z(x, y, z) = \frac{\mu_0}{2} \int_{-\infty}^{\infty} \int_{-\infty}^{\infty} & \left[j_x^{(1)}(k_x, k_z)e^{-k_y(y-b)} + j_x^{(2)}(k_x, k_z)e^{-k_y(y+b)} \right. \\ & \left. + j_x^{(s1)}(k_x, k_z)e^{-k_y(y-d)} + j_x^{(s2)}(k_x, k_z)e^{-k_y(y+d)}\right] \\ & \times e^{i(k_x x + k_z z)}\, dk_x\, dk_z \end{aligned} \tag{3.166}$$

and that for $y < -d$ is given by

$$\begin{aligned} B_z(x, y, z) = -\frac{\mu_0}{2} \int_{-\infty}^{\infty} \int_{-\infty}^{\infty} & \left[j_x^{(1)}(k_x, k_z)e^{k_y(y-b)} + j_x^{(2)}(k_x, k_z)e^{k_y(y+b)} \right. \\ & \left. + j_x^{(s1)}(k_x, k_z)e^{k_y(y-d)} + j_x^{(s2)}(k_x, k_z)e^{k_y(y+d)}\right] \\ & \times e^{i(k_x x + k_z z)}\, dk_x\, dk_z \end{aligned} \tag{3.167}$$

where $j_x^{(s1)}(k_x, k_z)$ and $j_x^{(s2)}(k_x, k_z)$ are the Fourier transforms of $J_x^{(s1)}$ and $J_x^{(s2)}$, respectively. It can be shown easily that these fields, as well as the other two components, vanish when $j_x^{(s1)}(k_x, k_z)$ and $j_x^{(s2)}(k_x, k_z)$ are chosen as

$$\begin{aligned} j_x^{(s1)}(k_x, k_z) = & -\text{csch}(2k_y d) \\ & \times \left\{j_x^{(1)}(k_x, k_z)\sinh[k_y(b+d)] + j_x^{(2)}(k_x, k_z)\sinh[k_y(d-b)]\right\} \end{aligned} \tag{3.168}$$

$$j_x^{(s2)}(k_x,k_z) = -\operatorname{csch}(2k_y d) \times \left\{ j_x^{(1)}(k_x,k_z)\sinh[k_y(d-b)] + j_x^{(2)}(k_x,k_z)\sinh[k_y(b+d)] \right\}. \tag{3.169}$$

The required currents $j_x^{(1)}(k_x,k_z)$ and $j_x^{(2)}(k_x,k_z)$ can be determined by applying the target field method to the field in the region of $-b < y < b$, which is given by

$$\begin{aligned} B_z(x,y,z) = &-\frac{\mu_0}{2}\int_{-\infty}^{\infty}\int_{-\infty}^{\infty}\Big[ j_x^{(1)}(k_x,k_z)e^{k_y(y-b)} + j_x^{(2)}(k_x,k_z)e^{-k_y(y+b)} \\ &+ j_x^{(s1)}(k_x,k_z)e^{k_y(y-d)} + j_x^{(s2)}(k_x,k_z)e^{-k_y(y+d)}\Big] \\ &\times e^{i(k_x x + k_z z)}\, dk_x\, dk_z. \end{aligned} \tag{3.170}$$

### 3.9.4 Minimization of Inductance and Power Dissipation

To minimize the inductance, we first have to derive an expression for it in terms of current. Consider again a bi-planar coil. The inductance of the coil is given by

$$L = \frac{\mu_0}{4\pi I^2}\int_{-\infty}^{\infty}\int_{-\infty}^{\infty}\int_{-\infty}^{\infty}\int_{-\infty}^{\infty}\frac{\mathbf{J}^{(1)}(x,z)\cdot\mathbf{J}^{(2)}(x',z')}{R}\, dx\, dz\, dx'\, dz'. \tag{3.171}$$

Substituting into the above the well-known expansion

$$\frac{1}{R} = \frac{1}{2\pi}\int_{-\infty}^{\infty}\int_{-\infty}^{\infty}\frac{1}{k_y}e^{ik_x(x-x')+ik_z(z-z')-k_y|y-y'|}dk_x\, dk_z \tag{3.172}$$

we obtain

$$\begin{aligned} L = \frac{\mu_0}{8\pi^2 I^2}\int_{-\infty}^{\infty}\int_{-\infty}^{\infty}\frac{1}{k_y}\Big\{ &\left|\mathbf{j}^{(1)}(k_x,k_z)\right|^2 + \left|\mathbf{j}^{(2)}(k_x,k_z)\right|^2 \\ &+2\mathrm{Re}\left[\mathbf{j}^{(1)}(k_x,k_z)\cdot\mathbf{j}^{(2)}(-k_x,-k_z)\right] e^{-2k_y b}\Big\}\, dk_x\, dk_z. \end{aligned} \tag{3.173}$$

Applying Eq. (3.157) to the above yields

$$\begin{aligned} L = \frac{\mu_0}{8\pi^2 I^2}\int_{-\infty}^{\infty}\int_{-\infty}^{\infty}\frac{1}{k_y}\Big\{ &\left|j_x^{(1)}(k_x,k_z)\right|^2 + \left|j_x^{(2)}(k_x,k_z)\right|^2 \\ &+2\mathrm{Re}\left[j_x^{(1)}(k_x,k_z)\cdot j_x^{(2)}(-k_x,-k_z)\right] e^{-2k_y b}\Big\}\left(1+\frac{k_x^2}{k_z^2}\right)\, dk_x\, dk_z. \end{aligned} \tag{3.174}$$

Neglecting the cross term, we obtain

$$L \approx \frac{\mu_0}{8\pi^2 I^2} \int_{-\infty}^{\infty} \int_{-\infty}^{\infty} \frac{1}{k_y} \left\{ \left| j_x^{(1)}(k_x, k_z) \right|^2 + \left| j_x^{(2)}(k_x, k_z) \right|^2 \right\} \times \left(1 + \frac{k_x^2}{k_z^2}\right) dk_x \, dk_z \tag{3.175}$$

or

$$L \approx \frac{\mu_0}{8\pi^2 I^2} \int_{-\infty}^{\infty} \int_{-\infty}^{\infty} \frac{k_y}{k_z^2} \left\{ \left| j_x^{(1)}(k_x, k_z) \right|^2 + \left| j_x^{(2)}(k_x, k_z) \right|^2 \right\} dk_x \, dk_z . \tag{3.176}$$

To find the current distribution that minimizes the inductance and, at the same time, produces a desired field, we consider the expression

$$U = L[j_x^{(1)}(k_x, k_z), j_x^{(2)}(k_x, k_z)] + \frac{1}{I} \sum_{n=1}^{N} \lambda_n \left\{ B_n^{\text{desired}} - B_n[j_x^{(1)}(k_x, k_z), j_x^{(2)}(k_x, k_z)] \right\} \tag{3.177}$$

and differentiate it with respect to $j_x^{(1)}(k_x, k_z)$ and $j_x^{(2)}(k_x, k_z)$ and set the resultant expressions to zero:

$$\frac{\partial U}{\partial j_x^{(m)}} = \frac{\partial L}{\partial j_x^{(m)}} - \frac{1}{I} \sum_{n=1}^{N} \lambda_n \frac{\partial B_n}{\partial j_x^{(m)}} = 0 \qquad (m = 1, 2) \tag{3.178}$$

where

$$\frac{\partial L}{\partial j_x^{(m)}} = \frac{\mu_0}{4\pi^2 I^2} \int_{-\infty}^{\infty} \int_{-\infty}^{\infty} \frac{k_y}{k_z^2} j_x^{(m)}(k_x, k_z) \, dk_x \, dk_z \qquad (m = 1, 2) \tag{3.179}$$

and

$$\frac{\partial B_n}{\partial j_x^{(1)}} = -\frac{\mu_0}{2} \int_{-\infty}^{\infty} \int_{-\infty}^{\infty} e^{k_y(y_n - b)} \, e^{i(k_x x_n + k_z z_n)} dk_x dk_z \tag{3.180}$$

$$\frac{\partial B_n}{\partial j_x^{(2)}} = \frac{\mu_0}{2} \int_{-\infty}^{\infty} \int_{-\infty}^{\infty} e^{-k_y(y_n + b)} \, e^{i(k_x x_n + k_z z_n)} dk_x dk_z \tag{3.181}$$

where we used Eq. (3.161), which is for the case without a shield. For shielded coils, Eq. (3.170) should be used. Substituting Eqs. (3.179)–(3.181) into Eqs. (3.178), we obtain

$$j_x^{(1)}(k_x, k_z) = -2\pi^2 I \frac{k_z^2}{k_y} \sum_{n=1}^{N} \lambda_n e^{i(k_x x_n + k_z z_n)} e^{k_y(y_n - b)} \tag{3.182}$$

$$j_x^{(2)}(k_x, k_z) = 2\pi^2 I \frac{k_z^2}{k_y} \sum_{n=1}^{N} \lambda_n e^{i(k_x x_n + k_z z_n)} e^{-k_y(y_n + b)}. \tag{3.183}$$

To determine the Lagrange multipliers, we substitute these into Eq. (3.161) to find

$$B_z(x,y,z) = \pi^2 \mu_0 I \sum_{n=1}^{N} \lambda_n \int_{-\infty}^{\infty} \int_{-\infty}^{\infty} \frac{k_z^2}{k_y} \left[ e^{k_y(y+y_n-2b)} + e^{-k_y(y+y_n+2b)} \right] \times e^{i[k_x(x+x_n)+k_z(z+z_n)]} dk_x dk_z. \tag{3.184}$$

Applying this at the specified points, we obtain a matrix equation given by

$$[A]\{\lambda\} = \{b\} \tag{3.185}$$

where $\{\lambda\} = [\lambda_1, \lambda_2, \ldots, \lambda_N]^T$, $\{b\} = [B_1^{\text{desired}}, B_2^{\text{desired}}, \ldots, B_N^{\text{desired}}]^T$, and

$$A_{mn} = \pi^2 \mu_0 I \int_{-\infty}^{\infty} \int_{-\infty}^{\infty} \frac{k_z^2}{k_y} \left[ e^{k_y(y_m+y_n-2b)} + e^{-k_y(y_m+y_n+2b)} \right] \times e^{i[k_x(x_m+x_n)+k_z(z_m+z_n)]} dk_x dk_z. \tag{3.186}$$

Finally, we note that for most cases there is a certain relation between $j_x^{(1)}(k_x, k_z)$ and $j_x^{(2)}(k_x, k_z)$; hence, one can be expressed in terms of the other. In that case, Eq. (3.177) is a function of either $j_x^{(1)}(k_x, k_z)$ or $j_x^{(2)}(k_x, k_z)$ and the formulation can then be simplified.

The same method can be applied to the minimization of power dissipation. The power dissipated in a bi-planar coil can be expressed as

$$P_d = \frac{\rho_r}{t} \int_{-\infty}^{\infty} \int_{-\infty}^{\infty} \left[ \mathbf{J}^{(1)}(x,z) \cdot \mathbf{J}^{(1)}(x,z) + \mathbf{J}^{(2)}(x,z) \cdot \mathbf{J}^{(2)}(x,z) \right] dx\, dz \tag{3.187}$$

which can also be written as

$$P_d = \frac{\rho_r}{(2\pi)^2 t} \int_{-\infty}^{\infty} \int_{-\infty}^{\infty} \left[ \mathbf{j}^{(1)}(k_x, k_z) \cdot \mathbf{j}^{(1)}(k_x, k_z) + \mathbf{j}^{(2)}(k_x, k_z) \cdot \mathbf{j}^{(2)}(k_x, k_z) \right] dk_x dk_z. \tag{3.188}$$

By repeating the procedure of the inductance minimization with $L$ replaced by $P_d/I^2$, we can find the desired current distribution that minimizes power dissipation. One can also minimize both inductance and power dissipation by defining a properly weighted quantity of the two.

## 3.A Modified Bessel Functions

Modified Bessel functions, denoted by $I_n(x)$ and $K_n(x)$, are the two linearly independent solutions of the second-order differential equation

$$x^2 \frac{d^2y}{dx^2} + x\frac{dy}{dx} - (x^2 + n^2)y = 0 \tag{3.189}$$

which is called the modified Bessel's equation. They can be expressed explicitly as

$$I_n(x) = \sum_{m=0}^{\infty} \frac{(x/2)^{2m+n}}{m!\,(m+n)!} \tag{3.190}$$

and

$$\begin{aligned} K_n(x) = & \frac{1}{2}\sum_{m=0}^{n-1}(-1)^m \frac{(n-m-1)!}{m!}\left(\frac{x}{2}\right)^{2m-n} \\ & + (-1)^{n+1}\sum_{m=0}^{\infty}\frac{(x/2)^{2m+n}}{m!\,(m+n)!}\left(\ln\frac{x}{2} + \gamma - \frac{1}{2}\sum_{k=1}^{m}\frac{1}{k} - \frac{1}{2}\sum_{k=1}^{m+n}\frac{1}{k}\right) \end{aligned} \tag{3.191}$$

where $\gamma \approx 0.5772156649$ denotes Euler's constant.

The modified Bessel functions satisfy the recurrence relations given by

$$I_{n-1}(x) - I_{n+1}(x) = \frac{2n}{x} I_n(x) \tag{3.192}$$

$$K_{n-1}(x) - K_{n+1}(x) = -\frac{2n}{x} K_n(x) \tag{3.193}$$

and their differentiation formulas are given by

$$I_n'(x) = I_{n-1}(x) - \frac{n}{x} I_n(x) \tag{3.194}$$

$$K_n'(x) = -K_{n-1}(x) - \frac{n}{x} K_n(x). \tag{3.195}$$

They also satisfy the Wronskian relation given by

$$I_n(x)K_{n+1}(x) + I_{n+1}(x)K_n(x) = \frac{1}{x}. \tag{3.196}$$

The modified Bessel functions have many other mathematical properties, which are summarized in Abramowitz and Stegun (1964). For example, for negative orders, we have

$$I_{-n}(x) = I_n(x), \qquad K_{-n}(x) = K_n(x). \tag{3.197}$$

For a fixed $n$, when $x \to 0$,

$$I_0(x) \sim 1, \qquad I_n(x) \sim \frac{(x/2)^n}{n!} \qquad (n > 0) \tag{3.198}$$

$$K_0(x) \sim -\ln x, \qquad K_n(x) \sim \frac{n!}{2n}\left(\frac{x}{2}\right)^{-n} \qquad (n > 0). \tag{3.199}$$

For a fixed $n$, when $x \to \infty$,

$$I_n(x) \sim \frac{1}{\sqrt{2\pi x}}e^x, \qquad K_n(x) \sim \sqrt{\frac{\pi}{2x}}e^{-x}. \tag{3.200}$$

For a fixed $x$, when $n \to \infty$,

$$I_n(x) \sim \frac{1}{\sqrt{2\pi n}}\left(\frac{ex}{n}\right)^n, \qquad K_n(x) \sim \sqrt{\frac{\pi}{2n}}\left(\frac{n}{ex}\right)^n. \tag{3.201}$$

The numerical evaluation of the modified Bessel functions is described in Zhang and Jin (1996). The following is a FORTRAN program for computing $I_n(x)$ and $K_n(x)$ and their first derivative.

```
        SUBROUTINE IKNX(N,X,NM,BI,DI,BK,DK)
C
C       ============================================================
C       Purpose: Compute modified Bessel functions In(x) and Kn(x),
C                and their derivatives
C       Input:   x --- Argument of In(x) and Kn(x) ( 0 < x < 700 )
C                n --- Order of In(x) and Kn(x)
C       Output:  BI(n) --- In(x)
C                DI(n) --- In'(x)
C                BK(n) --- Kn(x)
C                DK(n) --- Kn'(x)
C                NM --- Highest order computed
C       Routines called:
C                MSTA1 and MSTA2 for computing the starting
C                point for backward recurrence
C       ============================================================
C
        IMPLICIT DOUBLE PRECISION (A-H,O-Z)
        DIMENSION BI(0:N),DI(0:N),BK(0:N),DK(0:N)
        PI=3.141592653589793D0
        EL=0.57721566490153D0
        NM=N
        IF (X.LT.1.0D-100) THEN
           DO 10 K=0,N
```

```
            BI(K)=0.0D0
            BK(K)=1.0D+300
            DI(K)=0.0D0
10          DK(K)=-1.0D+300
         BI(0)=1.0D0
         DI(1)=0.5D0
         RETURN
      ENDIF
      IF (N.EQ.0) NM=1
      M=MSTA1(X,200)
      IF (M.LT.NM) THEN
         NM=M
      ELSE
         M=MSTA2(X,NM,15)
      ENDIF
      BS=0.0D0
      SK0=0.0D0
      F0=0.0D0
      F1=1.0D-100
      DO 15 K=M,0,-1
         F=2.0D0*(K+1.0D0)*F1/X+F0
         IF (K.LE.NM) BI(K)=F
         IF (K.NE.0.AND.K.EQ.2*INT(K/2)) SK0=SK0+4.D0*F/K
         BS=BS+2.0D0*F
         F0=F1
15       F1=F
      S0=DEXP(X)/(BS-F)
      DO 20 K=0,NM
20       BI(K)=S0*BI(K)
      IF (X.LE.8.D0) THEN
         BK(0)=-(DLOG(.5D0*X)+EL)*BI(0)+S0*SK0
         BK(1)=(1.0D0/X-BI(1)*BK(0))/BI(0)
       ELSE
         A0=DSQRT(PI/(2.0D0*X))*DEXP(-X)
         K0=16
         IF (X.GE.25.0) K0=10
         IF (X.GE.80.0) K0=8
         IF (X.GE.200.0) K0=6
         DO 30 L=0,1
            BKL=1.0D0
            VT=4.0D0*L
            R=1.0D0
            DO 25 K=1,K0
               R=0.125D0*R*(VT-(2.0*K-1.0)**2)/(K*X)
25             BKL=BKL+R
```

```
              BK(L)=A0*BKL
30          CONTINUE
        ENDIF
        G0=BK(0)
        G1=BK(1)
        DO 35 K=2,NM
           G=2.0D0*(K-1.0D0)/X*G1+G0
           BK(K)=G
           G0=G1
35         G1=G
        DI(0)=BI(1)
        DK(0)=-BK(1)
        DO 40 K=1,NM
           DI(K)=BI(K-1)-K/X*BI(K)
40         DK(K)=-BK(K-1)-K/X*BK(K)
        RETURN
        END

        INTEGER FUNCTION MSTA1(X,MP)
        IMPLICIT DOUBLE PRECISION (A-H,O-Z)
        A0=DABS(X)+1.0D-10
        N0=INT(1.1*A0)
        F0=ENVJ(N0,A0)-MP
        N1=N0+5
        F1=ENVJ(N1,A0)-MP
        DO 10 IT=1,20
           NN=N1-(N1-N0)/(1.0D0-F0/F1)
           F=ENVJ(NN,A0)-MP
           IF(ABS(NN-N1).LT.1) GO TO 20
           N0=N1
           F0=F1
           N1=NN
 10        F1=F
 20     MSTA1=NN+4
        RETURN
        END
        REAL*8 FUNCTION ENVJ(N,X)
        DOUBLE PRECISION X
        ENVJ=.5D0*DLOG10(6.28D0*N)-N*DLOG10(1.36D0*X/N)
        RETURN
        END

        INTEGER FUNCTION MSTA2(X,N,MP)
        IMPLICIT DOUBLE PRECISION (A-H,O-Z)
        A0=DABS(X)+1.0D-10
```

```
      HMP=0.5D0*MP
      EJN=ENVJ(N,A0)
      IF(EJN.LE.HMP) THEN
         OBJ=MP
         N0=INT(1.1*A0)
      ELSE
         OBJ=HMP+EJN
         N0=N
      ENDIF
      F0=ENVJ(N0,A0)-OBJ
      N1=N0+5
      F1=ENVJ(N1,A0)-OBJ
      DO 10 IT=1,20
         NN=N1-(N1-N0)/(1.0D0-F0/F1)
         F=ENVJ(NN,A0)-OBJ
         IF(ABS(NN-N1).LT.1) GO TO 20
         N0=N1
         F0=F1
         N1=NN
10       F1=F
20    MSTA2=NN+4
      RETURN
      END
```

## 3.B Alternative Derivation of Equation (3.66)

Equation (3.66) can also be derived with the aid of a vector potential, which is defined as

$$\mathbf{A}(\mathbf{r}) = \frac{\mu_0}{4\pi} \iiint_V \frac{\mathbf{J}(\mathbf{r}')}{R}\, dv'. \tag{3.202}$$

In this case, we are interested in the magnetic field produced by a cylindrical surface current, which has no radial component. Thus,

$$\mathbf{J}(\mathbf{r}') = [\hat{\phi}' J_\phi(\phi', z') + \hat{z} J_z(\phi', z')]\delta(\rho' - a) \tag{3.203}$$

where $\delta(\rho' - a)$ denotes the Dirac delta function. Substituting this into Eq. (3.202) and taking the dot product with $\hat{\rho}$, $\hat{\phi}$, and $\hat{z}$, we obtain

$$A_\rho = \frac{\mu_0}{4\pi} \int_{-\infty}^{\infty} \int_0^{2\pi} J_\phi(\phi', z') \sin(\phi - \phi') \frac{1}{R} a\, d\phi' dz' \tag{3.204}$$

$$A_\phi = \frac{\mu_0}{4\pi} \int_{-\infty}^{\infty} \int_0^{2\pi} J_\phi(\phi', z') \cos(\phi - \phi') \frac{1}{R} a\, d\phi' dz' \tag{3.205}$$

$$A_z = \frac{\mu_0}{4\pi}\int_{-\infty}^{\infty}\int_0^{2\pi} J_z(\phi', z')\frac{1}{R}a\, d\phi' dz'. \tag{3.206}$$

Using the well-known expansion

$$\frac{1}{|\mathbf{r}-\mathbf{r}'|} = \frac{1}{\pi}\int_{-\infty}^{\infty}\sum_{m=-\infty}^{\infty} e^{im(\phi-\phi')}e^{ik(z-z')}I_m(|k|\,\rho_<)K_m(|k|\,\rho_>)dk \tag{3.207}$$

where

$$\rho_< = \begin{cases} \rho & \rho < \rho' \\ \rho' & \rho' < \rho \end{cases} \quad \text{and} \quad \rho_> = \begin{cases} \rho & \rho > \rho' \\ \rho' & \rho' > \rho. \end{cases}$$

and substituting Eq. (3.207) into Eqs. (3.204)–(3.206), we obtain for $\rho < a$ (inside the cylinder)

$$A_\rho = -\frac{i\mu_0 a}{4\pi}\int_{-\infty}^{\infty}\sum_{m=-\infty}^{\infty} j_\phi^m(k)e^{im\phi}e^{ikz}$$
$$\times\left[I_{m-1}(|k|\,\rho)K_{m-1}(|k|\,a) - I_{m+1}(|k|\,\rho)K_{m+1}(|k|\,a)\right]dk \tag{3.208}$$

$$A_\phi = \frac{\mu_0 a}{4\pi}\int_{-\infty}^{\infty}\sum_{m=-\infty}^{\infty} j_\phi^m(k)e^{im\phi}e^{ikz}$$
$$\times\left[I_{m-1}(|k|\,\rho)K_{m-1}(|k|\,a) + I_{m+1}(|k|\,\rho)K_{m+1}(|k|\,a)\right]dk \tag{3.209}$$

$$A_z = \frac{\mu_0 a}{2\pi}\int_{-\infty}^{\infty}\sum_{m=-\infty}^{\infty} j_z^m(k)e^{im\phi}e^{ikz}I_m(|k|\,\rho)K_m(|k|\,a)dk \tag{3.210}$$

where $j_z^{(m)}(k)$ and $j_\phi^{(m)}(k)$ are defined by Eqs. (3.62) and (3.63). Since $\mathbf{B} = \nabla\times\mathbf{A}$, from Eqs. (3.208)–(3.210) we obtain

$$B_z(\rho,\phi,z) = -\frac{\mu_0 a}{2\pi}\int_{-\infty}^{\infty}\sum_{m=-\infty}^{\infty} e^{im\phi}e^{ikz}\,|k|\,j_\phi^{(m)}(k)I_m(|k|\,\rho)K_m'(|k|\,a)\,dk$$
$$(\rho \le a) \tag{3.211}$$

where we have simplified the result using the recurrence and Wronskian relations of the modified Bessel functions. Equation (3.211) is the same as Eq. (3.66).

## Problems

3.1 Consider the $RL$-circuit in Fig. 3.1. Find the waveform of the input voltage such that the current in the circuit decreases in the form

$$i(t) = \frac{V}{R}e^{-q(R/L)t}$$

3.2 Calculate the efficiency of the Maxwell coil pair and that of the gradient coil made of two coil pairs whose position and current are given in Eq. (3.15).

3.3 Consider a coil made of $2N$ circular loops carrying the same current in the same direction and placed symmetrically along the $z$-axis. The position of the loops can be chosen so that the magnetic field is most uniform around the origin. Find the position of the loops for $N = 1$, 2, and 3. Hint: Use an expression similar to Eq. (3.14).

3.4 Write a computer program based on Eqs. (3.17)–(3.19) and design a coil to produce a uniform magnetic field around the origin and another coil to produce a $z$-gradient using 10 loops.

3.5 Write a computer program to minimize the error defined in Eq. (3.20) by searching for the position of the loops whose current is a constant. Try a case for a coil with 10 loops.

3.6 Consider the configurations in Fig. 3.6. Assume that the distance of the four inner wires from the origin is $a$ and the distance of the four outer wires from the origin in configuration (a) is $2a$. Further, assume the length of the wires in the $x$-direction is $4a$. Calculate the efficiency of the two configurations.

3.7 Show that for the Golay coil sketched in Fig. 3.7, $\partial B_z/\partial y = \partial B_y/\partial z$ near the origin. Hint: Use one of Maxwell's equations. In fact, in Suits and Wilken (1989), the gradient to be optimized is $\partial B_y/\partial z$.

3.8 Choose a set of parameters and evaluate the integral in Eq. (3.100) with $t(k) = 1$ to find the required current distribution to produce a $z$-gradient. Repeat the calculation by using the $t(k)$ given in Eq. (3.93). Discuss the effect of the apodization length.

3.9 Choose a set of parameters and evaluate the integral in Eqs. (3.107) and (3.108) with $t(k) = 1$ to find the required current distribution to produce an $x$-gradient. Repeat the calculation by using the $t(k)$ given in Eq. (3.93). Discuss the effect of the apodization length.

3.10 Given a certain current distribution ($J_\phi$ and $J_z$) on a cylindrical surface, which could be the desired current distribution obtained using the target field method. If this continuous current distribution is to be modeled by a set of discrete wires, describe the procedure to calculate the shape and position of these wires. Hint: Consult Problem 2.9.

3.11 Calculate the current distribution on the shield of a single circular loop. Assume that the loop's radius is $a$ and the shield's radius is $1.5a$. If the shield is to be approximated by three loops carrying the same current, find the position of the loops.

3.12 Calculate the current distribution on the shield of a Helmholtz pair. Assume that the Helmholtz pair's radius is $a$ and the shield's radius is $1.5a$. If the shield is to be approximated by two loops carrying the same current, find the position of the loops.

3.13 Using Eq. (3.131), calculate the inductance of a single loop, a Helmholtz pair, and a Maxwell pair.

3.14 Rederive the result in Section 3.9.1 using $\mathbf{B} = \nabla \times \mathbf{A}$ and Eq. (3.172).

3.15 Using Eqs. (3.146) and (3.147), find the magnetic field produced by the four wires in Fig. 3.5(c).

3.16 Using Eqs. (3.145)–(3.147), find the magnetic field $B_z$ along the $y$-axis generated by a circular loop placed in the $xz$-plane and centered at the origin.

## References


M. Abramowitz and I. Stegun, Eds. (1964), *Handbook of Mathematical Functions*. Washington: National Bureau of Standards. Reprinted by Dover Publications, New York, 1968.

V. Bangert and P. Mansfield (1982), "Magnetic field gradient coils for NMR imaging," *J. Phys. E: Sci. Instrum.*, vol. 15, pp. 235–239.

R. Bowtell and P. Mansfield (1990), "Screened coil designs for NMR imaging in magnets with transverse field geometry," *Meas. Sci. Technol.*, vol. 1, pp. 431–439.

R. Bowtell and P. Mansfield (1991), "Gradient coil design using active magnetic screening," *Magn. Reson. Med.*, vol. 17, pp. 15–21.

J. W. Carlson (1987), "A convenient multipole expansion for magnetic fields of arcs and applications to the design of an asymmetric gradient coil," in *Book of Abstracts, 6th Annu. Mtg. Soc. Magn. Reson. Med.*, p. 397.

J. W. Carlson, K. A. Derby, K. C. Hawryszko, and M. Weideman (1992), "Design and evaluation of shielded gradient coils," *Magn. Reson. Med.*, vol. 26, pp. 191–206.

S. Crozier and D. M. Doddrell (1993), "Gradient-coil design by simulated annealing," *J. Magn. Reson.*, vol. 103, pp. 354–357.

T. A. Frenkiel, A. Jasinski, and P. G. Morris (1988), "Apparatus for generation of magnetic field gradient waveforms for NMR imaging," *J. Phys. E: Sci. Instrum.*, vol. 21, pp. 374–377.

M. J. E. Golay (1957), "Magnetic field control apparatus," U.S. Patent 3,515,979, Nov. 4, 1957. M. J. E. Golay (1970), "Coil arrangement for field homogenization in nuclear magnetic resonance apparatus," Ger. Offen Patent Number 1,946,059. Also, see M. J. E. Golay, U.S. Patent 3,569,823, 1971 and U.S. Patent 3,622,869, 1971.

E. D. Goldberg (1989), *Genetic Algorithms in Search, Optimization and Machine Learning.* Reading, MA: Addison-Wesley.

D. I. Hoult (1973), Ph.D. thesis, Oxford University, Oxford, U.K.

P. Mansfield and B. Chapman (1986a), "Active magnetic screening of coils in NMR imaging," *J. Magn. Reson.*, vol. 66, pp. 573–576.

P. Mansfield and B. Chapman (1986b), "Active magnetic screening of coils for static and time-dependent magnetic field generation in NMR imaging," *J. Phys. E: Sci. Instrum.*, vol. 19, pp. 540–545.

P. Mansfield and B. Chapman (1987), "Multishield active magnetic screening of coil structures in NMR," *J. Magn. Reson.*, vol. 72, pp. 211–223.

P. Mansfield and P. G. Morris (1982), *NMR Imaging in Biomedicine.* New York: Academic Press.

P. Mansfield, R. Turner, B. Chapman, and R. M. Bowley (1985), "Magnetic field screens," U.S. Patent 4,978,920.

M. A. Martens, L. S. Petropoulos, R. W. Brown, J. H. Andrews, M. A. Morich, and J. L. Patrick (1991), "Insertable biplanar gradient coil for MR imaging," *Rev. Sci. Instrum.*, vol. 62, pp. 2639–2645.

M. A. Morich, D. A. Lampman, W. R. Dannels, and F. T. Goldie (1988), "Exact temporal eddy current compensation in magnetic resonance imaging systems," *IEEE Trans. Med. Imaging*, vol. 7, pp. 247–254.

W. H. Press, S. A. Teukolsky, W. T. Vetterling, and B. P. Flannery (1992), *Numerical Recipes* (2nd edition). Cambridge: Cambridge Univ. Press.

P. B. Roemer and J. S. Hickey (1986), "Self-shielded gradient coils for nuclear magnetic resonance imaging," European Patent Application 87,101,198.

F. Romeo and D. I. Hoult (1984), "Magnetic field profiling: Analysis and correcting coil design," *Magn. Reson. Med.*, vol. 1, pp. 44–65.

H. Siebold (1990), "Gradient field coils for MR imaging with high spectral purity," *IEEE Trans. Magn.*, vol. 26, pp. 897–900.

B. H. Suits and D. E. Wilken (1989), "Improving magnetic field gradient coils for NMR imaging," *J. Phys. E: Sci. Instrum.*, vol. 22, pp. 565–573.

S. R. Thomas, L. J. Busse, and J. F. Schenck (1988), "Gradient coil technology," in *Magnetic Resonance Imaging*, Vol II. C. L. Partain *et al.* Eds. Philadelphia: W. B. Saunders Company.

R. Turner (1986), "A target field approach to optimal coil design," *J. Phys. D: Appl. Phys.*, vol. 19, pp. 147–151.

R. Turner (1988), "Minimum inductance coils," *J. Phys. E: Sci. Instrum.*, vol. 21, pp. 948–952.

R. Turner (1993), "Gradient coil design: A review of methods," *Magn. Reson. Imaging*, vol. 11, pp. 903–920.

R. Turner and R. M. Bowley (1986), "Passive screening of switched magnetic field gradients," *J. Phys. E: Sci. Instrum.*, vol. 19, pp. 876–879.

J. J. Van Vaals and A. H. Bergman (1990), "Optimization of eddy current compensation," *J. Magn. Reson.*, vol. 90, pp. 52–70.

E. Wong, A. Jesmanowicz, and J. S. Hyde (1991), "Coil optimization for MRI by conjugate gradient descent," *Magn. Reson. Med.*, vol. 21, pp. 39–48.

K. Yoda (1990), "Analytic design method of self-shielded planar coils," *J. Appl. Phys.*, vol. 67, pp. 4349–4353.

S. Zhang and J. Jin (1996), *Computation of Special Functions.* New York: Wiley.

I. Zupancic (1962), "Current shims for high-resolution nuclear magnetic resonance on the problem of correcting magnetic field inhomogeneities," *J. Sci. Instrum.*, vol. 39, pp. 621–624.

I. Zupancic and J. Pirs (1976), "Coils producing a magnetic field gradient for diffusion measurements with NMR," *Phys. E: Sci. Instrum.*, vol. 9, pp. 79–80.

# Chapter 4

# Analysis and Design of RF Coils

## 4.1 Introduction

Radiofrequency (RF) coils, also known as RF resonators and RF probes, are key components in a magnetic resonance imaging (MRI) system. They serve two purposes. The first is to generate RF pulses at the Larmor frequency to excite the nuclei in the object to be imaged. When a coil is used for this purpose, it is often called an RF transmit coil. The second is to pick up RF signals emitted by the nuclei at the same frequency. When a coil is used for this purpose, it is called an RF receive coil. The magnetic field of the RF pulse generated by an RF transmit coil is referred to in the MRI literature as the $B_1$ field, whose direction is perpendicular to the direction of the main magnetic field—the $B_0$ field. To obtain high quality MRI images, RF coils must satisfy two basic requirements. First, an RF coil, when used for transmission, must be able to produce a homogeneous $B_1$ field in the volume of interest at the Larmor frequency so that the nuclei can be excited uniformly. Second, an RF coil, when used for reception, must have a high signal-to-noise ratio (SNR) and, meanwhile, must be able to pick up RF signals with the same gain at any point in the volume of interest. In view of the well-known reciprocity of electromagnetic fields, if the receive coil is used as a transmit coil, it must be able to produce a homogeneous $B_1$ field in the volume of interest, as will be shown in the next section. In many applications, an RF coil is used both for transmission and reception. In this case, the coil must have good $B_1$ field homogeneity and a high SNR as well. In addition to the two basic requirements described above, there are other requirements related to the safety and comfort of RF coils. Although these requirements are also important for practical applications, they will not be discussed here.

Because the direction of the $B_1$ field is not the same as the $B_0$ and

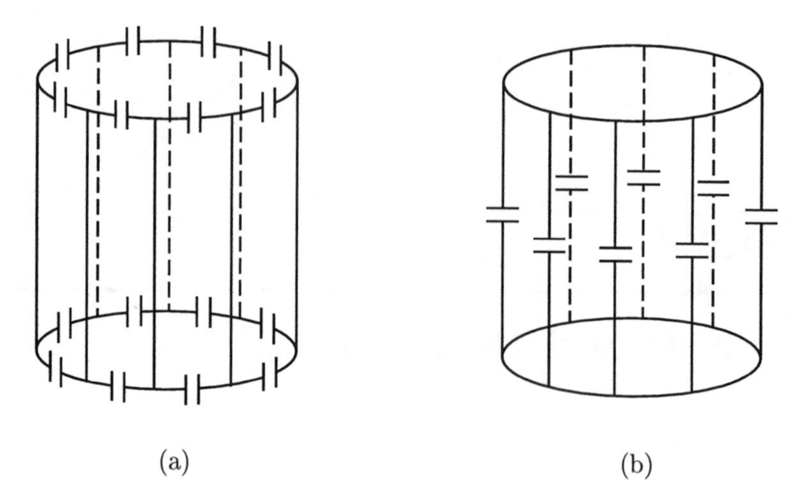


**Figure 4.1.** Illustration of birdcage coils. (a) Highpass birdcage coil. (b) Lowpass birdcage coil.

gradient fields, the design of RF coils is fundamentally different than the design of the magnet, shim coils, and gradient coils. Over the past decade, many different RF coils have been developed and, according to their shapes, they can be categorized into two groups. The first group is called volume coils, which include Helmholtz coils, saddle coils, and highpass and lowpass birdcage coils (Fig. 4.1). Of these coils, the birdcage coils are most popular because they can produce a very homogeneous $B_1$ field over a large volume within the coil (Hayes *et al.* 1985). These coils are often used both for transmission and reception. The second group is called surface coils, which include single-loop and multiple-loop coils of various shapes (Fig. 4.2). These coils are usually much smaller than the volume coils and, hence, have higher SNR because they receive noises only from nearby regions (Bendall 1988). However, they have a relatively poor $B_1$ field homogeneity and, thus, are mainly used as receive coils.

In this chapter, we introduce the concepts of resonance and reciprocity to illustrate the basic requirements of RF coils. We then describe a simple analysis of RF coils, which models an RF coil with an equivalent lumped-circuit. This is followed by a description of a method to incorporate the effects of RF shields into the analysis of RF coils. After that, we apply the method to analyze the field inhomogeneity of birdcage coils and develop a rigorous method for RF coil analysis, which can be especially useful for coils at high frequencies. The chapter concludes with a review of some special purpose RF coils.

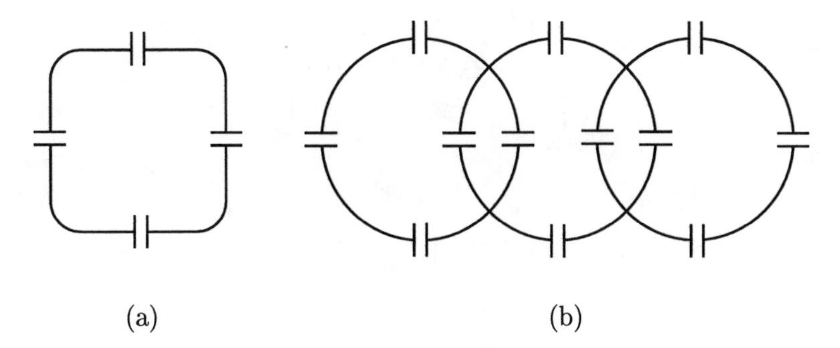


**Figure 4.2.** Illustration of surface coils. (a) A single-loop coil. (b) A surface coil array.

## 4.2 Concepts of Resonance and Reciprocity

To understand the concept of resonance and why RF coils must be resonators for MRI applications, we consider the $RLC$ circuit illustrated in Fig. 4.3. In accordance with Kirchhoff's law, we obtain

$$RI + \frac{i}{\omega C}I - i\omega L = V \tag{4.1}$$

where $\omega$ denotes the angular frequency and $i = \sqrt{-1}$. Hence, the current is given by

$$I = V\left(R + \frac{i}{\omega C} - i\omega L\right)^{-1}. \tag{4.2}$$

If $R = 0$, this reduces to

$$\begin{aligned} I &= V\left(\frac{i}{\omega C} - i\omega L\right)^{-1} \\ &= V\left[\frac{L}{i\omega}\left(\omega^2 - \frac{1}{LC}\right)\right]^{-1} \end{aligned} \tag{4.3}$$

from which it is obvious that $I \to \infty$ when

$$\omega = \omega_r = \frac{1}{\sqrt{LC}}. \tag{4.4}$$

This phenomenon is called resonance and $\omega_r$ is called the resonant frequency. Of course, in practice, the resistance $R$ cannot vanish completely and, therefore, the magnitude of the current cannot be infinity.

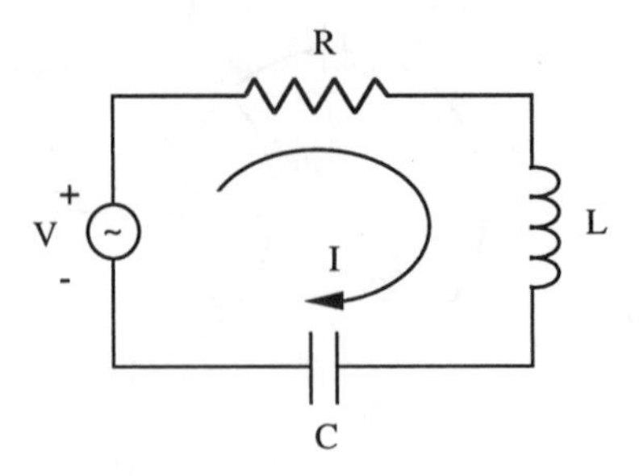


**Figure 4.3.** An *RLC*-circuit.

Nevertheless, the current would be maximum at the resonant frequency. Since the magnetic field produced by the current is directly proportional to the magnitude of the current, an RF coil can produce a desired magnetic field strength with a relatively low input voltage when it operates at the resonant frequency.

When the resistance is not zero, some energy will be dissipated in the circuit and the quality of the circuit is decreased. To provide a quantitative measure of the quality, we can define a quality factor as

$$Q = 2\pi \frac{\text{maximum energy stored}}{\text{total energy dissipated per period}}. \tag{4.5}$$

For the circuit in Fig. 4.3, the quality factor can be found easily as

$$Q = \frac{1}{R}\sqrt{\frac{L}{C}}. \tag{4.6}$$

For a complex circuit, it can be difficult to find the values for $R$, $L$, and $C$ of the equivalent circuit. In that case, the quality factor can be more conveniently obtained as

$$Q = \frac{\omega_r}{\Delta\omega} \tag{4.7}$$

where $\Delta\omega$ denotes the bandwidth, which can be measured easily. We note that the quality factor is an important parameter in the design of RF coils in MRI. It is often used in the calculation of the coil's and sample's resistance and thus the SNR of the received signal (Hoult and Richards 1976, Chen *et al.* 1986).

To understand the concept of reciprocity and the relationship between the transmitting and receiving properties of an RF coil, we consider two problems illustrated in Fig. 4.4. The first problem, illustrated in Fig. 4.4(a),

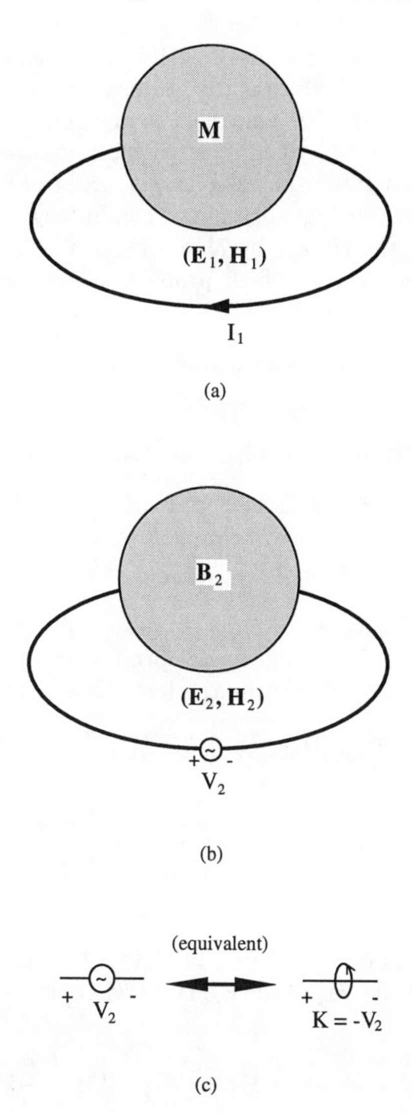


**Figure 4.4.** (a) A magnetization (**M**) in an object induces a current ($I_1$) in an RF coil. (b) A voltage source ($V_2$) produces a magnetic field ($\mathbf{B}_2$) inside an object through an RF coil. (c) The voltage can be modeled as a small loop of magnetic current ($K$).

concerns the current induced in an RF coil by the magnetization vector $\mathbf{M}$ in the object to be imaged which is the source of NMR signals. The second problem, shown in Fig. 4.4(b), concerns the magnetic field produced in the object by the same RF coil when it is fed by a voltage source $V_2$. It can be shown (Harrington 1961) that a voltage source can be represented by a small loop of magnetic current encircling a conducting wire whose magnetic current is related to the voltage by $K = -V_2$, as illustrated in Fig. 4.4(c).

Denote the fields in the first problem as $(\mathbf{E}_1, \mathbf{H}_1)$, which satisfy Maxwell's equations

$$\nabla \times \mathbf{E}_1 = i\omega\mu_0\mathbf{H}_1 + i\omega\mu_0\mathbf{M} \tag{4.8}$$

$$\nabla \times \mathbf{H}_1 = -i\omega\epsilon\mathbf{E}_1. \tag{4.9}$$

Denote the fields in the second problem as $(\mathbf{E}_2, \mathbf{H}_2)$, which satisfy Maxwell's equations

$$\nabla \times \mathbf{E}_2 = i\omega\mu_0\mathbf{H}_2 - \mathbf{J}_m \tag{4.10}$$

$$\nabla \times \mathbf{H}_2 = -i\omega\epsilon\mathbf{E}_2. \tag{4.11}$$

where $\mathbf{J}_m$ denotes the magnetic current density of the small loop carrying the magnetic current $K$. Taking the dot product of Eq. (4.8) with $\mathbf{H}_2$ and Eq. (4.10) with $\mathbf{H}_1$ and subtracting the latter from the former, we obtain

$$\mathbf{H}_2 \cdot \nabla \times \mathbf{E}_1 - \mathbf{H}_1 \cdot \nabla \times \mathbf{E}_2 = \mathbf{H}_1 \cdot \mathbf{J}_m + i\omega\mathbf{B}_2 \cdot \mathbf{M} \tag{4.12}$$

which becomes

$$\mathbf{H}_2 \cdot \nabla \times \left(\frac{i}{\omega\epsilon}\nabla \times \mathbf{H}_1\right) - \mathbf{H}_1 \cdot \nabla \times \left(\frac{i}{\omega\epsilon}\nabla \times \mathbf{H}_2\right) = \mathbf{H}_1 \cdot \mathbf{J}_m + i\omega\mathbf{B}_2 \cdot \mathbf{M} \tag{4.13}$$

upon the substitution of Eqs. (4.9) and (4.11). Integrating Eq. (4.13) over the entire volume of $(\mathbf{E}_1, \mathbf{H}_1)$ and $(\mathbf{E}_2, \mathbf{H}_2)$ and applying the second Green's vector theorem

$$\iiint_V \left[\mathbf{H}_2 \cdot \nabla \times \left(\frac{i}{\omega\epsilon}\nabla \times \mathbf{H}_1\right) - \mathbf{H}_1 \cdot \nabla \times \left(\frac{i}{\omega\epsilon}\nabla \times \mathbf{H}_2\right)\right] dv$$

$$= \oiint_S \frac{i}{\omega\epsilon}\left[\mathbf{H}_1 \times (\nabla \times \mathbf{H}_2) - \mathbf{H}_2 \times (\nabla \times \mathbf{H}_1)\right] \cdot \hat{n}\, ds \tag{4.14}$$

which can be easily derived from the divergence theorem in Eq. (2.2), we obtain

$$\oiint_S (\mathbf{H}_1 \times \mathbf{E}_2 - \mathbf{H}_2 \times \mathbf{E}_1) \cdot \hat{n}\, ds = \iiint_V (\mathbf{H}_1 \cdot \mathbf{J}_m + i\omega\mathbf{B}_2 \cdot \mathbf{M})\, dv \tag{4.15}$$

where $S$ denotes the surface enclosing the volume $V$. Since $V$ is an infinite volume, $S$ can be considered as a spherical surface whose radius approaches infinity. At any point of this surface, $(\mathbf{E}_1, \mathbf{H}_1)$ and $(\mathbf{E}_2, \mathbf{H}_2)$ can be considered as plane waves whose electric and magnetic fields are related by

$$\mathbf{E}_1 = Z_0 \mathbf{H}_1 \times \hat{n} \quad \text{and} \quad \mathbf{E}_2 = Z_0 \mathbf{H}_2 \times \hat{n} \tag{4.16}$$

where $Z_0 = \sqrt{\mu_0/\epsilon_0}$ denotes the free-space wave impedance. Substituting Eq. (4.16) into Eq. (4.15), we find that the surface integral at the left-hand side of Eq. (4.15) vanishes. Hence, Eq. (4.15) becomes

$$\iiint_V \mathbf{H}_1 \cdot \mathbf{J}_m \, dv = -i\omega \iiint_V \mathbf{B}_2 \cdot \mathbf{M} \, dv \tag{4.17}$$

whose left-hand side can be written as

$$\iiint_V \mathbf{H}_1 \cdot \mathbf{J}_m \, dv = K \oint_c \mathbf{H}_1 \cdot d\mathbf{l} = K I_1 = -V_2 I_1 \tag{4.18}$$

where $c$ denotes the small loop that models the voltage source. From Eqs. (4.17) and (4.18), we finally obtain the current induced in the RF coil by the magnetization as

$$I_1 = \frac{i\omega}{V_2} \iiint_V \mathbf{B}_2 \cdot \mathbf{M} \, dv. \tag{4.19}$$

From Eq. (4.19), we can draw two conclusions. First, since $I_1$ is proportional to $\mathbf{B}_2$ which is the magnetic field produced by the RF coil for a given $V_2$, an efficient transmit coil is also an efficient receive coil. Since a resonator is an efficient magnetic field generator, it is also a highly sensitive receiver. Second, if an RF coil, when used for transmission, can generate a homogeneous $\mathbf{B}_2$ field inside the object to be imaged, when used for reception, it can pick up signals produced by the magnetization with the same gain at any point in the object.

Finally, we note that Eq. (4.19) can also be written as

$$V_1 = \frac{i\omega}{I_2} \iiint_V \mathbf{B}_2 \cdot \mathbf{M} \, dv \tag{4.20}$$

where $V_1$ denotes the voltage induced in the coil by magnetization $\mathbf{M}$ and $I_2$ denotes the current in the coil that produces the magnetic field $\mathbf{B}_2$. Equation (4.20) is more familiar to the MRI community due to the work by Hoult and Richards (1976).

## 4.3 Equivalent Circuit Analysis

RF coils are usually made of conducting wires or conducting strips and capacitors. Because of their relatively complicated structures, it is difficult and time consuming to analyze them exactly based on Maxwell's equations. However, for RF coils whose size is a small fraction of a wavelength, we can employ the so-called equivalent circuit method to analyze them. The basic principle of this method is, first, to establish an equivalent lumped-circuit for the coil by modeling a conducting wire or strip as an inductor, then to analyze the equivalent circuit using the well-known Kirchhoff's voltage and current laws and, finally, to calculate the $B_1$ field using Biot-Savart's law. This method is highly efficient, reasonably accurate, and thus very practical for the design of RF coils. The method can be applied to any RF coils and to illustrate the procedure of analysis, we first consider a simple example and then proceed to the analysis of both highpass and lowpass birdcage and open coils.

### 4.3.1 A Simple Example

The first step of the equivalent circuit method is to establish an equivalent lumped-circuit for the coil to be analyzed. To illustrate this step, consider the simple example shown in Fig. 4.5(a). This is a surface coil made of either circular wires or thin strips with a capacitor. By modeling the conducting wires or strips as inductors, the coil can be represented by an equivalent circuit illustrated in Fig. 4.5(b). The values of the inductances can be calculated from their length and radius (or width for strips). The appropriate formulas for calculating the inductances are given in Eq. (2.82) for circular wires and in Eq. (2.85) for strips, which are repeated here for convenience:

$$L = 0.002l\left(\ln\frac{2l}{a} - 1\right) \quad (\mu\text{H}) \tag{4.21}$$

where $l$ and $a$ denote the length and radius (in cm) of a circular wire, and

$$L = 0.002l\left(\ln\frac{2l}{w} + \frac{1}{2}\right) \quad (\mu\text{H}) \tag{4.22}$$

where $l$ and $w$ denote, respectively, the length and width (in cm) of a strip.

The equivalent circuit can then be easily analyzed using Kirchhoff's voltage law. In accordance with this law, we have

$$\frac{i}{\omega C}I - 2i\omega L_1 I + 2i\omega M_1 I - 2i\omega L_2 I + 2i\omega M_2 I = 0 \tag{4.23}$$

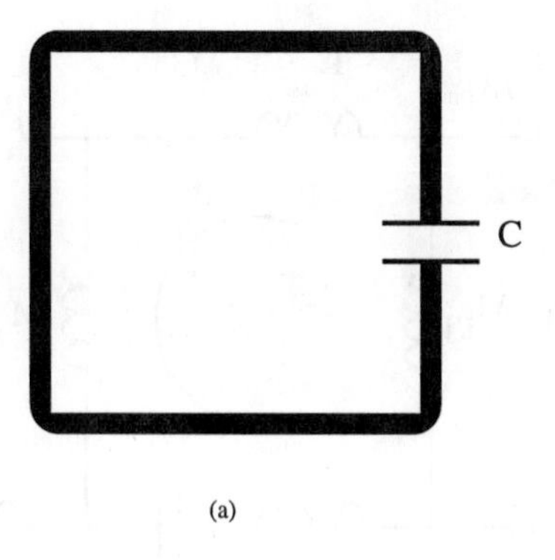


(a)

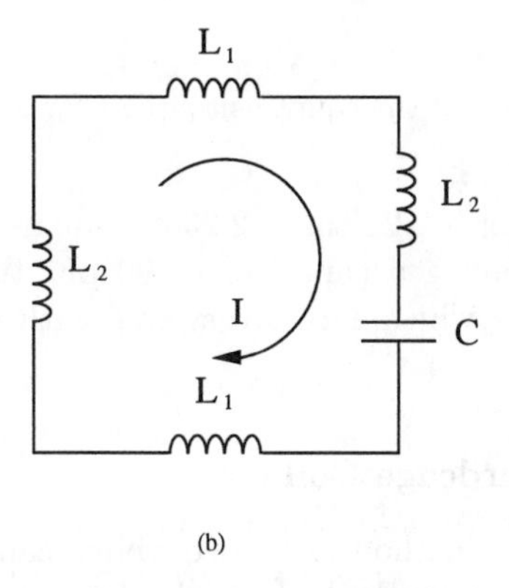


(b)

**Figure 4.5.** (a) A physical coil. (b) The equivalent circuit.

where $M_1$ denotes the mutual inductance between the two horizontal wires and $M_2$ denotes the mutual inductance between the two vertical wires. Their values can be calculated using Eq. (2.91), which is repeated here for convenience

$$M = 0.002l \left[ \ln\left( \frac{l}{d} + \sqrt{1 + \frac{l^2}{d^2}} \right) - \sqrt{1 + \frac{d^2}{l^2}} + \frac{d}{l} \right] \quad (\mu\text{H}) \tag{4.24}$$

where $d$ denotes the distance (in cm) between the two wires. Note that there is no mutual inductance between two wires perpendicular to each other. From Eq. (4.23), we find the resonant frequency as

$$\omega_r = \frac{1}{\sqrt{2(L_1 + L_2 - M_1 - M_2)C}}. \tag{4.25}$$

The current in the coil is constant since there is only a single loop.

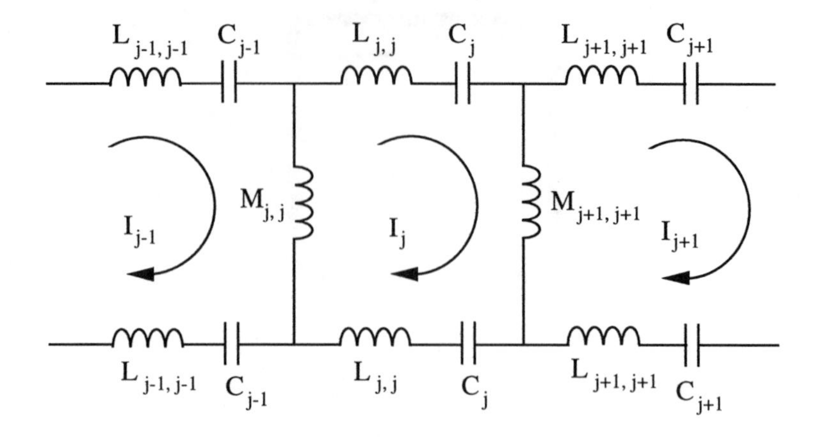


**Figure 4.6.** A segment of the equivalent circuit for a highpass birdcage coil.

As an example, for a 2.25 cm × 2.25 cm square loop made of a 0.143-cm wide strip and having a capacitor of 90 pF, the calculated resonant frequency is 67.1 MHz which agrees very well with the measured result of 67.4 MHz.

### 4.3.2 Highpass Birdcage Coil

The equivalent circuit method described above can be extended to more complicated coils. Consider the highpass birdcage coil shown in Fig. 4.1(a). This coil is made of several equi-spaced conductors (wires or strips) on a cylindrical surface, whose ends are connected by several capacitors. For the convenience of description, we use word "leg" or "rung" to represent the parallel conductors on the cylindrical surface and use word "end-ring" to denote the end loop consisting of capacitors. By modeling the conductors as inductors, the highpass birdcage coil can be modeled by a highpass ladder network, a segment of which is given in Fig. 4.6. Specifically, in this figure, $M_{j,j}$ denotes the self-inductance of the $j$th leg, $C_j$ denotes the capacitance of the capacitor connected between the $j$th and $(j+1)$th legs, and $L_{j,j}$ denotes the self-inductance of the conductors used to connect the capacitor. Although not shown in the figure, we denote the mutual inductance between the $j$th leg and the $k$th leg as $M_{j,k}$ or $M_{k,j}$, the mutual inductance between the conductor connecting the $j$th capacitor and the conductor connecting the $k$th capacitor in the same end-ring as $L_{j,k}$ or $L_{k,j}$, and the mutual inductance between the conductor connecting the $j$th capacitor and the conductor connecting the $k$th capacitor in the different end-rings as $\tilde{L}_{j,k}$ or $\tilde{L}_{k,j}$.

With the values for the inductance and capacitance, the circuit in Fig. 4.6 is completely defined. Before presenting a general analysis, it is instructive to examine a simplified case where we neglect the mutual inductance and assume $C_1 = C_2 = \cdots = C$, $L_1 = L_2 = \cdots = L$, and $M_{11} = M_{22} = \cdots = M$. Assume that the birdcage coil has $N$ parallel legs. In accordance with Kirchhoff's voltage law, for the loop consisting of the $j$th and $(j+1)$th legs and the $j$th capacitors, we have

$$-i\omega M(I_j - I_{j-1}) - i\omega M(I_j - I_{j+1}) - 2i\omega L I_j + \frac{2i}{\omega C} I_j = 0 \qquad (j = 1, 2, \ldots, N) \quad (4.26)$$

where $I_j$ denotes the current in this loop. This equation can be written as

$$M(I_{j+1} + I_{j-1}) + 2\left(\frac{1}{\omega^2 C} - L - M\right) I_j = 0 \quad (j = 1, 2, \ldots, N). \quad (4.27)$$

Because of cylindrical symmetry, the current $I_j$ must satisfy the periodic condition $I_{j+N} = I_j$. Therefore, the $N$ linearly independent solutions (or modes) of Eq. (4.27) have the form

$$(I_j)_m = \begin{cases} \cos \dfrac{2\pi m j}{N} & m = 0, 1, 2, \ldots, \dfrac{N}{2} \\ \sin \dfrac{2\pi m j}{N} & m = 1, 2, \ldots, \dfrac{N}{2} - 1 \end{cases} \quad (4.28)$$

where $(I_j)_m$ denotes the value of $I_j$ in the $m$th solution. The current in the $j$th leg is then given by

$$(I_j)_m - (I_{j-1})_m = \begin{cases} -2 \sin \dfrac{\pi m}{N} \sin \dfrac{2\pi m (j - \frac{1}{2})}{N} & m = 0, 1, 2, \ldots, \dfrac{N}{2} \\ 2 \sin \dfrac{\pi m}{N} \cos \dfrac{2\pi m (j - \frac{1}{2})}{N} & m = 1, 2, \ldots, \dfrac{N}{2} - 1. \end{cases} \quad (4.29)$$

Apparently, the solutions of $m = 1$ provide a current variation similar to $\sin\phi$ or $\cos\phi$. According to the analysis in Section 2.7, such a current distribution produces a very uniform transverse magnetic field inside the coil.

To determine the characteristic (resonant) frequency for each solution, we substitute Eq. (4.28) into Eq. (4.27) and obtain

$$M \cos \frac{2\pi m}{N} + \left(\frac{1}{\omega^2 C} - L - M\right) = 0 \quad (4.30)$$

from which we find

$$\omega_m = \left[C\left(L + 2M\sin^2\frac{\pi m}{N}\right)\right]^{-1/2} \quad \left(m = 0, 1, 2, \ldots, \frac{N}{2}\right). \quad (4.31)$$

Examining this result, we observe three points. First, the highest resonant frequency occurs for the mode $m = 0$ and, from Eqs. (4.28) and (4.29), we see that this mode has a constant current in the end-rings and no current in the legs. This is often referred to as the end-ring resonance, whose resonant frequency is $\omega_0 = 1/\sqrt{LC}$. Second, for the two modes having the same $m$, their resonant frequencies are the same. These two modes are called the degenerate modes and they produce the magnetic fields perpendicular to each other. Third, the modes of $m = 1$ have the second highest resonant frequency. As mentioned above, these two modes are capable of producing a uniform magnetic field and, thus, are useful for MRI applications.

Now, let us consider a more general and accurate analysis, which includes the effect of mutual inductance. In accordance with Kirchhoff's voltage law, for the loop consisting of the $j$th and $(j+1)$th legs and the $j$th capacitors, we have

$$\sum_{k=1}^{N} i\omega M_{j,k}(I_k - I_{k-1}) + \sum_{k=1}^{N} i\omega M_{j+1,k}(I_{k-1} - I_k) + \sum_{k=1}^{N} 2i\omega(L_{j,k} - \tilde{L}_{j,k})I_k - \frac{2i}{\omega C_j}I_j = 0 \quad (j = 1, 2, \ldots, N) \quad (4.32)$$

which can be written as

$$\sum_{k=1}^{N}(M_{j,k} - M_{j+1,k})(I_k - I_{k-1}) + 2\sum_{k=1}^{N}(L_{j,k} - \tilde{L}_{j,k})I_k = \frac{2\lambda}{C_j}I_j \quad (j = 1, 2, \ldots, N) \quad (4.33)$$

where $\lambda = 1/\omega^2$. To write Eq. (4.33) in matrix form, we first rewrite it as

$$\sum_{k=1}^{N}(M_{j,k} - M_{j+1,k})I_k - \sum_{k=1}^{N}(M_{j,k} - M_{j+1,k})I_{k-1} + 2\sum_{k=1}^{N}(L_{j,k} - \tilde{L}_{j,k})I_k = \frac{2\lambda}{C_j}I_j \quad (j = 1, 2, \ldots, N) \quad (4.34)$$

and then manipulate the indices to find

$$\sum_{k=1}^{N}(M_{j,k} - M_{j+1,k})I_k - \sum_{k=0}^{N-1}(M_{j,k+1} - M_{j+1,k+1})I_k$$

$$+2\sum_{k=1}^{N}(L_{j,k}-\tilde{L}_{j,k})I_k = \frac{2\lambda}{C_j}I_j \quad (j=1,2,\ldots,N). \tag{4.35}$$

Equation (4.35) can be written in matrix form as

$$[K]\{I\} = \lambda[H]\{I\} \tag{4.36}$$

where $\{I\}$ denotes a column vector given by $\{I\} = [I_1,\ I_2,\ \ldots,\ I_N]^T$, and $[K]$ and $[H]$ are both $N \times N$ square matrices, whose elements are given by

$$K_{j,k} = M_{j,k} - M_{j+1,k} - M_{j,k+1} + M_{j+1,k+1} + 2(L_{j,k} - \tilde{L}_{j,k}) \tag{4.37}$$

$$H_{j,k} = 2\delta_{j,k}/C_j \tag{4.38}$$

where $\delta_{j,k}$ denotes the Kronecker delta defined by $\delta_{j,k} = 1$ for $j = k$ and $\delta_{j,k} = 0$ for $j \neq k$. Obviously, $[K]$ is a symmetric matrix and $[H]$ is a diagonal matrix.

To have a nontrivial solution of Eq. (4.36), the determinant of the matrix $[K - \lambda H]$ must vanish, that is,

$$\det[K - \lambda H] = 0. \tag{4.39}$$

Since this determinant is a polynomial of degree $N$, Eq. (4.39) has $N$ solutions $(\lambda_1,\ \lambda_2,\ \ldots,\ \lambda_N)$, which correspond to $N$ resonant frequencies. These $N$ solutions are called the eigenvalues or characteristic values of Eq. (4.36). For each $\lambda_m$, we can find a nontrivial solution for $\{I\}$ which can be denoted as $\{I\}_m$. Therefore, for $N$ solutions of $\lambda$, we have $N$ solutions for $\{I\}$: $\{I\}_1$, $\{I\}_2$, $\ldots$, $\{I\}_N$ and these are called the eigenvectors or characteristic modes. In mathematics, Eq. (4.36) is referred to as the generalized eigenvalue problem, and all the eigenvalues and eigenvectors can be calculated efficiently using some well-developed computer programs. Once $\{I\}_m$ is obtained, the magnetic field corresponding to each mode can be calculated using Biot-Savart's law.

The method described above is easy to implement. Table 4.1 gives typical results of the resonant frequencies for a 16-leg highpass birdcage coil calculated using the approximate formula given by Eq. (4.31) and those calculated using Eq. (4.39). It is evident that the neglect of mutual inductance can cause a significant error in the calculation of resonant frequencies. The $B_1$ field for each odd mode is given in Fig. 4.7 in the form of contour and density plots.

### 4.3.3 Lowpass Birdcage Coil

For the lowpass birdcage coil shown in Fig. 4.1(b), the equivalent circuit is given in Fig. 4.8. Neglecting the mutual inductance and assuming

**Table 4.1.** Typical Result of the Resonant Frequencies for a 16-Leg Highpass Birdcage Coil.

| Mode | Resonant Freq. (MHz) From Eq. (4.31) | Resonant Freq. (MHz) From Eq. (4.39) |
|---|---|---|
| $m = 0$ | 143.216 | 143.216 |
| 1 | 75.648 | 63.958 |
| 2 | 75.648 | 63.958 |
| 3 | 43.293 | 43.107 |
| 4 | 43.293 | 43.107 |
| 5 | 30.564 | 34.295 |
| 6 | 30.564 | 34.295 |
| 7 | 24.226 | 29.450 |
| 8 | 24.226 | 29.450 |
| 9 | 20.685 | 26.530 |
| 10 | 20.685 | 26.530 |
| 11 | 18.653 | 24.765 |
| 12 | 18.653 | 24.765 |
| 13 | 17.587 | 23.890 |
| 14 | 17.587 | 23.890 |
| 15 | 17.254 | 23.506 |

$C_1 = C_2 = \cdots = C$, $L_1 = L_2 = \cdots = L$, and $M_{11} = M_{22} = \cdots = M$, we obtain

$$\left(\frac{1}{\omega^2 C} - M\right)(I_{j+1} + I_{j-1}) - 2\left(\frac{1}{\omega^2 C} - L - M\right) I_j = 0 \qquad (j = 1, 2, \ldots, N). \tag{4.40}$$

Its solutions are also given in Eq. (4.28) and the corresponding resonant frequencies are found as

$$\omega_m = \left[C\left(M + L\Big/2\sin^2\frac{\pi m}{N}\right)\right]^{-1/2} \quad \left(m = 0, 1, 2, \ldots, \frac{N}{2}\right). \tag{4.41}$$

Clearly, the end-ring resonant mode ($m = 0$) has a resonant frequency of zero and the modes of $m = 1$ have the second lowest resonant frequencies. This is in contrast to the highpass birdcage coil for which the modes of $m = 1$ have the second highest resonant frequencies.

A more general and accurate analysis, which includes the mutual inductance, yields the same matrix equation as Eq. (4.36) except that $[H]$

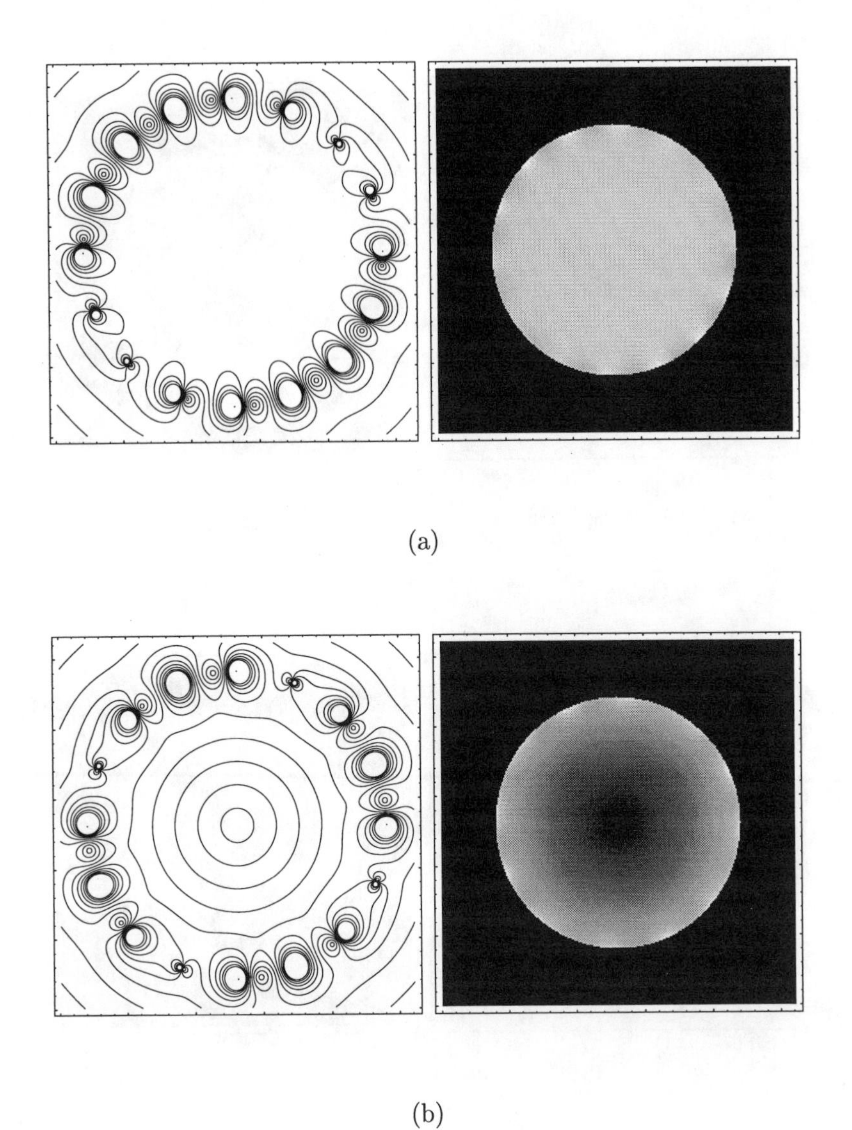

(a)

(b)

**Figure 4.7.** Contour and density plots of the $B_1$ field of a 16-leg highpass birdcage coil. (a) Mode 1. (b) Mode 3.

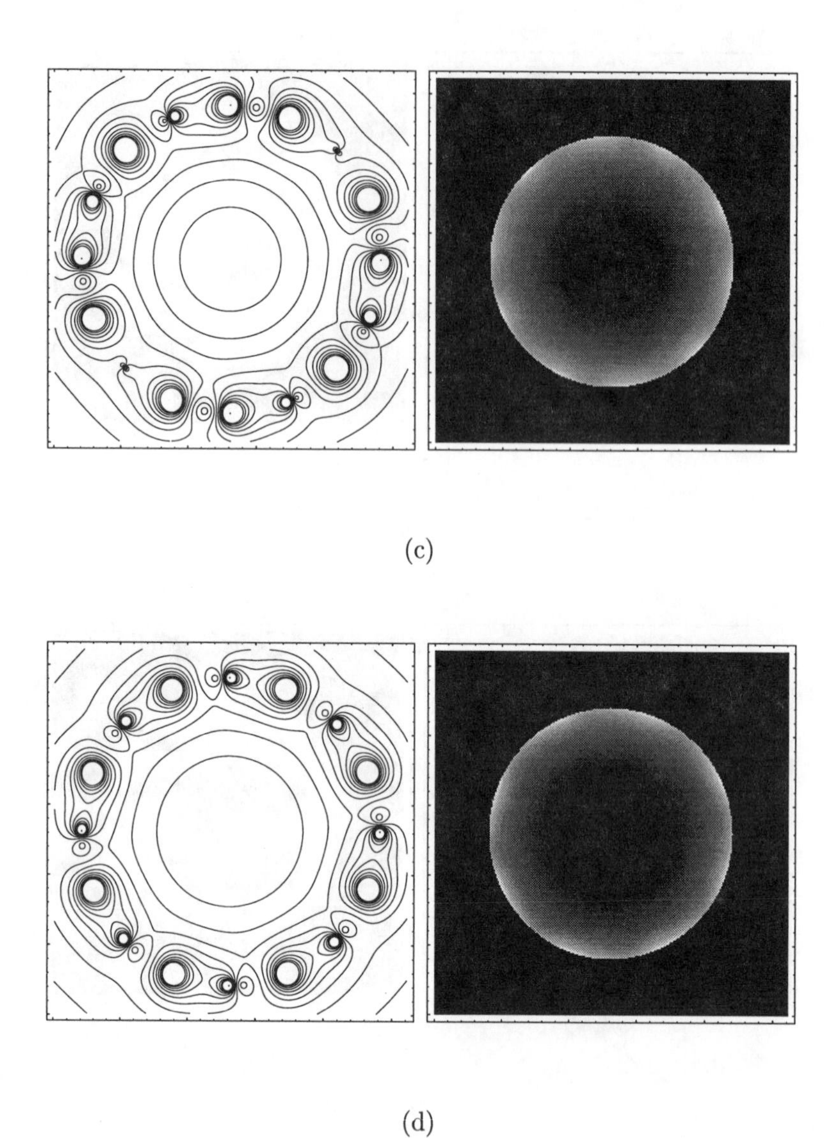

(c)

(d)

**Figure 4.7. (continued)** Contour and density plots of the $B_1$ field of a 16-leg highpass birdcage coil. (c) Mode 5. (d) Mode 7.

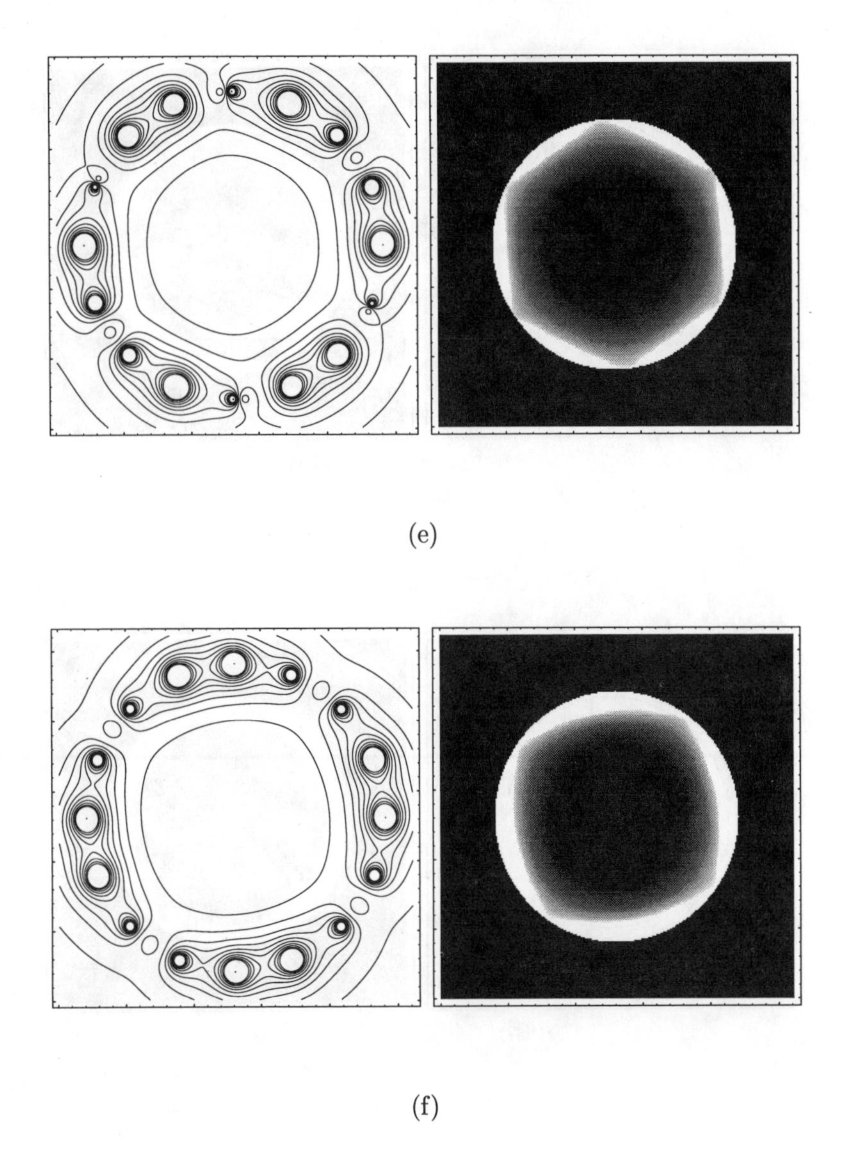

**Figure 4.7. (continued)** Contour and density plots of the $B_1$ field of a 16-leg highpass birdcage coil. (e) Mode 9. (f) Mode 11.

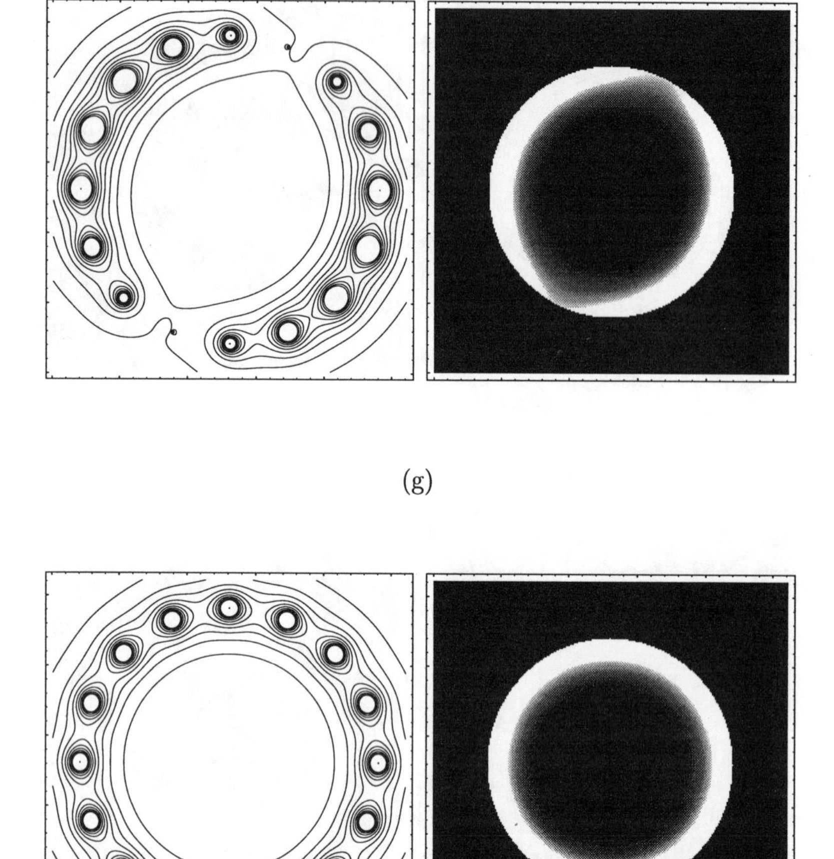

(g)

(h)

**Figure 4.7. (continued)** Contour and density plots of the $B_1$ field of a 16-leg highpass birdcage coil. (g) Mode 13. (h) Mode 15.

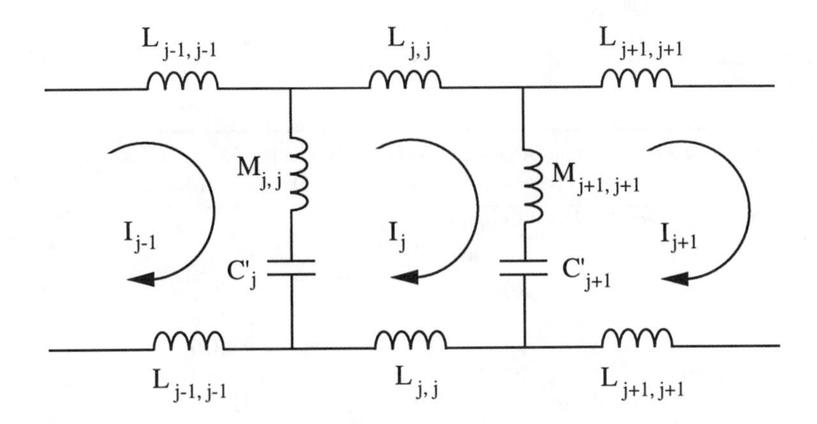


**Figure 4.8.** A segment of the equivalent circuit for a lowpass birdcage coil.

is now a tridiagonal matrix given by

$$\begin{aligned} H_{j,j-1} &= -1/C'_j, \qquad H_{j,j} = 1/C'_j + 1/C'_{j+1} \\ H_{j,j+1} &= -1/C'_{j+1}, \quad H_{j,k} = 0 \quad \text{for other } k. \end{aligned} \tag{4.42}$$

Table 4.2 gives typical results of the resonant frequencies for a 16-leg lowpass birdcage coil calculated using the approximate formula given by Eq. (4.41) and those calculated using Eq. (4.39) with Eq. (4.42). It is evident that the neglect of mutual inductance can cause a significant error in the calculation of resonant frequencies. The $B_1$ field for each mode is identical to those given in Fig. 4.7.

### 4.3.4 Hybrid Birdcage Coil

For a hybrid birdcage coil shown in Fig. 4.9, the equivalent circuit is given in Fig. 4.10. The simplified analysis yields solutions given in Eq. (4.28) and resonant frequencies given by

$$\omega_m = \left[\left(2M\sin^2\frac{\pi m}{N} + L\right)\Big/\left(\frac{2}{C'}\sin^2\frac{\pi m}{N} + \frac{1}{C}\right)\right]^{-1/2} \qquad \left(m = 0, 1, 2, \ldots, \frac{N}{2}\right). \tag{4.43}$$

Apparently, the resonant frequency for the end-ring resonant mode is $\omega_0 = 1/\sqrt{LC}$. Furthermore, the resonant frequencies for the modes of $m = 1$ are not necessarily the second lowest or the second highest. Finally,

**Table 4.2.** Typical Result of the Resonant Frequencies for a 16-Leg Lowpass Birdcage Coil.

| Mode | Resonant Freq. (MHz) From Eq. (4.41) | Resonant Freq. (MHz) From Eq. (4.39) |
|---|---|---|
| $m = 0$ | 0.000 | 0.000 |
| 1 | 73.090 | 63.961 |
| 2 | 73.090 | 63.961 |
| 3 | 89.370 | 89.016 |
| 4 | 89.370 | 89.016 |
| 5 | 93.761 | 104.556 |
| 6 | 93.761 | 104.556 |
| 7 | 95.428 | 115.171 |
| 8 | 95.428 | 115.171 |
| 9 | 96.204 | 122.511 |
| 10 | 96.204 | 122.511 |
| 11 | 96.597 | 127.366 |
| 12 | 96.597 | 127.366 |
| 13 | 96.787 | 130.147 |
| 14 | 96.787 | 130.147 |
| 15 | 96.844 | 131.053 |

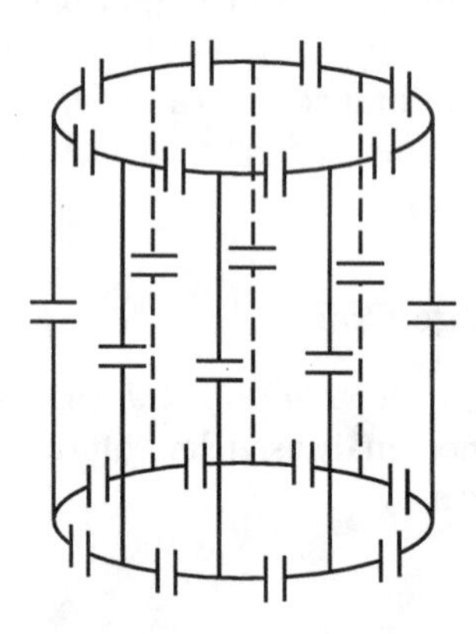

**Figure 4.9.** Illustration of a hybrid birdcage coil.

we note that Eq. (4.43) reduces to Eq. (4.31) when $C' \to \infty$ and to Eq. (4.41) when $C \to \infty$, as expected.

A more general and accurate analysis, which includes the mutual inductance, yields the same matrix equation as Eq. (4.36) except that $[H]$

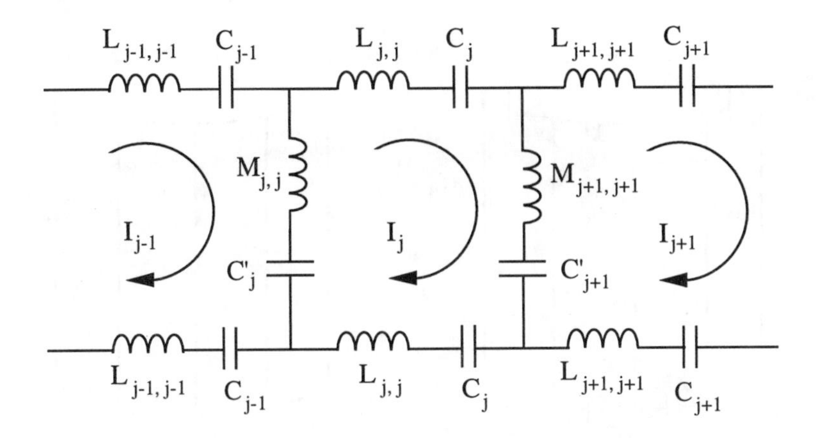


**Figure 4.10.** A segment of the equivalent circuit for a hybrid birdcage coil.

is now a tridiagonal matrix given by

$$\begin{aligned} H_{j,j-1} &= -1/C'_j, \qquad H_{j,j} = 2/C_j + 1/C'_j + 1/C'_{j+1} \\ H_{j,j+1} &= -1/C'_{j+1}, \quad H_{j,k} = 0 \quad \text{for other } k. \end{aligned} \tag{4.44}$$

### 4.3.5 Open Coils

The analysis described above can also be applied to open coils formed by a segment of ladder network, such as those shown in Fig. 4.11 (Ballon *et al.* 1990, Jin *et al.* 1993). If the number of legs parallel to the axis of the coil is $N$, there are $N-1$ independent loops. Applying Kirchhoff's voltage law to each loop and recognizing that $I_0 = I_N = 0$, we can obtain the same matrix equation as derived for the birdcage coils, except that $\{I\} = [I_1,\ I_2,\ \ldots,\ I_{N-1}]^T$, and both $[K]$ and $[H]$ are $(N-1)\times(N-1)$ square matrices.

It is also instructive to carry out the simplified analysis by neglecting the mutual inductance. Because of the conditions that $I_0 = I_N = 0$, the solution for the current in each loop has the form

$$(I_j)_m = \sin\frac{\pi m j}{N} \quad (m = 1, 2, \ldots, N-1) \tag{4.45}$$

and the current in each leg is then given by

$$(I_j)_m - (I_{j-1})_m = 2\sin\frac{\pi m}{2N}\cos\frac{\pi m(j-\frac{1}{2})}{N} \quad (m = 1, 2, \ldots, N-1). \tag{4.46}$$

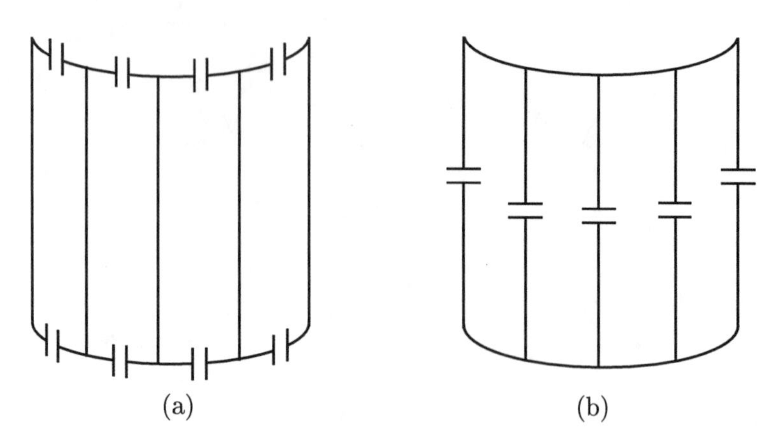


**Figure 4.11.** Illustration of open coils. (a) Highpass open coil. (b) Lowpass open coil.

The resonant frequencies for the highpass open coil are given by

$$\omega_m = \left[C\left(L + 2M\sin^2\frac{\pi m}{2N}\right)\right]^{-1/2} \quad (m = 1, 2, \ldots, N-1) \tag{4.47}$$

and those for the lowpass open coil are

$$\omega_m = \left[C\left(M + L\big/2\sin^2\frac{\pi m}{2N}\right)\right]^{-1/2} \quad (m = 1, 2, ..., N-1). \tag{4.48}$$

Table 4.3 gives the resonant frequencies of a 9-leg highpass open coil whose cross section and physical size are illustrated in Fig. 4.12. (At this moment we ignore the RF shield, whose effect is discussed in the next section.) The coil is 33.9 cm long and the legs used for its construction are 1.27 cm wide copper strips. The capacitors have a value of 60 pF for one case and 72 pF for another case. The calculated results are compared with the measured data. As can be seen, the agreement is within 5%, which can easily be compensated for by using a tuning capacitor. The small discrepancies are believed to be caused by the tolerances of the capacitors used. It is worthwhile to point out that the inductance of the strips used to connect the capacitors is very important for an accurate analysis of the resonant frequencies, and, therefore, it cannot be neglected. Without including this inductance, the calculated resonant frequency for the first mode is 133.4 MHz for the coil with 60 pF capacitors and 121.8 MHz for the coil with 72 pF capacitors, resulting in a significant error.

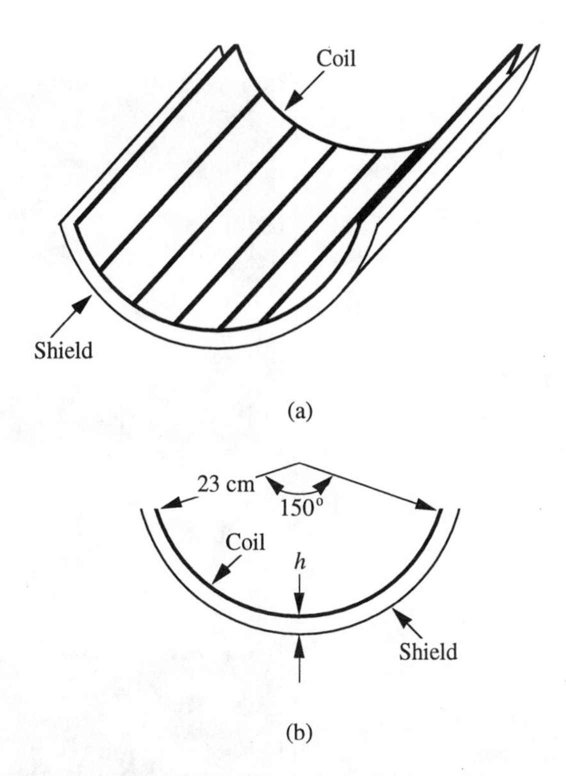


**Figure 4.12.** Illustration of an open coil having nine conducting strips parallel to its axis. (a) Three-dimensional sketch (the capacitors are not shown for the sake of clarity). (b) Cross-sectional view.

The $B_1$ field plots are given in Fig. 4.13. The density plot is given in a circular region, which has a diameter of 15.2 cm and is placed 5 cm above the bottom of the RF coil. As can be seen, the field homogeneity degrades quickly as the order of the mode increases.

In addition to predicting the resonant frequencies and the field distribution, the equivalent circuit method can also be used to find where to feed the coil so that one can achieve a good match and where to place a tuning capacitor so that one can tune the coil effectively. An examination of the current distribution of the fundamental mode of the open coil reveals that the current along the end-ring varies from zero at one end to maximum at the center, then to zero again at the other end. This results in a current distribution along the parallel legs which is maximum at the two

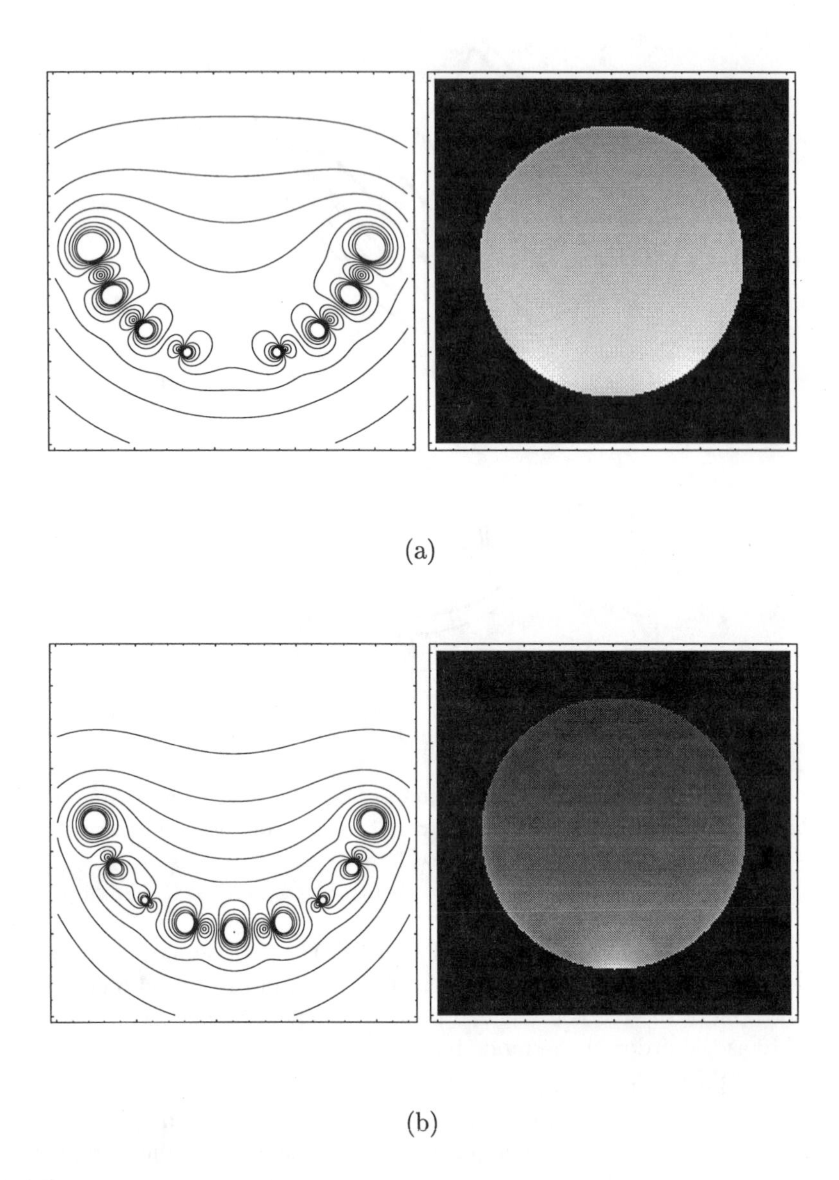

**Figure 4.13.** Contour and density plots of the $B_1$ field of a 9-leg highpass open coil. (a) Mode 1. (b) Mode 2.

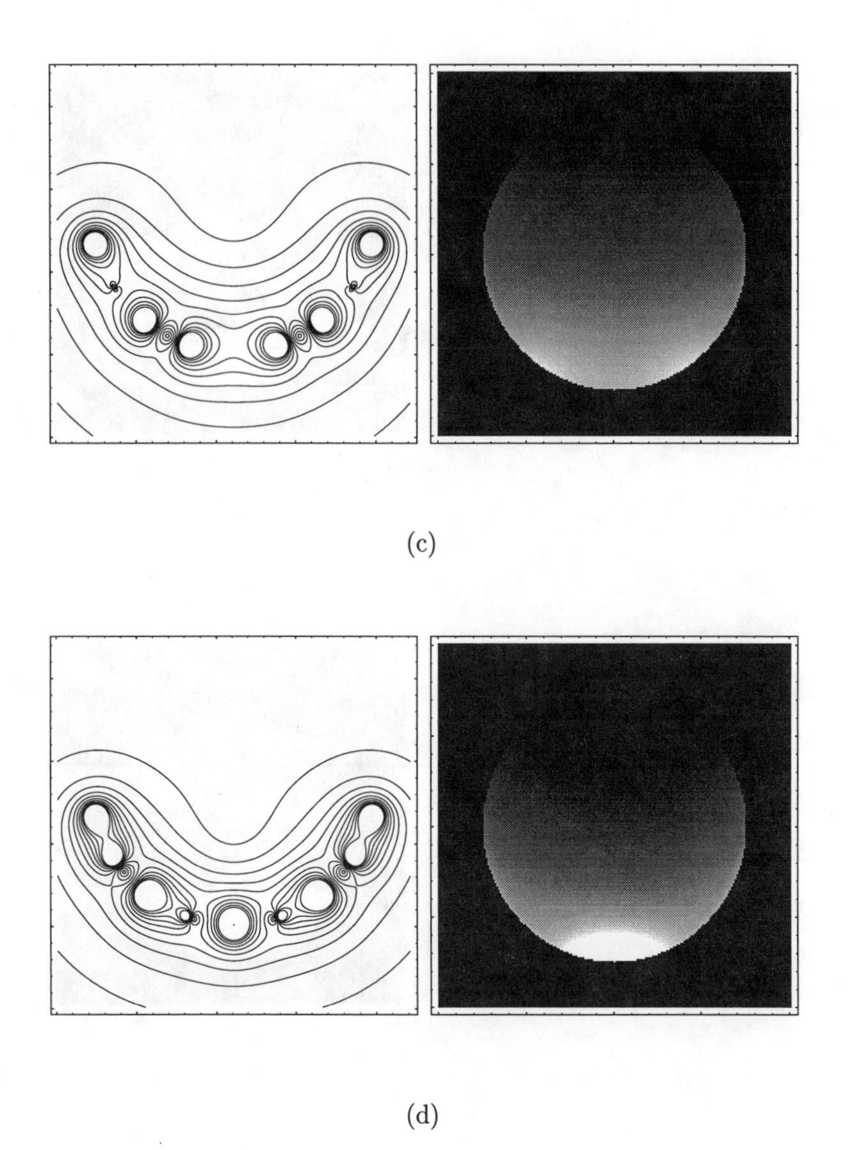

(c)

(d)

**Figure 4.13. (continued)** Contour and density plots of the $B_1$ field of a 9-leg highpass open coil. (c) Mode 3. (d) Mode 4.

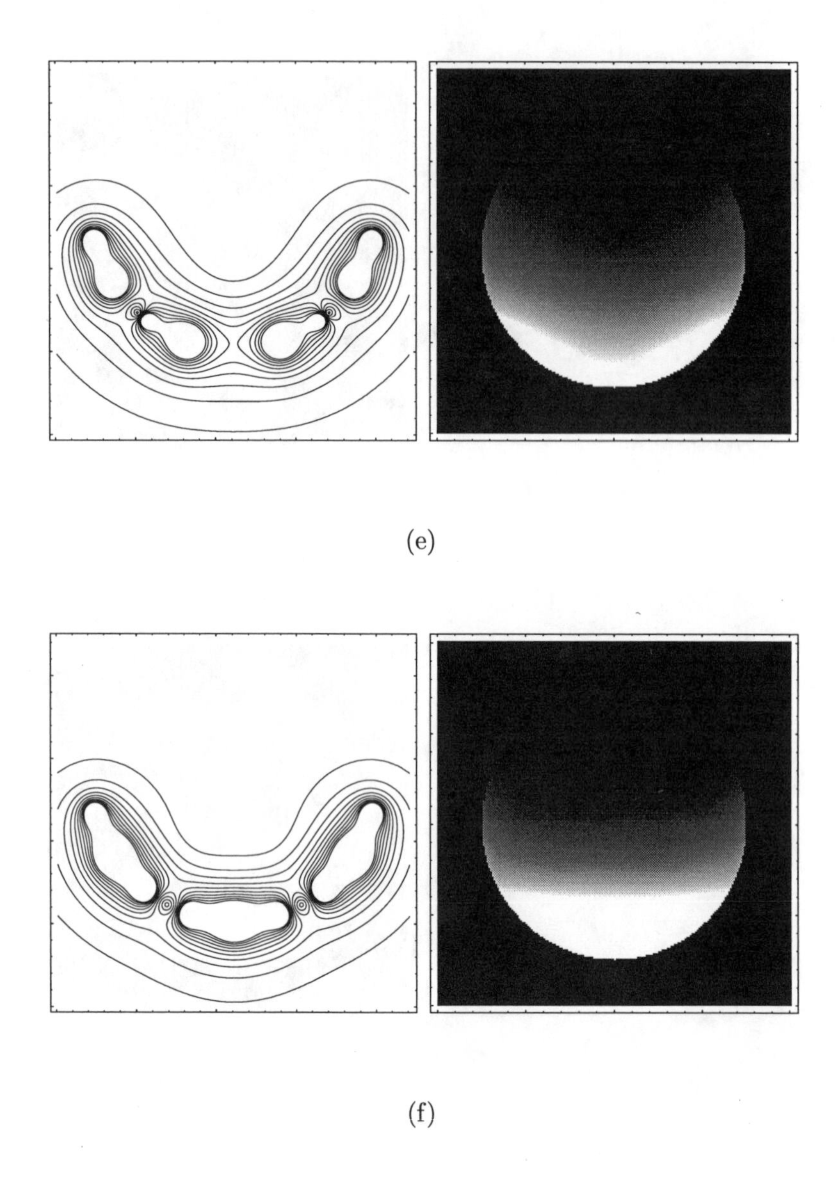

(e)

(f)

**Figure 4.13. (continued)** Contour and density plots of the $B_1$ field of a 9-leg highpass open coil. (e) Mode 5. (f) Mode 6.

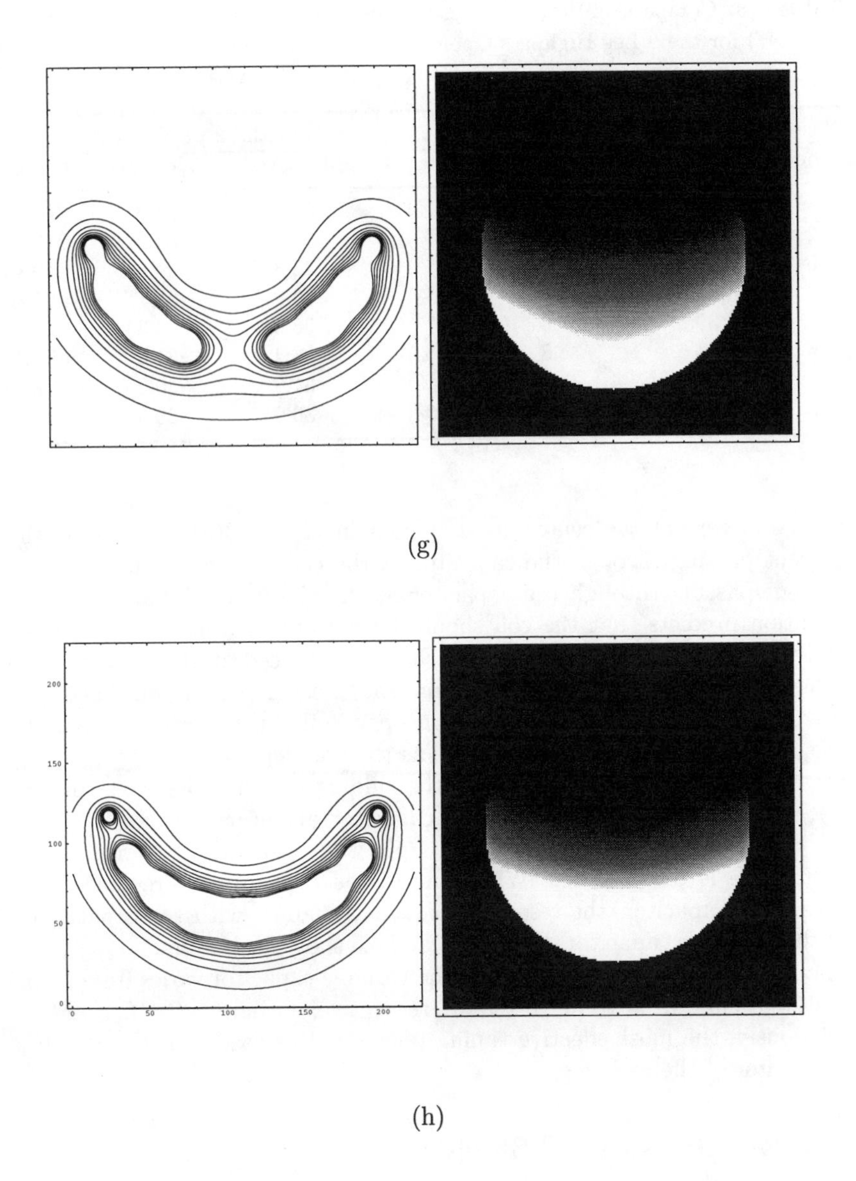

**Figure 4.13. (continued)** Contour and density plots of the $B_1$ field of a 9-leg highpass open coil. (g) Mode 7. (h) Mode 8.

**Table 4.3.** Comparison Between Measured and Calculated Resonant Frequencies (in MHz) for the 9-Leg Highpass Open Coil (Jin *et al.* 1993).

| Mode | With 60 pF Capacitors | | | With 72 pF Capacitors | | |
|---|---|---|---|---|---|---|
| | Measured | Calculated | (error) | Measured | Calculated | (error) |
| $m = 1$ | 72.1 | 75.4 | (4.6%) | 66.8 | 68.9 | (3.1%) |
| 2 | 58.0 | 58.2 | (0.3%) | 53.3 | 53.2 | (0.2%) |
| 3 | 49.5 | 48.1 | (2.8%) | 45.3 | 44.0 | (2.9%) |
| 4 | 43.5 | 41.8 | (3.9%) | 39.8 | 38.1 | (4.3%) |
| 5 | 39.0 | 37.6 | (3.6%) | 36.0 | 34.3 | (4.7%) |
| 6 | 36.6 | 34.8 | (4.9%) | 33.4 | 31.8 | (4.7%) |
| 7 | 34.6 | 33.1 | (4.3%) | 31.9 | 30.2 | (5.3%) |
| 8 | 33.5 | 32.1 | (4.2%) | 30.9 | 29.3 | (5.2%) |

sides and zero at the center, as is evident in Fig. 4.13(a). Therefore, the current passing through the capacitor at the center is maximum and the current passing through the capacitor at the side is minimum. Physical intuition predicts that the coil should be fed at the center of one of the end-rings and the tuning capacitor should be placed at the center of the other end-ring. Both the simulation and measurements confirmed this prediction. For example, consider an open coil consisting of ten parallel legs, whose cross section is the same as the one depicted in Fig. 4.12. For reference, denote the capacitor at the side as $C_1$, the one next to it as $C_2$, and so on. Consequently, the capacitor at the center is $C_5$. With all capacitors having a value of 100 pF, the resonant frequency of the first mode is 63.85 MHz. When one of the capacitors is replaced with a variable capacitor, the resonant frequency changes with the capacitance of that variable capacitor. Tables 4.4 and 4.5 show the minimum ($f_{\min}$) and maximum ($f_{\max}$) frequencies when the variable capacitor varies from 40 pF to 160 pF, and from 70 pF to 190 pF, respectively, where $\Delta f = f_{\max} - f_{\min}$. Obviously, the most effective tuning point for this case is at $C_5$, which is the center of the end-ring.

## 4.4 Analysis of RF Shields

As mentioned earlier, an MRI scanner uses a set of three gradient coils to obtain spatially selected information and a set of shim coils to achieve a high degree of homogeneity of the main magnetic field. These coils generally consist of multiple turns of wires whose total length may be on the order of

**Table 4.4.** Variation of Resonant Frequency When the Tuning Capacitor Varies from 40 pF to 160 pF.

| Tuning Capacitor | $f_{\min}$ (MHz) | $f_{\max}$ (MHz) | $\Delta f$ (MHz) |
|---|---|---|---|
| $C_1$ | 63.64 | 67.06 | 3.42 |
| $C_2$ | 63.18 | 72.55 | 9.37 |
| $C_3$ | 62.59 | 74.98 | 12.39 |
| $C_4$ | 62.02 | 75.98 | 13.96 |
| $C_5$ | 61.76 | 76.26 | 14.50 |

**Table 4.5.** Variation of Resonant Frequency When the Tuning Capacitor Varies from 70 pF to 190 pF.

| Tuning Capacitor | $f_{\min}$ (MHz) | $f_{\max}$ (MHz) | $\Delta f$ (MHz) |
|---|---|---|---|
| $C_1$ | 63.60 | 64.22 | 0.62 |
| $C_2$ | 63.05 | 65.19 | 2.14 |
| $C_3$ | 62.34 | 66.11 | 3.77 |
| $C_4$ | 61.63 | 66.68 | 5.05 |
| $C_5$ | 61.30 | 66.86 | 5.56 |

many meters. When RF fields, produced by an RF coil, impinge on these coils, numerous interactions occur which can degrade the performance of the RF coil. For example, the gradient and shim coils can cause losses to the RF coil, resulting in a low SNR in MR images. They can also give rise to spurious resonance which may displace and dampen the desired resonance of the coil. Therefore, an RF coil is often partially enclosed in an RF shield, as illustrated in Fig. 4.14, to prevent the RF fields from penetrating into the gradient and shim coils, reducing or eliminating the interactions between the RF coil and the gradient and shim coils. However, the presence of an RF shield has a dramatic effect on the resonant frequencies and field distribution of the RF coil. Therefore, an accurate analysis of RF coils must include the effects of the RF shield.

### 4.4.1 Analysis Using Image Method

As described in the preceding section, an RF coil can be analyzed using the method of equivalent circuits, which amounts to replacing the distributed structure with lumped elements. In this section, we use the method of

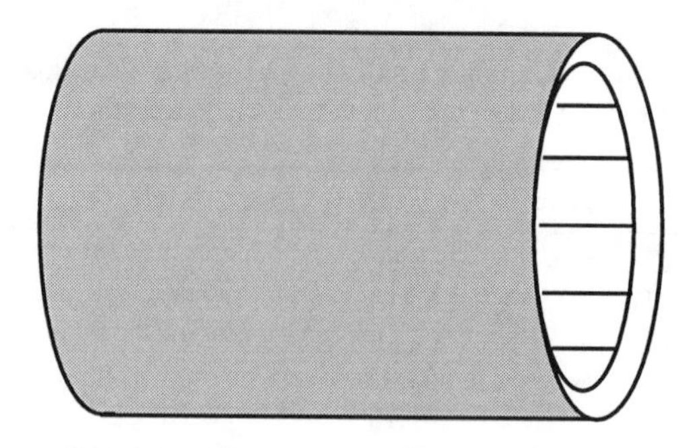

**Figure 4.14.** A birdcage coil enclosed by an RF shield.

images to effectively take into account the shield's effects in the analysis (Lu and Joseph 1991, Jin *et al.* 1995).

In accordance with the method of images, the field produced by the currents induced on a shield is identical to the field produced by the image of the original current. Since, in this case, the conductors are parallel to the shield, the image currents are in the opposite direction of the currents running on the conductors in order to satisfy the boundary condition on the shield, as sketched in Figs. 4.15 and 4.16. This results in a reduction in the values of the self- and mutual inductance, thus increasing the resonant frequencies. To be more specific, let $L'_{j,k}$ be the mutual inductance between the conductor used to connect the $j$th capacitor and the image of the conductor used to connect the $k$th capacitor in the same end-ring, $\tilde{L}'_{j,k}$ be the mutual inductance between the conductor used to connect the $j$th capacitor and the image of the conductor used to connect the $k$th capacitor in the different end-ring, and $M'_{j,k}$ be the mutual inductance between the $j$th leg and the image of the $k$th leg. To take the shield's effects into the analysis, $L_{j,k}$, $\tilde{L}_{j,k}$, and $M_{j,k}$ in the preceding section should be replaced by $L_{j,k} - L'_{j,k}$, $\tilde{L}_{j,k} - \tilde{L}'_{j,k}$, and $M_{j,k} - M'_{j,k}$, respectively. As a result, Eq. (4.37) becomes

$$K_{j,k} = M_{j,k} - M'_{j,k} - M_{j+1,k} + M'_{j+1,k} - M_{j,k+1} + M'_{j,k+1} + M_{j+1,k+1} - M'_{j+1,k+1} + 2(L_{j,k} - L'_{j,k} - \tilde{L}_{j,k} + \tilde{L}'_{j,k}). \quad (4.49)$$

With the formulation given above, we have to find the image for each conductor. Since the shield is of finite size, it is difficult, if not impossible, to determine the exact location of the image. However, if we introduce the approximation which assumes the shield to be of infinite size, the location of the image can be determined easily. For example, if the shield is locally flat, the location of the image would be on the other side of the shield whose

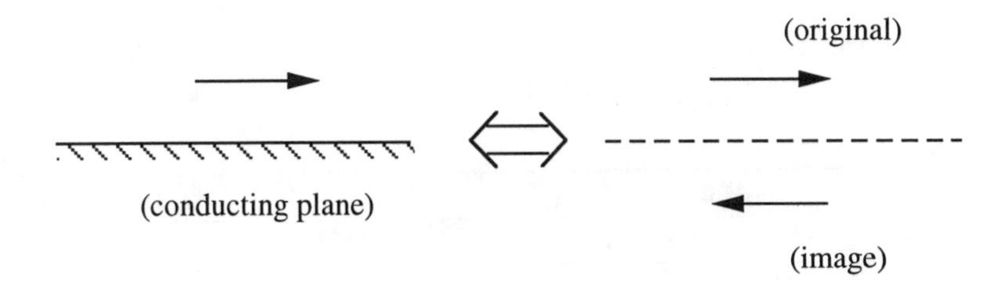


**Figure 4.15.** Illustration of the image theory. (a) Original problem. (b) Equivalent problem.

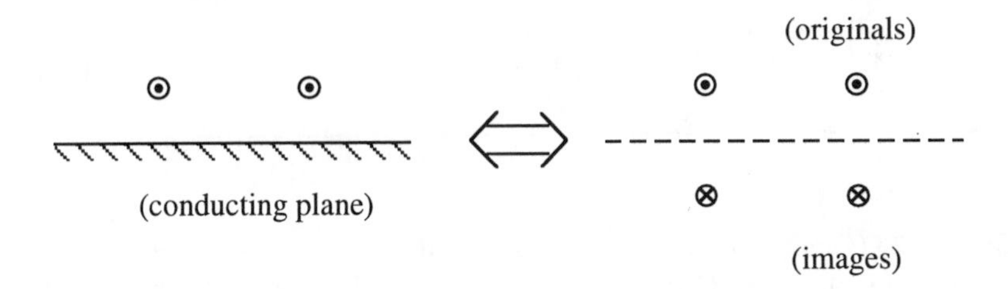


**Figure 4.16.** Illustration of the image theory. (a) Original problem. (b) Equivalent problem.

position is symmetric to the original current with respect to the shield. If the shield is locally a cylindrical surface and the original current is parallel to the axis of the shield, the location of the image would be on the other side of the shield whose distance from the shield is $d = R_i - R_s = R_s^2/R - R_s$ where $R_s$ is the radius of the shield and $R$ is the distance between the original current and the axis of the shield (Lu and Joseph 1991). Although the approximation described above seems to be rather simple, it is accurate enough since, in most designs, the shield is placed very close to the coil and extends beyond the ends of the coil.

To demonstrate the validity of the method, we consider the open coil illustrated in Fig. 4.12. Tables 4.6 and 4.7 give the calculated and measured resonant frequencies for the coil without the shield, with a shield placed 2.54 cm away from the coil, and with a shield placed 1.27 cm away from the coil. (When the shield is placed 2.54 cm away from the coil, the image currents are 2.82 cm away from the shield, and when the shield is placed 1.27 cm away from the coil, the image currents are 1.34 cm away from the shield.) All eight resonant frequencies are presented to ensure the validity of the simulation, although one is usually interested in only the first frequency which corresponds to the fundamental mode. As can be seen, the

**Table 4.6.** Comparison Between Measured and Calculated Resonant Frequencies (in MHz) for the Open Coil with 60 pF Capacitors (Jin *et al.* 1995).

| Mode | No shield | | | $h = 2.54$ cm | | | $h = 1.27$ cm | | |
|---|---|---|---|---|---|---|---|---|---|
| | Meas. | Cal. | (error) | Meas. | Cal. | (error) | Meas. | Cal. | (error) |
| 1 | 72.1 | 75.4 | (4.6%) | 90.4 | 89.4 | (1.1%) | 103.8 | 101.1 | (2.6%) |
| 2 | 58.0 | 58.2 | (0.3%) | 69.9 | 70.0 | (0.1%) | 80.4 | 79.7 | (0.7%) |
| 3 | 49.5 | 48.1 | (2.8%) | 56.5 | 56.1 | (0.7%) | 64.0 | 63.8 | (0.3%) |
| 4 | 43.5 | 41.8 | (3.9%) | 48.0 | 47.1 | (1.9%) | 53.5 | 53.3 | (0.4%) |
| 5 | 39.0 | 37.6 | (3.6%) | 42.0 | 41.3 | (1.7%) | 46.5 | 46.4 | (0.2%) |
| 6 | 36.6 | 34.8 | (4.9%) | 38.6 | 37.6 | (2.6%) | 42.0 | 41.9 | (0.2%) |
| 7 | 34.6 | 33.1 | (4.3%) | 36.0 | 35.2 | (2.2%) | 38.9 | 39.2 | (0.8%) |
| 8 | 33.5 | 32.1 | (4.2%) | 35.0 | 34.0 | (2.9%) | 38.0 | 37.6 | (1.1%) |

**Table 4.7.** Comparison Between Measured and Calculated Resonant Frequencies (in MHz) for the Open Coil with 72 pF Capacitors (Jin *et al.* 1995).

| Mode | No shield | | | $h = 2.54$ cm | | | $h = 1.27$ cm | | |
|---|---|---|---|---|---|---|---|---|---|
| | Meas. | Cal. | (error) | Meas. | Cal. | (error) | Meas. | Cal. | (error) |
| 1 | 66.8 | 68.9 | (3.1%) | 84.0 | 81.6 | (2.9%) | 95.0 | 92.3 | (2.8%) |
| 2 | 53.3 | 53.2 | (0.2%) | 65.6 | 63.9 | (2.6%) | 73.6 | 72.8 | (1.1%) |
| 3 | 45.3 | 44.0 | (2.9%) | 52.7 | 51.2 | (2.8%) | 58.6 | 58.2 | (0.7%) |
| 4 | 39.8 | 38.1 | (4.3%) | 44.1 | 43.0 | (2.5%) | 48.7 | 48.6 | (0.2%) |
| 5 | 36.0 | 34.3 | (4.7%) | 38.7 | 37.7 | (2.6%) | 42.6 | 42.4 | (0.5%) |
| 6 | 33.4 | 31.8 | (4.7%) | 35.7 | 34.3 | (3.9%) | 38.2 | 38.3 | (0.3%) |
| 7 | 31.9 | 30.2 | (5.3%) | 33.2 | 32.2 | (3.0%) | 35.7 | 35.7 | (0.0%) |
| 8 | 30.9 | 29.3 | (5.2%) | 32.2 | 31.0 | (3.7%) | 34.6 | 34.3 | (0.9%) |

agreement between the measured and calculated frequencies is within 5%, which can easily be compensated for by using a tuning capacitor. The small discrepancies are believed to be caused by the tolerances of the capacitors used.

To show the effect of the shield on the $B_1$ field homogeneity, Fig. 4.17 shows the $B_1$ contour and density plots for the coil without a shield and with a shield placed 2.54 cm away from the RF coil. The density plot is given in a circular region, which has a diameter of 15.2 cm and is placed 5 cm above the bottom of the RF coil. As can be expected, the presence of

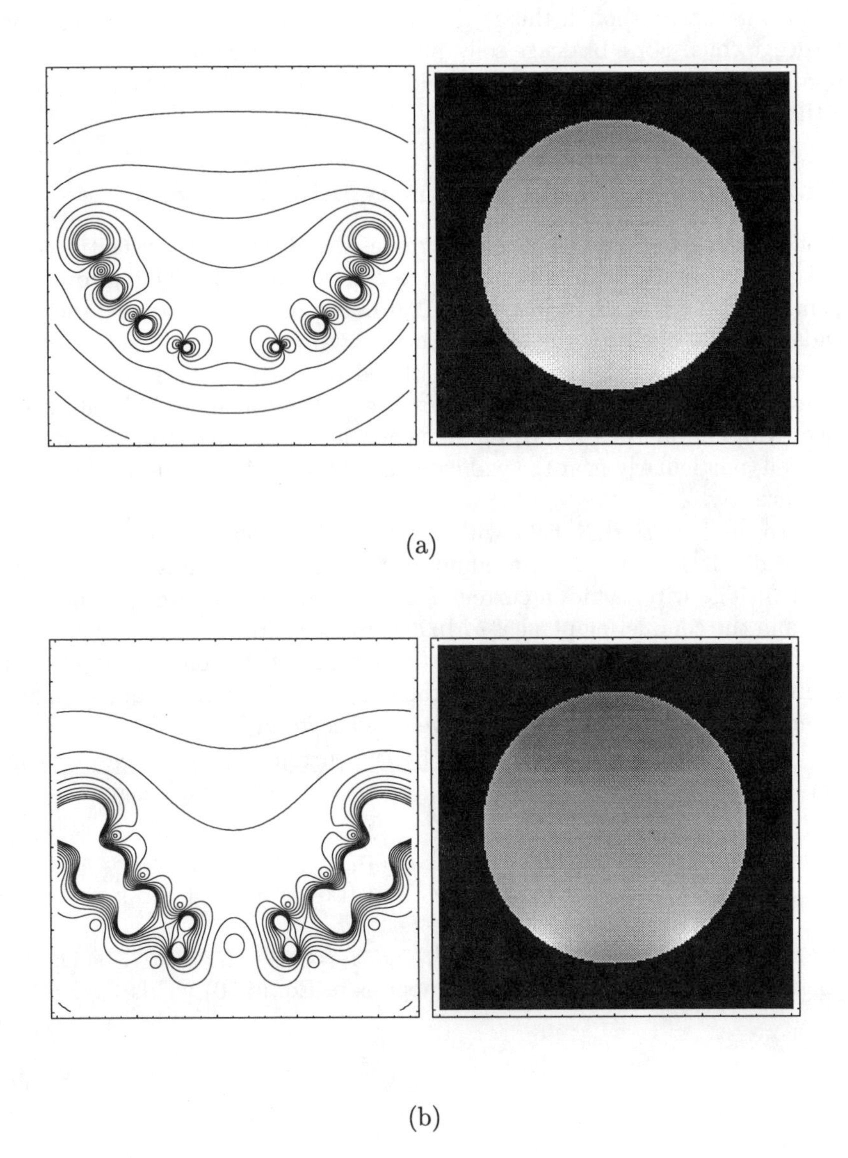

(a)

(b)

**Figure 4.17.** $B_1$ contour and density plots. (a) For the coil without a shield ($h = \infty$). (b) For the coil with a shield placed 2.54 cm away from the coil ($h = 2.54$ cm).

an RF shield decreases the homogeneity of the $B_1$ field. However, we must point out that, although this is the case for many coils, it is not true for birdcage coils. For a birdcage coil, the image is also a birdcage coil carrying opposing currents. Therefore, the field inside the coil is still homogeneous although its strength is reduced.

### 4.4.2 Improving Field Homogeneity Using End-Caps

Although in general an RF shield decreases the $B_1$ field homogeneity, when it is placed at the ends of a birdcage coil, it can actually improve the homogeneity of the $B_1$ field (Hayes 1986). For most applications, the two ends must be open for the sake of entry; however, for some coils such as head coils, one of the ends can be closed by a conducting sheet. This conducting sheet acts as a mirror for the coil and effectively doubles its electrical length. As a result, the homogeneity of the field produced inside the coil, particularly near the end capped with the mirror, can be improved significantly.

To analyze the $B_1$ field with a mirror, consider first a wire placed perpendicularly in front of an infinite conducting plane, illustrated in Fig. 4.18(a). The wire carries a current $I$ and the distance between its nearest end and the conducting plane is $\delta$. In accordance with the theory of images, the field produced by the current in the presence of the conducting plane is equivalent to the field produced by the current and its image in free space where the conducting plane is removed, as shown in Fig. 4.18(b).

To compute the field produced by the current and its image, we can apply Biot-Savart's law. Specifically, the field at point $(\rho, z)$ is given by

$$\mathbf{B}(\rho, z) = \hat{\phi}\frac{\mu_0 I}{4\pi}\left[\int_{z_1}^{z_2} + \int_{z_3}^{z_4}\right]\frac{\rho\, dz'}{[(z-z')^2+\rho^2]^{3/2}} \tag{4.50}$$

where $\rho = \sqrt{x^2+y^2}$, $z_3 = z_2 + 2\delta$, and $z_4 = z_3 + L$, with $L$ being the length of the wire. Evaluating the integrals in Eq. (4.50) yields

$$\mathbf{B}(\rho, z) = \hat{\phi}\frac{\mu_0 I}{4\pi\rho} f(\rho, z) \tag{4.51}$$

where

$$\begin{aligned} f(\rho, z) = {} & \frac{z_2 - z}{\sqrt{\rho^2 + (z_2 - z)^2}} - \frac{z_1 - z}{\sqrt{\rho^2 + (z_1 - z)^2}} \\ & + \frac{z_4 - z}{\sqrt{\rho^2 + (z_4 - z)^2}} - \frac{z_3 - z}{\sqrt{\rho^2 + (z_3 - z)^2}}. \end{aligned} \tag{4.52}$$

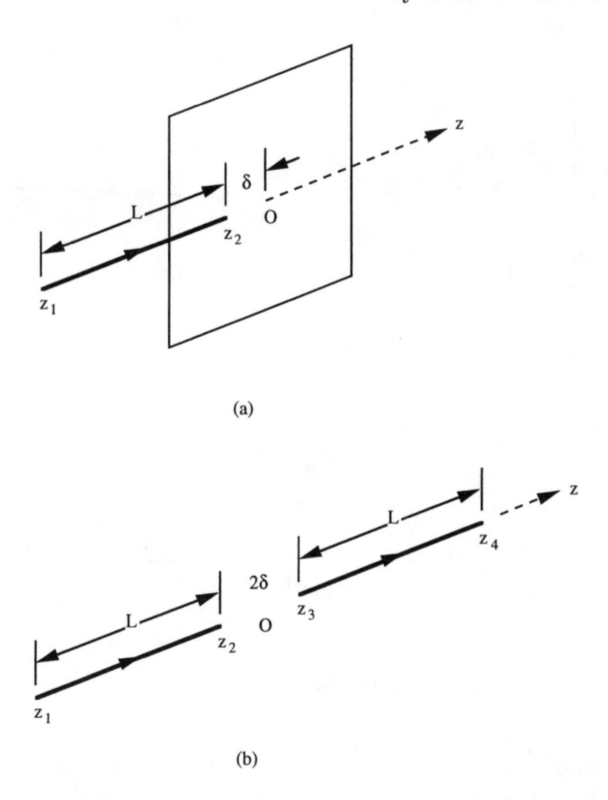


**Figure 4.18.** Illustration of the theory of images. (a) A wire placed perpendicularly in front of a conducting plane. (b) The equivalent problem.

For a coil consisting of $N$ wires parallel to its axis, the field produced by these wires in the presence of the conducting plane is then

$$\mathbf{B}(\rho, z) = \frac{\mu_0}{4\pi} \sum_{i=1}^{N} \frac{I_i}{\rho_i} f(\rho_i, z) \hat{\phi}_i \tag{4.53}$$

where $I_i$ denotes the current on the $i$th wire and

$$\rho_i = \sqrt{(x_i - x)^2 + (y_i - y)^2}$$
$$\hat{\phi}_i = \frac{y_i - y}{\rho_i} \hat{x} - \frac{x_i - x}{\rho_i} \hat{y}$$

with $(x_i, y_i)$ being the position of the $i$th wire.

To demonstrate the effect of the mirror on the field homogeneity, consider a birdcage coil consisting of 16 legs. The length of the coil is

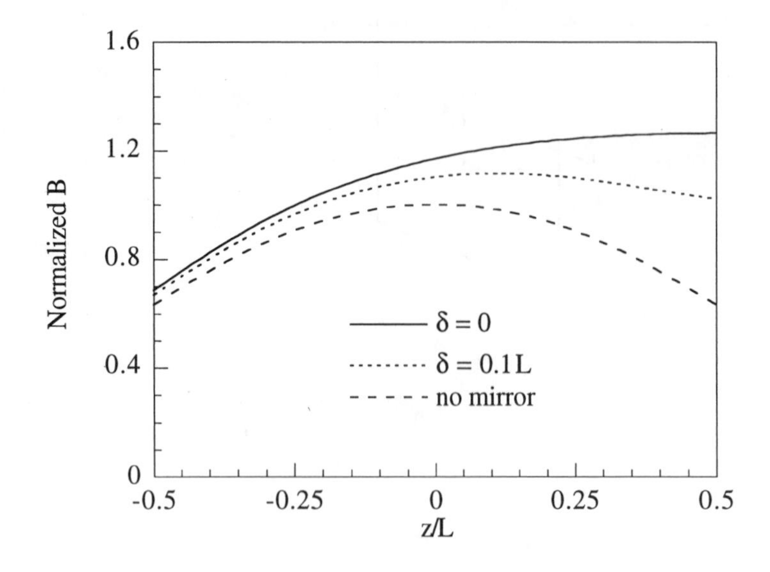


**Figure 4.19.** The $B_1$ field along the axis of the coil.

$L$ and the diameter of the coil is $D$. Figure 4.19 shows the $B_1$ field along the axis of the coil for $L = D$ and $\delta = 0$ and $0.1L$, compared with the result for the same coil without the mirror. The $B_1$ field distributions are shown in Fig. 4.20 for $\delta = 0.1L$ within the region having the same length as the coil and a diameter of $0.72D$.

A birdcage coil consists of not only the legs parallel to its axis, but also two end-rings. The currents on these end-rings also produce a magnetic field, which is destructive to the $B_1$ field homogeneity and thus is undesirable. While a mirror has a negligible effect on the field produced by the end-ring at the other end of the coil, it can significantly reduce the field produced by the end-ring near the mirror. The analysis is simple and is left to the reader as an exercise.

### 4.4.3 Design of RF Shield

Before considering the design of an RF shield, we first have to specify the requirements for the RF shield. Generally speaking, an RF shield should provide effective decoupling between the RF coil and gradient and shim coils without significantly degrading the coils' performance. To achieve this, an RF shield should act as a lowpass filter which should be transparent to

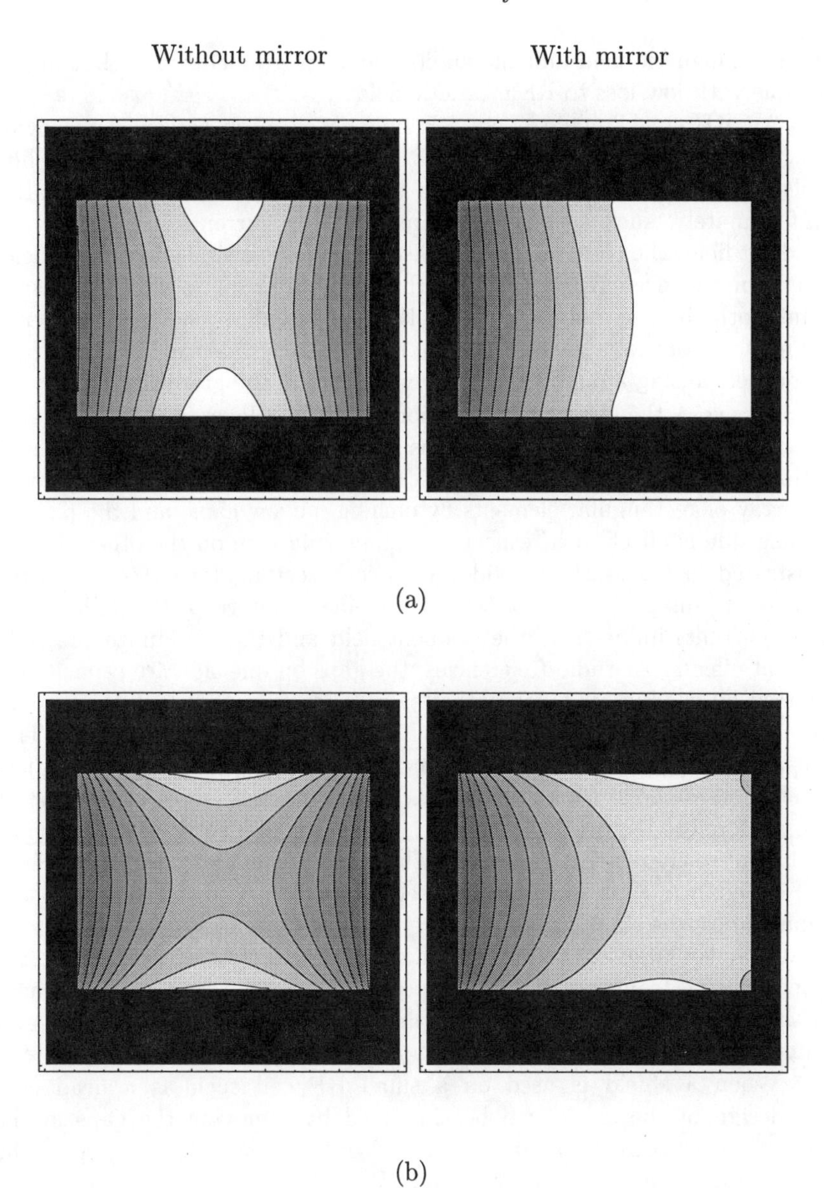


**Figure 4.20.** $B_1$ contour and density plots. (a) In the plane perpendicular to the $B_1$ field. (b) In the plane parallel to the $B_1$ field.

the DC magnetic field and the audio-frequency gradient fields, but highly opaque with low loss to RF magnetic fields.

An RF shield made of an RF opaque or mesh screen can provide effective decoupling between the RF coil and the gradient and shim coils provided that the screen has a thickness of several RF skin-depths. Unfortunately, such a shield can support eddy currents induced by the gradient field, thus lengthening the rise time of the switched gradient field. Furthermore, even if the shield is thin compared to its audio-frequency skin-depth, it may not be completely transparent to the high-frequency components of the gradient field and, thus, can degrade the high-frequency response, causing a distortion in the waveform of the gradient field.

To avoid the drawbacks mentioned above, Hayes and Eash (1987) suggested a shield design, which consists of copper sheets on both sides of a thin dielectric layer (0.005 inch thick). Each copper sheet is divided into an array of rectangular elements by etching narrow gaps, and the pattern on one side is offset with respect to a similar pattern on the other side, as illustrated in Fig. 4.21. Provided that each rectangular element is made sufficiently small, the gaps between the elements interrupt the paths of the eddy currents induced by the gradient field and thus minimize the eddy current effects. At radio frequencies, the gaps on one side are capacitively shorted by conductors on the other side. Therefore, the shield appears to be a single continuous conductor, which is opaque to the RF field. This phenomenon can also be understood using the circuit concept. The shield can be considered as a number of capacitors in parallel, whose capacitance is proportional to the overlapping area between the double sided copper sheet and is inversely proportional to the thickness of the dielectric layer. Since the impedance of the shield is inversely proportional to the frequency and capacitance, the shield will be opaque (small impedance) if the capacitance is sufficiently large at the radio frequencies. For the same capacitance, the shield will be transparent (large impedance) at audio frequencies because of the reduced frequency. For example, a shield having an impedance of 1 Ohm at 64 MHz would have an impedance of 6400 Ohms at 10 KHz.

When a shield is used on a small RF coil such as a head coil, the design of the shield can be simplified by removing the gaps in the circumferential direction (Hayes and Eash 1987, Shen 1992) because, at the center of the gradient coils, where the RF coil is placed, the gradient field is dominated by its $z$-component and the induced eddy current flows mainly in the circumferential direction. Therefore, the gaps in the circumferential direction do not interrupt the eddy current path and, as a result, they have no effect on the eddy current and can be removed. In fact, these gaps interrupt the path of the current induced by the RF field and reduce the effectiveness of the RF shield and therefore should be removed.

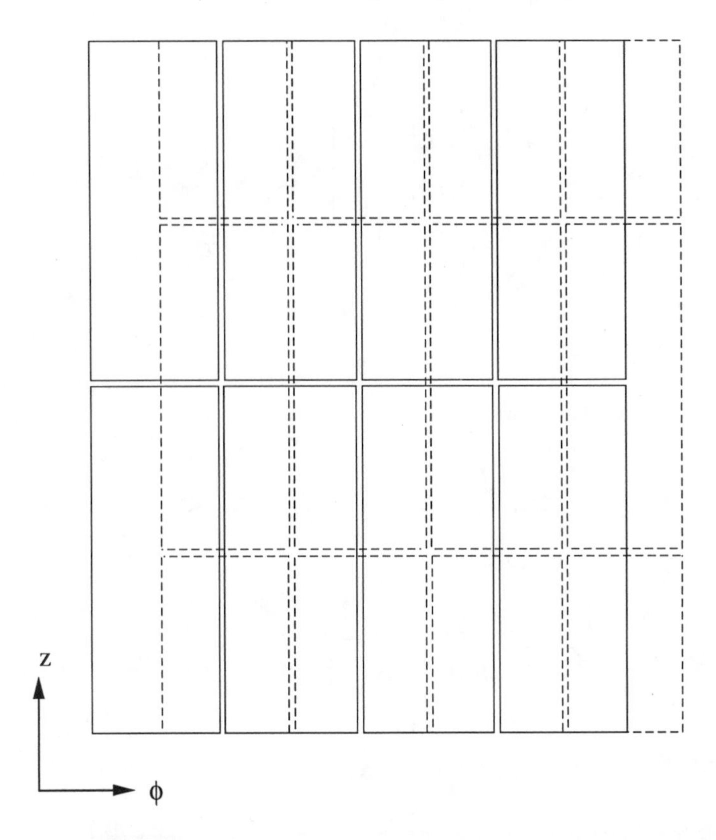


**Figure 4.21.** Illustration of a double-sided shield design. The copper patches on one side are illustrated using solid lines, whereas those on the other side are sketched using dashed lines.

## 4.5 Field Inhomogeneity of Birdcage Coils

Since their introduction in 1985, birdcage coils have been widely used for clinical NMR imaging. Ideally, as shown previously, a birdcage coil, whose capacitors each have the same value of capacitance, can produce a highly homogeneous $B_1$ field over a large volume within the coil. In practice, this is not the case because of the variation in the capacitance introduced by tune, balance, and drive mechanisms, as illustrated in Fig. 4.22. This figure depicts the end-ring configuration of a 16-leg quadrature birdcage coil having five additional variable capacitors. Two variable capacitors, $C_{m1}$ and $C_{m2}$, are used to achieve good matching between the feeds and the coil to minimize the reflected power. Another two variable capacitors, $C_{t1}$ and

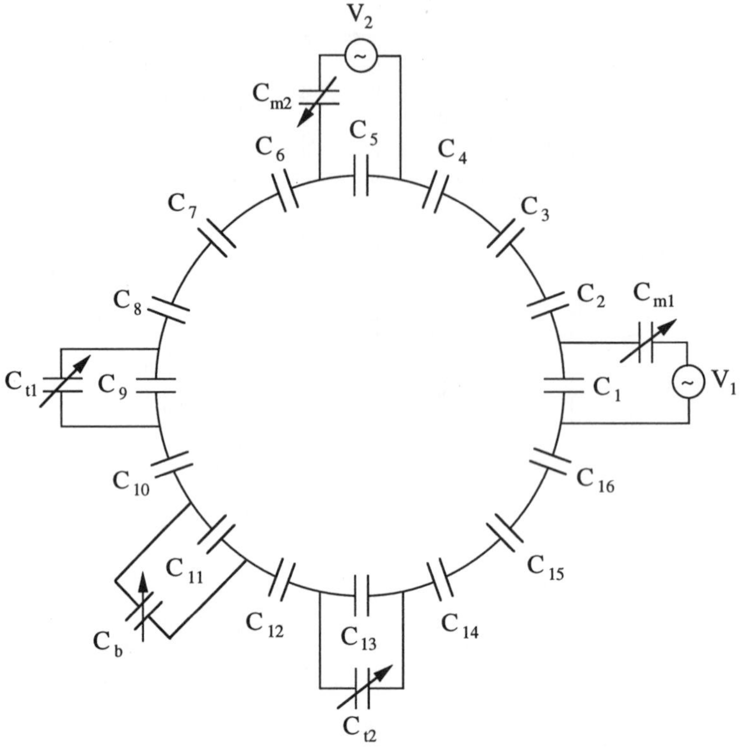

**Figure 4.22.** The end-ring configuration of a birdcage coil with match, tune, and balance capacitors.

$C_{t2}$, are used to achieve fine tuning because, in practice, capacitors with a desired value of capacitance are often unavailable and the constructed coil often has a resonant frequency that is different from the desired operating frequency. The fifth variable capacitor $C_b$ is used to achieve good balance between the two quadrature modes. The use of all these variable capacitors inevitably changes the capacitance of the associated capacitors, leading to a non-ideal birdcage coil with an inhomogeneous $B_1$ field. Such field inhomogeneity can cause severe performance problems when advanced techniques, such as multiple echo spin echo and fast spin echo, are attempted. It is, therefore, very important to identify the specific causes of the field inhomogeneity and then eliminate or reduce them as much as possible. In this section, we employ the equivalent circuit method to study this problem, based on the paper by Jin *et al.* (1994).

Although in the equivalent circuit method all capacitors are allowed

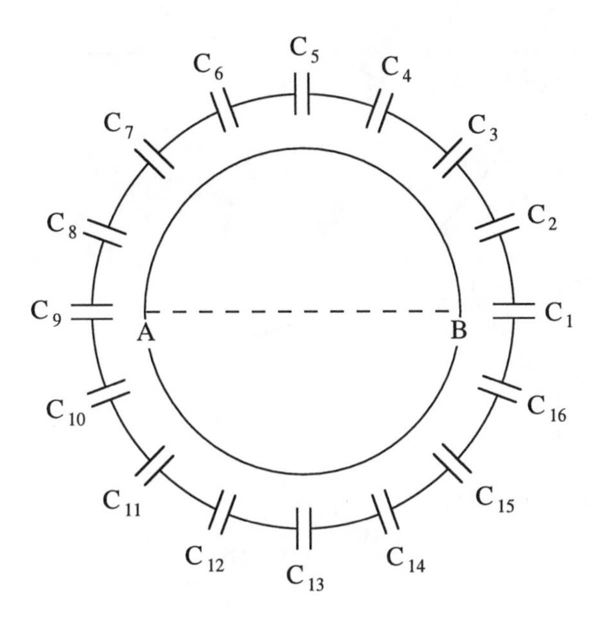


**Figure 4.23.** End-ring configuration of the birdcage coil used for simulation study.

to have different values, to render easily interpretable results, we consider a configuration in which only $C_1$ is variable and the rest are fixed with equal values. This is meaningful since changing the capacitance of a single capacitor is also a way to tune a birdcage coil.

The specific geometry (Fig. 4.23) employed in this simulation study has a radius of 14.0 cm and consists of 16 legs which are 1.27 cm wide and 38.1 cm long copper strips. The capacitors between two adjacent legs have a capacitance of 120 pF, except for $C_1$ which varies from 60 pF to 180 pF. The resonant frequency affected by this capacitor is shown in Fig. 4.24 from which it is seen that, as $C_1$ changes from 120 pF to 60 pF, the resonant frequency increases from 63.9 MHz to 68.4 MHz (4.5 MHz difference). In contrast, when $C_1$ changes from 120 pF to 180 pF, the resonant frequency decreases from 63.9 MHz to 62.65 MHz (1.25 MHz difference). Therefore, reducing the capacitance has a more pronounced effect on the resonant frequency. This is similar to what we have already seen in the case of open coils (see Tables 4.4 and 4.5).

Next, let us examine the change in the $B_1$ field caused by a change in $C_1$. Figure 4.25 plots the normalized $B_1$ field strength across the circular region having a radius of 10.2 cm for various values of $C_1$. As can be seen,

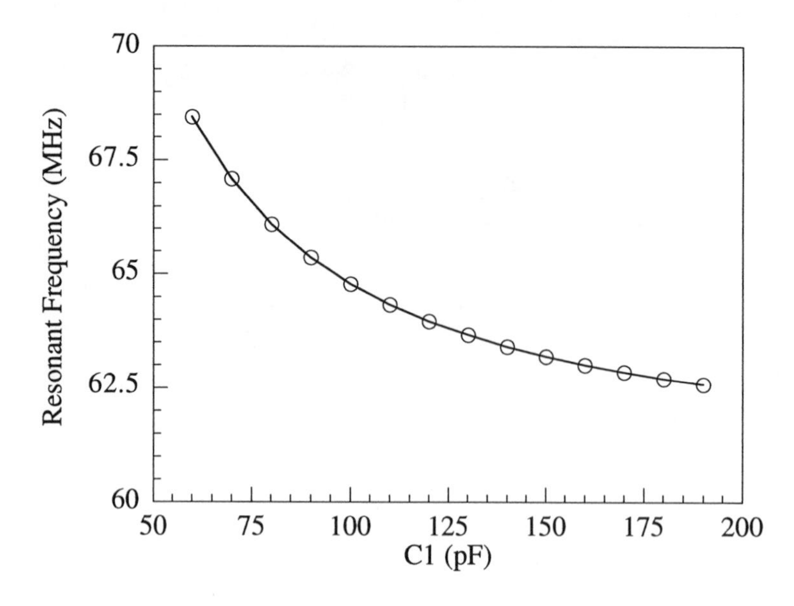


**Figure 4.24.** The resonant frequency as a function of $C_1$ value.

the field along the line AB (Fig. 4.23) changes drastically whereas the field along the line perpendicular to AB (not shown) varies rather slowly (less than 5%). Also, a decrease in $C_1$ has a more pronounced effect on the field homogeneity than an increase. To further investigate the correlation between the field inhomogeneity and the frequency shift shown in Fig. 4.24, we plot in Fig. 4.26 the maximum and average (over the entire circular region) deviation of the $B_1$ field as a function of the relative frequency shift. This frequency shift is defined as

$$\Delta f = 100 \times \frac{f - f_0}{f_0} \quad (\%) \tag{4.54}$$

where $f_0$ denotes the resonant frequency when $C_1$ has the same capacitance as the rest of capacitors and $f$ denotes the frequency after we change $C_1$. It is found that the $B_1$ field inhomogeneity is linearly proportional to the frequency shift:

$$\text{Maximum deviation in } B_1 \text{ field} \approx 7\Delta f \quad (\%) \tag{4.55}$$

and

$$\text{Average deviation in } B_1 \text{ field} \approx \Delta f \quad (\%). \tag{4.56}$$

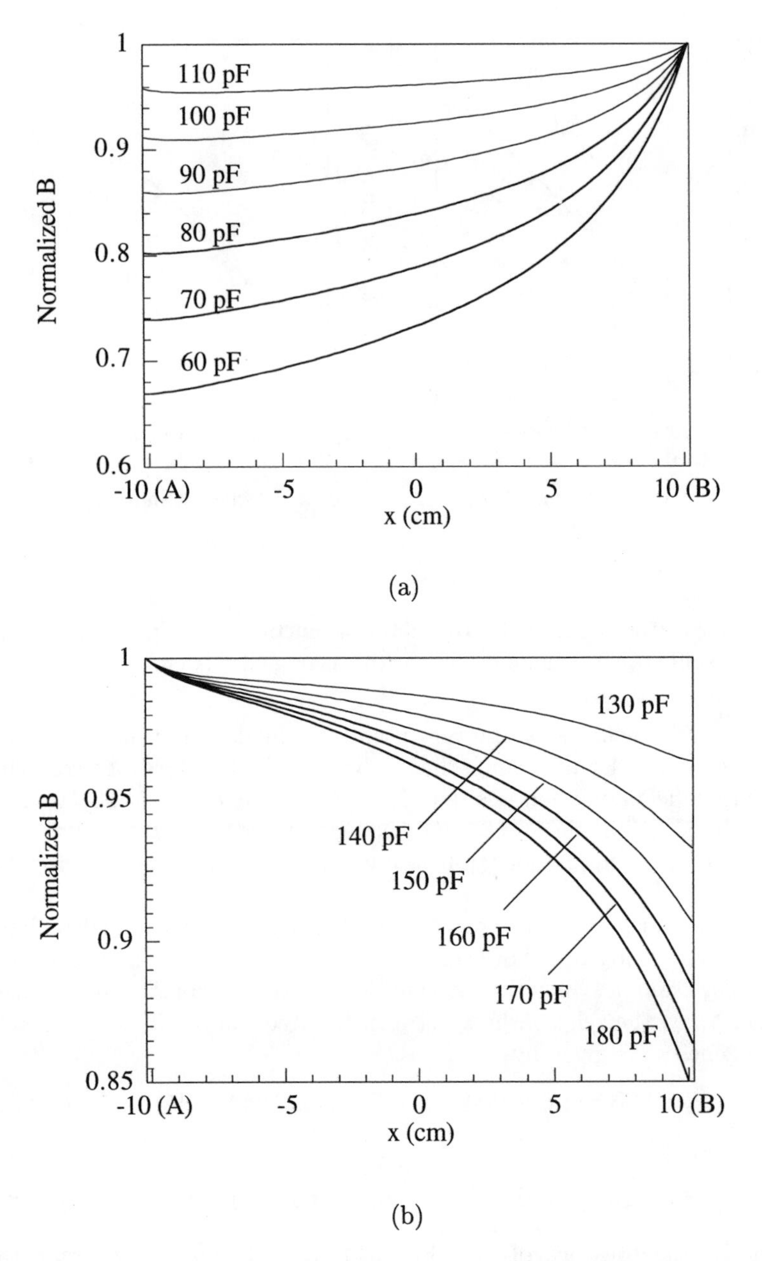


**Figure 4.25.** Normalized $B_1$ field along the dashed line AB shown in Fig. 4.23. (a) For $C_1$ from 120 pF to 60 pF. (b) For $C_1$ from 120 pF to 180 pF.

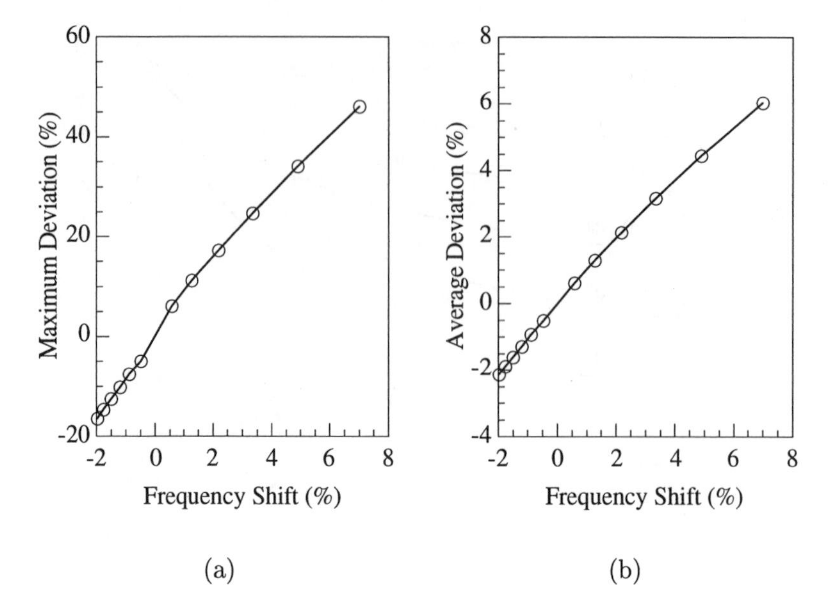


**Figure 4.26.** Deviation of the $B_1$ field as a function of the relative resonant frequency shift. (a) Maximum deviation. (b) Average deviation.

These two relationships can be very useful for the design of birdcage coils. To illustrate this, let us assume that we wish to build a birdcage coil with a maximum field deviation less than 20%. According to Eq. (4.55), we first have to build a coil whose resonant frequency is within $20/7 = 2.9\%$ from the desired operating frequency before we can use a variable capacitor for fine tuning.

The results presented above are pertinent to a birdcage coil without a shield. The study can, however, be extended to the coils having an RF shield. For example, when the coil considered above has an RF shield placed 2.54 cm away, the relationships between the frequency shift and the field inhomogeneity are given by

$$\text{Maximum deviation in } B_1 \text{ field} \approx 20\Delta f \ \ (\%) \tag{4.57}$$

and

$$\text{Average deviation in } B_1 \text{ field} \approx 2\Delta f \ \ (\%). \tag{4.58}$$

Obviously, the presence of an RF shield can substantially degrade the homogeneity of the $B_1$ field of an imperfect birdcage coil. However, the homogeneity requirement can still be satisfied if the coil can be constructed such that $\Delta f$ is sufficiently small.

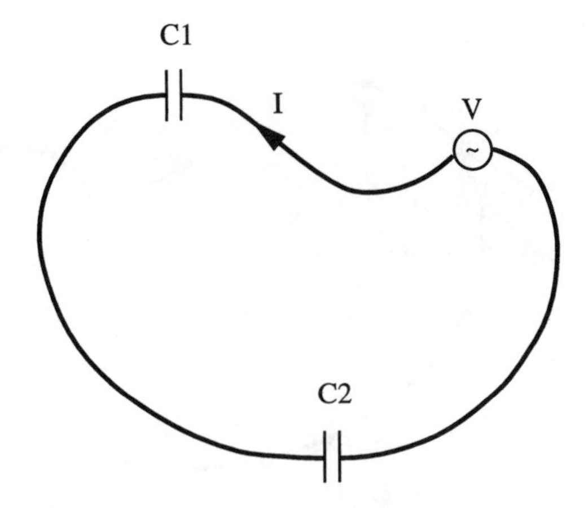


**Figure 4.27.** A generic RF coil.

Finally, we note that a random capacitance variation of ±5% on the capacitors does not cause any substantial changes in the field homogeneity. Our calculations showed a trivial degradation of less than 2% in the field homogeneity for this case.

## 4.6 Method of Moments Analysis

As mentioned earlier, the equivalent circuit method is an approximate analysis. It is applicable to RF coils whose size is a small fraction of the RF wavelength. For coils that are not small compared to the wavelength, its use would result in a significant error. In this section, we describe an accurate analysis, which is based on the integral equation formulation of the problem (Harrington 1993).

### 4.6.1 Unshielded Coil

Consider an RF coil made of wires carrying an electric current $I$, illustrated in Fig. 4.27. The electric field produced by the current can be expressed as

$$\mathbf{E}(\mathbf{r}) = i\omega\mathbf{A}(\mathbf{r}) - \nabla\Phi(\mathbf{r}) \tag{4.59}$$

where

$$\mathbf{A}(\mathbf{r}) = \mu_0 \int_C \mathbf{I}(\mathbf{r}')G(\mathbf{r},\mathbf{r}')\,dl' \tag{4.60}$$

$$\Phi(\mathbf{r}) = \frac{1}{i\omega\epsilon_0}\int_C \frac{dI(\mathbf{r}')}{dl'}G(\mathbf{r},\mathbf{r}')\,dl' \tag{4.61}$$

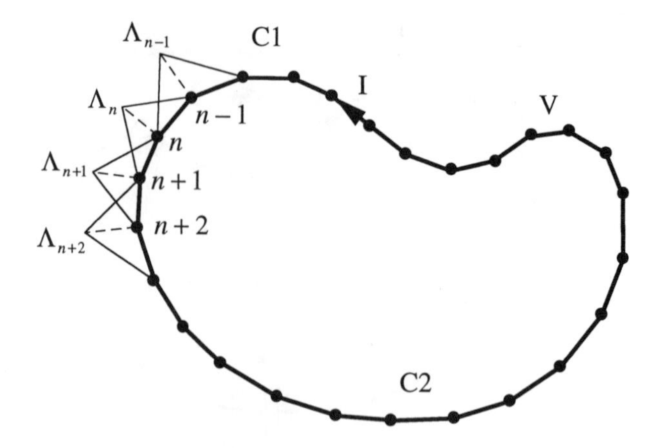


**Figure 4.28.** Discretized coil and the triangular basis functions.

where $C$ denotes the path of the wires and

$$G(\mathbf{r},\mathbf{r}') = \frac{e^{ik_0|\mathbf{r}-\mathbf{r}'|}}{4\pi|\mathbf{r}-\mathbf{r}'|} \tag{4.62}$$

which is called the free-space Green's function.

For a numerical discretization of Eq. (4.59), we first break $C$ into a number of short segments, as shown in Fig. 4.28. For good accuracy, the segments should be no longer than one fifth of a wavelength. The electric current $I$ can then be expanded in terms of basis functions. To evaluate Eq. (4.61), we have to choose basis functions that can be differentiated at least once. The simplest function that satisfies this requirement is the linear function. Therefore, we may expand the current as

$$\mathbf{I}(\mathbf{r}') = \sum_{n=1}^{N} \hat{l}_n \Lambda_n I_n \tag{4.63}$$

where $\Lambda_n$ denotes the triangular basis function spanning the $(n-1)$th and $n$th segments, and $\hat{l}_n$ denotes the direction of the current. Figure 4.28 shows $\Lambda_n$. Note that on a curved wire, $\hat{l}_n$ can be a function of position. Apparently, $I_n$ represents the current at the point between the $(n-1)$th and $n$th segments and $N$ denotes the total number of such points. Substituting Eq. (4.63) into Eqs. (4.61) and (4.62), we obtain

$$\mathbf{A}(\mathbf{r}) = \mu_0 \sum_{n=1}^{N} I_n \int_{C_n} \hat{l}_n \Lambda_n G(\mathbf{r},\mathbf{r}')\, dl' \tag{4.64}$$

$$\Phi(\mathbf{r}) = \frac{1}{i\omega\epsilon_0}\sum_{n=1}^{N} I_n \int_{C_n} \frac{d\Lambda_n}{dl'} G(\mathbf{r},\mathbf{r}')\, dl' \tag{4.65}$$

where $C_n$ denotes the $(n-1)$th and $n$th segments.

To solve for $I_n$, we use Galerkin's method. To be more specific, we take the dot product of Eq. (4.59) with $\hat{l}_m \Lambda_m$ and integrate along $C$ to obtain

$$\int_{C_m} \mathbf{E}(\mathbf{r})\cdot \hat{l}_m \Lambda_m dl = i\omega \int_{C_m} \mathbf{A}(\mathbf{r})\cdot \hat{l}_m \Lambda_m dl - \int_{C_m} \Lambda_m \frac{d\Phi(\mathbf{r})}{dl}\, dl. \tag{4.66}$$

Substituting Eqs. (4.64) and (4.65) into Eq. (4.66), we obtain a matrix equation, which can be written as

$$[Z]\{I\} = \{V\} \tag{4.67}$$

where $\{I\} = [I_1, I_2, \ldots, I_N]^T$, $\{V\} = [V_1, V_2, \ldots, V_N]^T$ are column vectors, and $[Z]$ is an $N \times N$ square matrix. The elements of $[Z]$ and $\{V\}$ are given by

$$\begin{aligned} Z_{mn} = {} & i\omega\mu_0 \int_{C_m} \Lambda_m \hat{l}_m \cdot \int_{C_n} \hat{l}_n \Lambda_n G(\mathbf{r},\mathbf{r}')\, dl'\, dl \\ & - \frac{1}{i\omega\epsilon_0} \int_{C_m} \Lambda_m \frac{d}{dl} \int_{C_n} \frac{d\Lambda_n}{dl'} G(\mathbf{r},\mathbf{r}')\, dl'\, dl \end{aligned} \tag{4.68}$$

$$V_m = \int_{C_m} \mathbf{E}(\mathbf{r})\cdot \hat{l}_m \Lambda_m\, dl. \tag{4.69}$$

Let us first consider the evaluation of $Z_{mn}$. Denote $C_{n^-}$ as the $(n-1)$th segment whose unit tangential vector is $\hat{l}_{n^-}$, and $C_{n^+}$ as the $n$th segment whose unit tangential vector is $\hat{l}_{n^+}$. The first term of Eq. (4.68) can be written as

$$\begin{aligned} Z_{mn}^{(1)} = i\omega\mu_0 \Big[ & \hat{l}_{m^-}\cdot \hat{l}_{n^-}\xi(m^-,n^-) + \hat{l}_{m^-}\cdot \hat{l}_{n^+}\xi(m^-,n^+) \\ & + \hat{l}_{m^+}\cdot \hat{l}_{n^-}\xi(m^+,n^-) + \hat{l}_{m^+}\cdot \hat{l}_{n^+}\xi(m^+,n^+) \Big] \end{aligned} \tag{4.70}$$

where

$$\xi(m^-,n^-) = \int_{C_{m^-}} \Lambda_m \int_{C_{n^-}} \Lambda_n G(\mathbf{r},\mathbf{r}')\, dl'\, dl \tag{4.71}$$

and the other three terms are similarly defined. When $C_{m^-}$ and $C_{n^-}$ are not the same segments, $\xi(m^-,n^-)$ can be evaluated using the midpoint approximation. When $C_{m^-}$ and $C_{n^-}$ are the same segment, $\xi(m^-, n^-)$ can be evaluated by subdividing the segment into smaller subsegments and approximating $\Lambda_n$ within each subsegment as a constant. In this case, we have to evaluate the integral

$$\psi = \int_{\Delta l}\int_{\Delta l} G(\mathbf{r}, \mathbf{r}')\, dl'\, dl = \frac{1}{4\pi}\int_{\Delta l}\int_{\Delta l} \frac{e^{ik_0 R}}{R}\, dl'\, dl \tag{4.72}$$

where $\Delta l$ denotes a short segment and $R = \sqrt{a^2 + (l - l')^2}$ with $a$ being the radius of the wire. Expanding the exponential in a Maclaurin series, we obtain

$$\psi = \frac{1}{4\pi}\int_{\Delta l}\int_{\Delta l} \left(\frac{1}{R} + ik_0 - \frac{k_0^2}{2}R + \cdots\right) dl'\, dl. \tag{4.73}$$

By keeping only the first two terms, Eq. (4.72) can be evaluated to give

$$\psi = \frac{\Delta l}{2\pi}\left[\ln\left(\frac{\Delta l}{a} + \sqrt{1 + \frac{(\Delta l)^2}{a^2}}\right) - \sqrt{1 + \frac{a^2}{(\Delta l)^2}} + \frac{a}{\Delta l}\right] + \frac{ik_0}{4\pi}(\Delta l)^2 \tag{4.74}$$

which can be simplified to

$$\psi = \frac{\Delta l}{2\pi}\left(\ln\frac{2\Delta l}{a} - 1\right) + \frac{ik_0}{4\pi}(\Delta l)^2 \tag{4.75}$$

when $\Delta l >> a$. By using integration by parts, the second term of Eq. (4.68) can be written as

$$Z_{mn}^{(2)} = \frac{1}{i\omega\epsilon_0}\int_{C_m} \frac{d\Lambda_m}{dl}\int_{C_n} \frac{d\Lambda_n}{dl'} G(\mathbf{r}, \mathbf{r}')\, dl'\, dl \tag{4.76}$$

which can be further written as

$$\begin{aligned} Z_{mn}^{(2)} = \frac{1}{i\omega\epsilon_0}\Bigg[&\frac{1}{l_{m^-}l_{n^-}}\zeta(m^-, n^-) - \frac{1}{l_{m^+}l_{n^-}}\zeta(m^+, n^-) \\ &- \frac{1}{l_{m^-}l_{n^+}}\zeta(m^-, n^+) + \frac{1}{l_{m^+}l_{n^+}}\zeta(m^+, n^+)\Bigg] \end{aligned} \tag{4.77}$$

where

$$\zeta(m^-, n^-) = \int_{C_{m^-}}\int_{C_{n^-}} G(\mathbf{r}, \mathbf{r}')\, dl'\, dl \tag{4.78}$$

and the other three terms are similarly defined. When $C_{m^-}$ and $C_{n^-}$ are not the same segments, $\zeta(m^-, n^-)$ can be evaluated using the midpoint approximation. When $C_{m^-}$ and $C_{n^-}$ are the same segment, $\zeta(m^-, n^-)$ can be evaluated using Eq. (4.75).

Now, let us consider the integral in Eq. (4.69). Since $\mathbf{E}(\mathbf{r})\cdot\hat{l}_m$ represents the electric field tangential to $C$, it must be zero because of the boundary condition, except at the locations of capacitors and feeds. Therefore, $V_m = 0$ when there is no capacitor and feed at point $m$. When there is a capacitor at point $m$, $V_m$ becomes the voltage across this capacitor, which is related to the current by

$$V_m = \frac{i}{\omega C'_m} I_m \tag{4.79}$$

where $C'_m$ denotes the capacitance of the capacitor at point $m$. Apparently, this term can be moved to the left-hand side of Eq. (4.67). When there is a feed or voltage at point $m$,

$$V_m = -V_m^{\text{ex}} \tag{4.80}$$

where $V_m^{\text{ex}}$ denotes the applied voltage at point $m$. As a result, the right-hand side of Eq. (4.67) contains only the applied voltage. Solving Eq. (4.67), we obtain the current in the coil from which the magnetic field can be evaluated from

$$\mathbf{B}(\mathbf{r}) = \nabla \times \mathbf{A}(\mathbf{r}) \tag{4.81}$$

where $\mathbf{A}(\mathbf{r})$ is given in Eq. (4.60) or Eq. (4.64).

We note that if the RF coil is made of conducting strips of width $w$, the formulation described above is still valid provided that Eq. (4.75) is replaced by

$$\psi = \frac{\Delta l}{2\pi}\left(\ln\frac{2\Delta l}{w} + \frac{1}{2}\right) + \frac{ik_0}{4\pi}(\Delta l)^2. \tag{4.82}$$

### 4.6.2 Shielded Coil

The above formulation is described for a coil without a shield and an end-cap; however, it can be extended to shielded and end-capped coils by including the effect of the currents on the shield and the end-cap in Eqs. (4.60) and (4.61). In this case, Eqs. (4.60) and (4.61) become

$$\mathbf{A}(\mathbf{r}) = \mu_0 \int_C \mathbf{I}(\mathbf{r}')G(\mathbf{r},\mathbf{r}')\,dl' + \mu_0 \iint_S \mathbf{J}(\mathbf{r}')G(\mathbf{r},\mathbf{r}')\,ds' \tag{4.83}$$

$$\Phi(\mathbf{r}) = \frac{1}{i\omega\epsilon_0}\int_C \frac{dI(\mathbf{r}')}{dl'}G(\mathbf{r},\mathbf{r}')\,dl' + \frac{1}{i\omega\epsilon_0}\iint_S \nabla'\cdot\mathbf{J}(\mathbf{r}')G(\mathbf{r},\mathbf{r}')\,ds' \tag{4.84}$$

where $S$ denotes the surface of the shield and/or end-cap and $\mathbf{J}$ denotes the surface current on $S$. For a numerical discretization, we divide $S$ into small rectangular or triangular patches. The current on $S$ can then be expanded as

$$\mathbf{J}(\mathbf{r}') = \sum_{n=1}^{N_s} J_n \mathbf{f}_n(\mathbf{r}') \tag{4.85}$$

where $\mathbf{f}_n(\mathbf{r}')$ denotes the chosen basis functions, which can be rooftop functions for rectangular patches (Ochi *et al.* 1994) and Rao-Wilton-Glisson functions for triangular patches (Rao *et al.* 1982). Also, $J_n$ denotes the unknown expansion coefficients and $N_s$ denotes the total number of the expansion coefficients. Following a similar procedure described earlier, we obtain a matrix equation

$$\begin{bmatrix} Z_{cc} & Z_{cs} \\ Z_{sc} & Z_{ss} \end{bmatrix} \begin{Bmatrix} I \\ J \end{Bmatrix} = \begin{Bmatrix} V \\ 0 \end{Bmatrix} \tag{4.86}$$

where $\{I\}$ and $\{V\}$ are the same as those in Eq. (4.67), $[Z_{cc}]$ is the same matrix as $[Z]$ in Eq. (4.67), and $\{J\} = [J_1, J_2, \ldots, J_{N_s}]^T$ is the unknown column vector. Also, $[Z_{cs}]$, $[Z_{sc}]$, and $[Z_{ss}]$ are the $N \times N_s$, $N_s \times N$, and $N_s \times N_s$ matrices, respectively, whose elements are given by

$$\begin{aligned}[Z_{cs}]_{mn} = {} & i\omega\mu_0 \int_{C_m} \hat{l}_m \Lambda_m \cdot \iint_{S_n} \mathbf{f}_n(\mathbf{r}') G(\mathbf{r}, \mathbf{r}')\, ds'\, dl \\ & + \frac{1}{i\omega\epsilon_0} \int_{C_m} \frac{d\Lambda_m}{dl} \iint_{S_n} \nabla' \cdot \mathbf{f}_n(\mathbf{r}') G(\mathbf{r}, \mathbf{r}')\, ds'\, dl \end{aligned} \tag{4.87}$$

$$\begin{aligned}[Z_{ss}]_{mn} = {} & i\omega\mu_0 \iint_{S_m} \mathbf{f}_m(\mathbf{r}) \cdot \iint_{S_n} \mathbf{f}_n(\mathbf{r}') G(\mathbf{r}, \mathbf{r}')\, ds'\, ds \\ & + \frac{1}{i\omega\epsilon_0} \iint_{S_m} \nabla \cdot \mathbf{f}_m(\mathbf{r}) \iint_{S_n} \nabla' \cdot \mathbf{f}_n(\mathbf{r}') G(\mathbf{r}, \mathbf{r}')\, ds'\, ds \end{aligned} \tag{4.88}$$

and $[Z_{sc}]_{mn} = [Z_{cs}]_{nm}$, where $S_m$ and $S_n$ denotes the surface covered by $\mathbf{f}_m(\mathbf{r})$ and $\mathbf{f}_n(\mathbf{r})$, respectively. The integrals in Eqs. (4.87) and (4.88) can be evaluated using numerical integration with a special treatment for the singularity in the Green's function. Clearly, $[Z_{cs}]$ and $[Z_{sc}]$ couple the currents in the coil to those on the shield and/or end-cap. Solving Eq. (4.86), we obtain the currents in the coil and the shield and/or end-cap.

### 4.6.3 Numerical Simulation

In the following, we present two numerical examples to demonstrate the capability of the method. One example is for a highpass birdcage coil

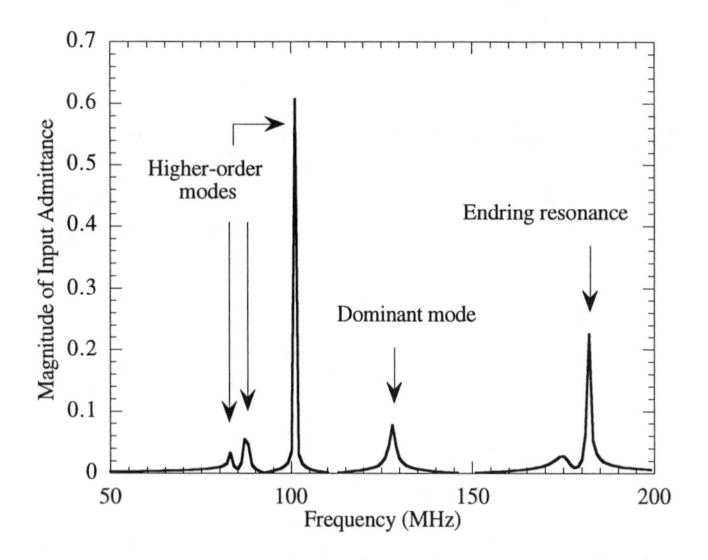


**Figure 4.29.** Magnitude of the input admittance of a highpass birdcage coil. Reproduced from Chen *et al.* (1998), ©1998 IEEE.

and the other is for a lowpass birdcage coil. Both are 26 cm long, have a diameter of 26 cm, have eight legs, and are made of wires of radius 0.2 cm. The capacitors in the highpass birdcage coil have a value of 2.98 pF and those in the lowpass birdcage coil have a value of 2.06 pF. The magnitude of the input admittance of the highpass birdcage coil is shown in Fig. 4.29. Five resonant modes are observed and the dominant mode has the second highest resonant frequency. The currents of the dominant mode in the end-rings are given in Fig. 4.30, from which we see that the current distribution is very close to the cosine function, as predicted in the equivalent circuit method. The currents in the legs are displayed in Fig. 4.31 and, apparently, they are very close to the sine function. The $B_1$ field in the three planes are shown in Fig. 4.32.

The corresponding results for the lowpass birdcage coil are given in Figs. 4.33 to 4.36. Four resonant modes are observed because the lowest (fifth) one has a resonant frequency of zero. A sine function distribution is observed in the currents in the end-ring and a cosine function distribution is observed in the currents in the legs. A nonuniform current distribution is also observed in the legs due to the effect of the capacitors. However, this does not have a significant effect on the homogeneity of the $B_1$ field, as shown in Fig. 4.36.

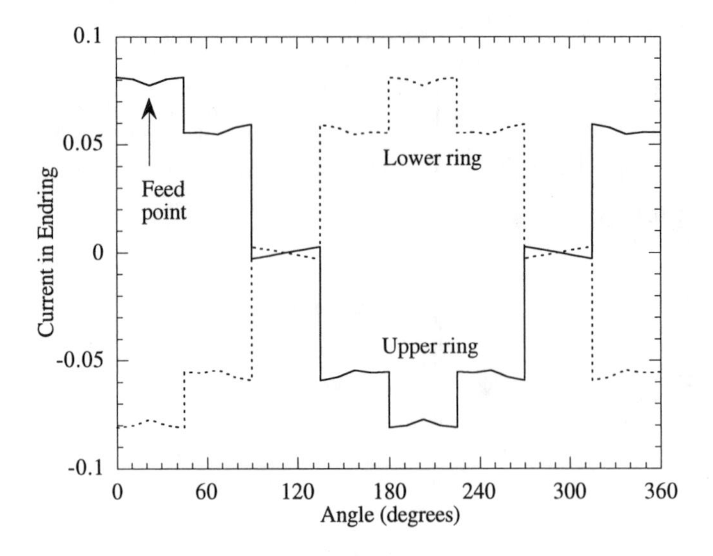


**Figure 4.30.** Currents of the dominant mode in the end-rings of a highpass birdcage coil. Reproduced from Chen *et al.* (1998), ©1998 IEEE.

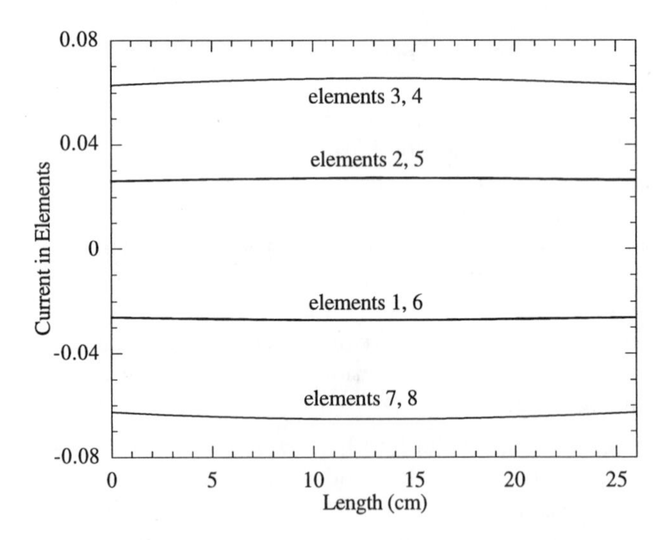


**Figure 4.31.** Currents of the dominant mode in the legs of a highpass birdcage coil. Reproduced from Chen *et al.* (1998), ©1998 IEEE.

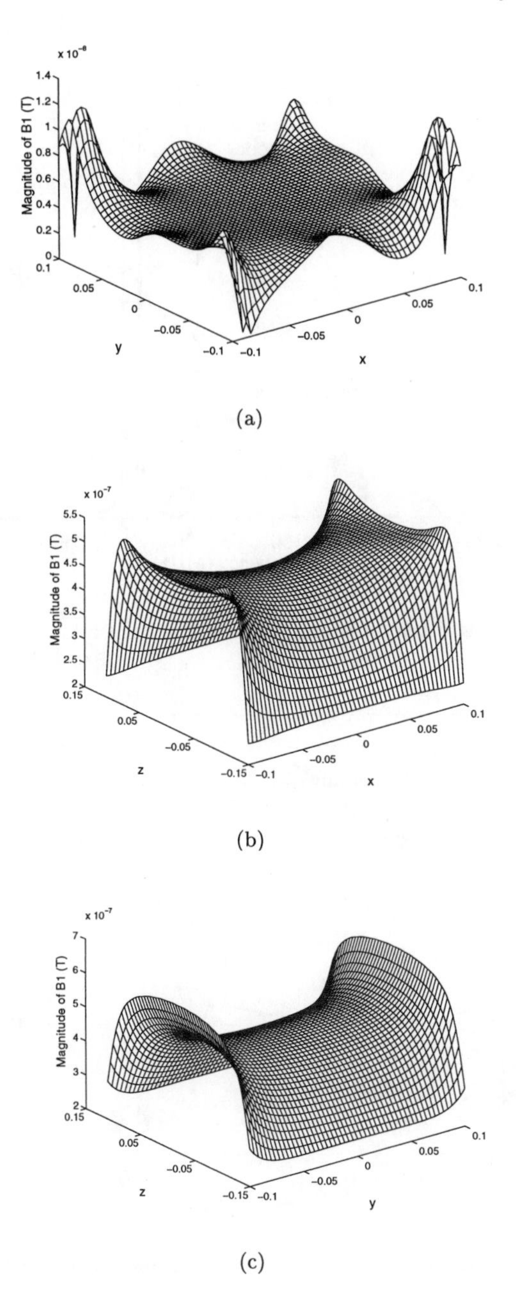


**Figure 4.32.** $B_1$ field of a highpass birdcage coil. (a) In the $xy$-plane. (b) In the $xz$-plane. (c) In the $yz$-plane.

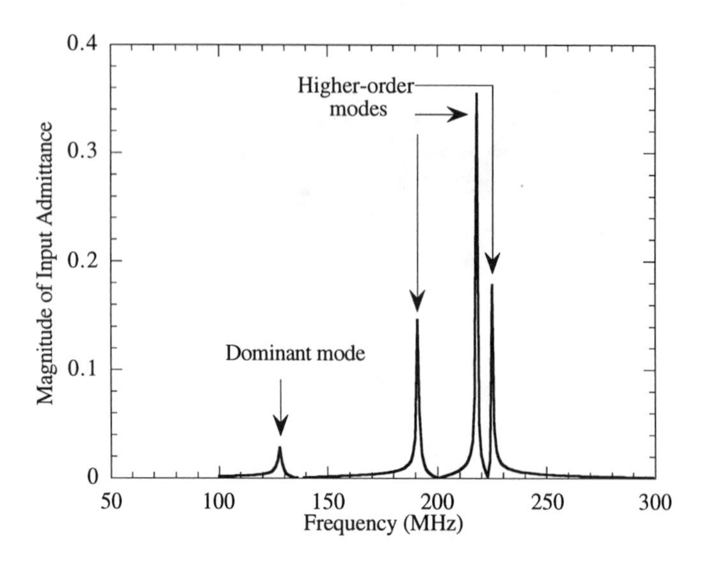


**Figure 4.33.** Magnitude of the input admittance of a lowpass birdcage coil.

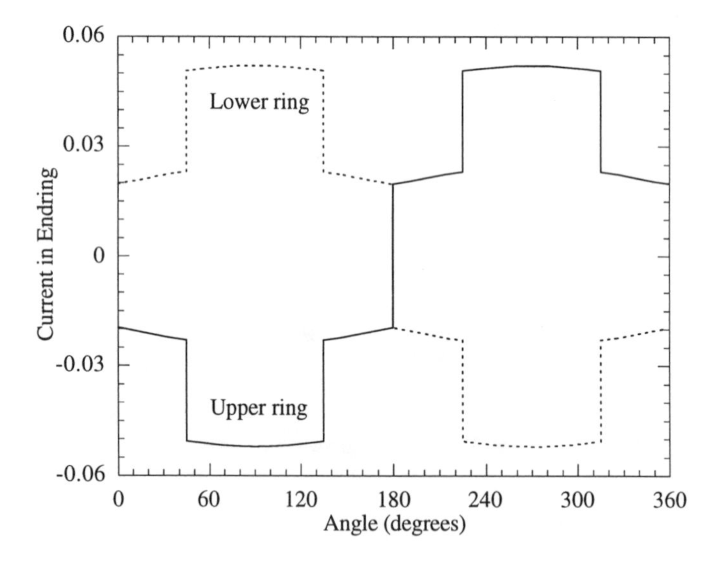


**Figure 4.34.** Currents of the dominant mode in the end-rings of a lowpass birdcage coil.

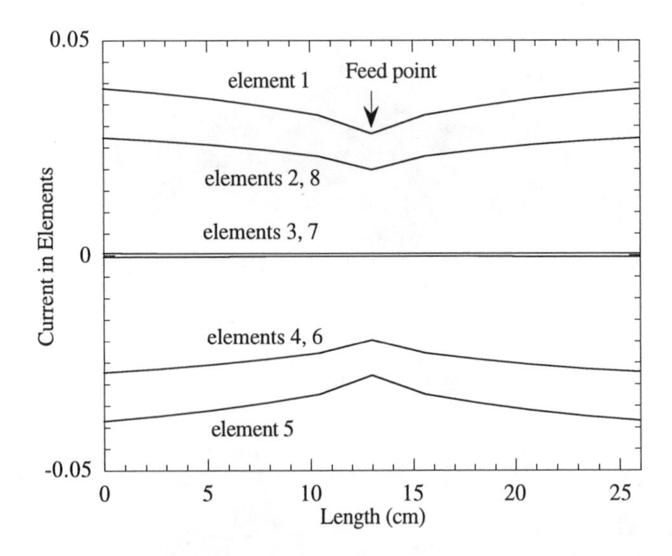


**Figure 4.35.** Currents of the dominant mode in the legs of a lowpass birdcage coil.

The last example gave a quantitative comparison between the calculated and the measured resonant frequencies of the flat ladder coil sketched in Fig. 4.37. The coil is made of 0.0562-inch wide conducting strips and is designed for skin imaging. The calculated and measured resonant frequencies are given in Table 4.8, which shows a good agreement. Note that because of its small size, this coil can also be analyzed using the equivalent circuit method, yielding results similar to those given in Table 4.8.

## 4.7 Miscellaneous Topics

Over the past two decades, many RF coils have been designed for many different applications. In this section, we briefly review several of them. A detailed treatment of these topics is beyond the scope of this chapter and the reader is referred to the references listed at the end of the chapter.

### 4.7.1 Brief History of Birdcage Coils

The lowpass birdcage coil was first developed by Hayes *et al.* (1985) for whole-body NMR imaging at 1.5 T. It was observed that the birdcage coil produces an RF field whose homogeneity is significantly better than that of a saddle coil or slotted tube resonator. It was further observed

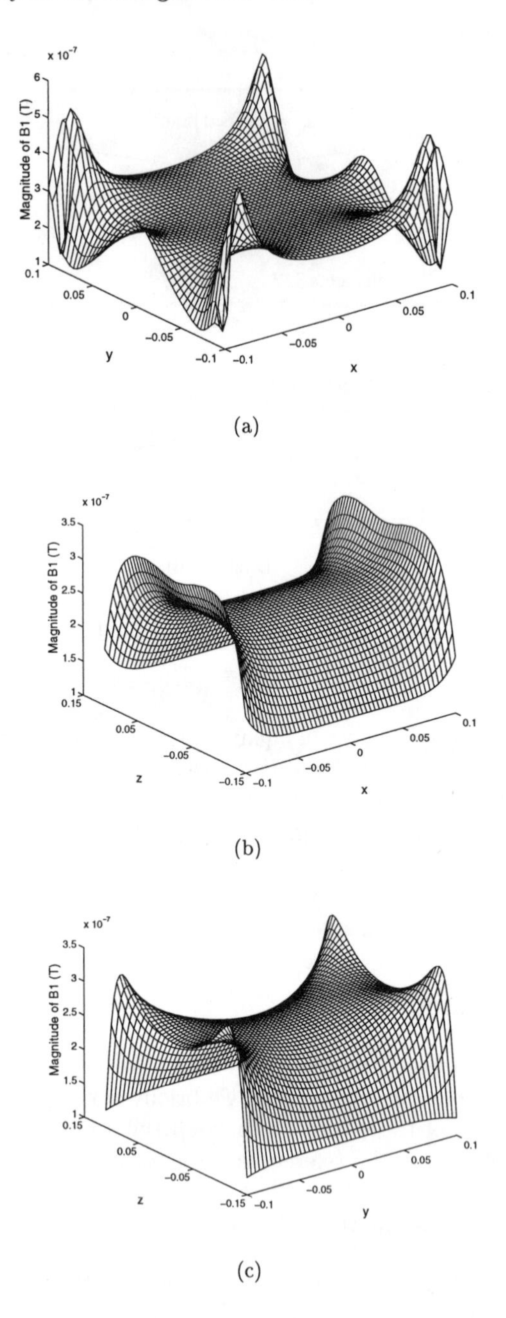


**Figure 4.36.** $B_1$ field of a lowpass birdcage coil. (a) In the $xy$-plane. (b) In the $xz$-plane. (c) In the $yz$-plane.

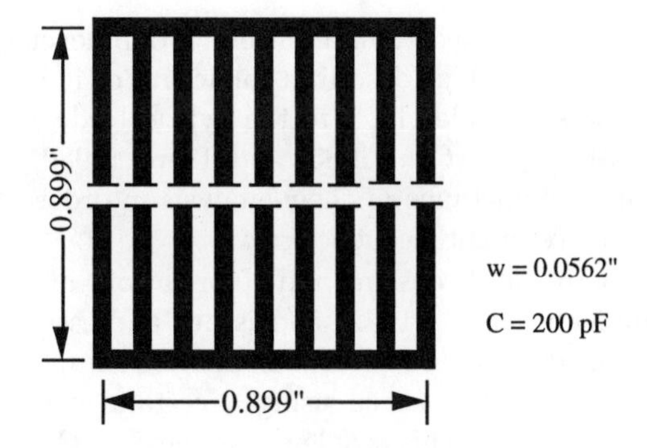


**Figure 4.37.** A flat lowpass ladder coil.

**Table 4.8.** Comparison Between Measured and Calculated Resonant Frequencies (in MHz) for the Flat Ladder Coil.

| Mode | Measured | Calculated | Error |
|---|---|---|---|
| 1 | 48.2 | 47.6 | 1.2% |
| 2 | 75.5 | 75.2 | 0.4% |
| 3 | 93.8 | 93.8 | 0.0% |
| 4 | 107.2 | 107.2 | 0.0% |
| 5 | 117.5 | 117.6 | 0.1% |
| 6 | 125.1 | 125.4 | 0.2% |
| 7 | 130.2 | 130.6 | 0.3% |
| 8 | 133.7 | 133.8 | 0.1% |

that the coil's cylindrical symmetry allows quadrature drive and reception which decreases RF power requirements by a factor of two and increases SNR by a factor of $\sqrt{2}$. A simplified analysis based on a lumped element equivalent circuit and Biot-Savart's law was presented for the evaluation of the resonant frequencies and the $B_1$ field. Hayes (1986) further showed that the homogeneity of the $B_1$ field in a birdcage coil can be improved by placing a conducting end-cap on the coil and a similar idea was employed by Wong *et al.* (1992) in the design of an elliptical birdcage coil. Instead of using a lowpass ladder network, one can also use a highpass ladder network to construct a so-called highpass birdcage coil (Hayes *et al.* 1986, Watkins and Fukushima 1988). A more detailed theoretical analysis of lowpass birdcage coils was presented by Tropp (1989), also based on a lumped element equivalent circuit model, and by Pascone *et al.* (1991) based on the transmission line theory. In addition, Tropp developed a theory of the driven birdcage coil, which describes capacitive or inductive drive schemes. The analysis was extended later to the hybrid birdcage coil (Tropp 1992). Note that both Hayes *et al.* (1985) and Tropp (1989, 1992) neglected the effect of mutual inductance in their analysis in order to obtain analytical solutions to the resonant frequencies.

The experimental design and fabrication of birdcage coils was discussed by Vullo *et al.* (1992) and issues addressed include inductance measurements, determination of resonant modes, and coil evaluation. When a birdcage coil is tuned using a certain capacitor, its cylindrical symmetry is destroyed. This problem was alleviated by Pimmel and Briguet (1992) in the design of a hybrid birdcage coil. This design uses two sets of capacitors, as shown in Fig. 4.9. Whereas the capacitors in the end-rings have fixed capacitance chosen to make the resonant frequency close to the desired frequency, the capacitors in the legs can be modified simultaneously, thus maintaining the cylindrical symmetry of the coil. To realize this, the capacitors in the legs are formed by two sets of conducting strips separated by a sheet of Teflon and their capacitance can be adjusted by changing the overlapping areas between the two sets of the conducting strips. A similar idea was also employed by Marro *et al.* (1992) in the design of a highpass birdcage coil, where the variable tuning capacitors are built into one of the end-rings. Recently, Vaughan *et al.* (1993, 1994) designed a shielded lowpass birdcage coil using distributed capacitance, which can be used for NMR imaging at high frequencies such as 256 MHz.

Even though there are techniques to tune the capacitors in the end-ring or in the legs simultaneously, changing the capacitance of a particular capacitor is still a commonly practiced method to tune a birdcage coil. The $B_1$ field inhomogeneity caused by such tuning was studied by Jin *et al.* (1994) using the equivalent circuit method, which includes the effect of mutual inductance. Guidelines were derived for constructing coils with a specified $B_1$ field homogeneity. This was discussed in Section 4.5.

### 4.7.2 Quadrature Coils

When an RF coil operates in a way that its $B_1$ field at a fixed point in space always points in a certain direction, the coil is called a linear coil and the $B_1$ field is called a linearly polarized field. As is well known, a linearly polarized $B_1$ field can be decomposed into two counter-rotating or circularly polarized components. For example, a linearly polarized $B_1$ field in the $x$ direction can be written as

$$\mathbf{B} = \hat{x} B_1 \cos \omega t$$

$$= \tfrac{1}{2}B_1(\hat{x}\cos\omega t + \hat{y}\sin\omega t) + \tfrac{1}{2}B_1(\hat{x}\cos\omega t - \hat{y}\sin\omega t) \qquad (4.89)$$

where the first term in the right-hand side represents a right-hand circularly polarized field and the second term represents a left-hand circularly polarized field, both having a magnitude of $B_1/2$. Among the two components, only one component that rotates in the same sense as spins precess excites the magnetization and the other is wasted. Such a waste can be avoided by a quadrature RF coil that directly produces a circularly polarized $B_1$ field. Doing so, the RF power requirement can be reduced by a factor of two. Similarly, the RF signal emitted by spins is a circularly polarized field. A circularly polarized field can be decomposed into two orthogonal linearly polarized components. When a linear coil is used for reception, only one component can be detected by the coil and the other component is wasted. Such a waste can also be avoided by using a quadrature coil for reception. Doing so, the SNR of the received signal can be increased by a factor of $\sqrt{2}$.

The use of a quadrature coil for excitation and detection was first proposed by Chen *et al.* (1983). A comparison of quadrature coils to linear coils was carried out by Glover *et al.* (1985). In addition to the verification of the decreased power and increased SNR as predicted, it was further observed that the use of quadrature excitation and detection can reduce the intensity of artifacts caused by dielectric standing wave effects and conduction currents. Whereas quadrature excitation and detection can be realized easily in birdcage coils, it is a more difficult task in other coils such as surface coils. As a result, many researchers have attempted to develop quadrature surface coils (Boskamp *et al.* 1992, Fayad *et al.* 1995, Fitzsimmons and Beck 1992, Hyde *et al.* 1987, Kuan and Leu 1992, Lee *et al.* 1990). Problem 4.5 shows one design of a surface quadrature coil.

### 4.7.3 Double-Tuned Coils

A double-tuned coil is a coil that can operate at two different frequencies. It has found applications in the integration of MR spectroscopy with MR imaging. A double-tuned coil can be easily realized using a cylindrical birdcage coil. For an ideal highpass birdcage coil, the current in the end-rings for the two dominant degenerate modes that produce a uniform $B_1$ field is given by

$$I_j^{(c)} = \cos\frac{2\pi j}{N} \qquad (4.90)$$

and

$$I_j^{(s)} = \sin\frac{2\pi j}{N} \qquad (4.91)$$

where $j$ denotes the position of the capacitors in the end-ring and $N$ denotes the total number of capacitors in the end-ring. Consider the first dominant mode in Eq. (4.90). It is clear that the current is maximum in the $(N/2)$th and $N$th capacitors and zero in the $(N/4)$th and $(3N/4)$th capacitors. Therefore, the resonant frequency of this mode is mostly affected by the $(N/2)$th and $N$th capacitors and will not be influenced by the $(N/4)$th and $(3N/4)$th capacitors. However, for the second dominant mode in Eq. (4.91), the current is maximum in the $(N/4)$th and $(3N/4)$th capacitors and zero in the $(N/2)$th and $N$th capacitors. Hence, the resonant frequency of this mode is mostly affected by the $(N/4)$th and $(3N/4)$th capacitors and will not be influenced by the $(N/2)$th and $N$th capacitors. As a result, we may decrease the resonant frequency of the first mode by increasing the capacitance in the $(N/2)$th and $N$th capacitors without affecting the current distribution of the second mode. Similarly, we may increase the resonant frequency of the second mode by reducing the capacitance in the $(N/4)$th and $(3N/4)$th capacitors without changing the current distribution of the first mode. However, an increase in the capacitance in the $(N/2)$th and $N$th capacitors does affect the current distribution of the first mode and a decrease in the capacitance in the $(N/4)$th and $(3N/4)$th capacitors also changes the current distribution of the second mode. To minimize these effects, we can distribute the changes in capacitance to all the capacitors according to the formula:

$$C_j = C + \Delta C \left| \cos \frac{2\pi j}{N} \right| - \Delta C \left| \sin \frac{2\pi j}{N} \right| \tag{4.92}$$

or (Joseph and Lu 1989)

$$C_j = C + \Delta C \cos \frac{4\pi j}{N} \tag{4.93}$$

where $C_j$ denotes the capacitance of the $j$th capacitor, and $C$ denotes the capacitance of the unperturbed coil, whose unsplit resonant frequency is in between the two desired frequencies, and $\Delta C$ denotes the maximum change in the capacitance, which is chosen to split the resonant frequency to the desired frequencies. A similar idea can be applied to a lowpass and a hybrid birdcage coil. As demonstrated by Joseph and Lu (1989), provided that the two desired frequencies are not far apart, the field inhomogeneity introduced by the perturbation in Eq. (4.92) or (4.93) is insignificant.

Whereas the method described above is simple and effective, it has a major disadvantage in that the coil constructed can generate only a linearly polarized field. One solution to this problem is proposed by Lu and Joseph (1991), which is based on the fact that the resonant frequency of a coil can be affected by the presence of an RF shield. As discussed in Section 4.4.1, the effect of a shield is to reduce the inductance and thus increase the resonant frequency and the degree of this effect is mainly determined by the distance between the coil and the shield. Therefore, a shield of a different radius will shift the resonant frequency differently. Based on this observation, Lu and Joseph (1991) designed a birdcage coil with two shields. The larger shield shifts the resonant frequency to 100.5 MHz and the smaller shield shifts the resonant frequency to 109.2 MHz. Of course, in this case, it is necessary to slide in or slide out the smaller shield between different imaging and, therefore, simultaneous imaging is impossible. Also, the difference between the two desired frequencies must be sufficiently small.

Another method to obtain a double-tuned quadrature birdcage coil is to use two birdcage coils arranged in a coaxial manner (Fitzsimmons *et al.* 1993). One coil is used at one frequency and the other is used at a different frequency. To reduce the mutual coupling between the two coils, which can cause a significant loss to the received signal, the two coils are rotated into a position so that the legs of one coil are placed midway between the legs of the other coil. Also, one coil is made shorter than the other to minimize the mutual coupling in the end-rings. It is observed that such a configuration is nearly ideal in the low frequency mode and is somewhat inefficient in the high frequency mode (Fitzsimmons *et al.* 1993). However, even at the high frequency, the quadrature gain is better than in the linear mode. This design may be improved by using a lowpass coil for the high frequency and a highpass coil for the low frequency to further reduce the mutual coupling between the two coils.

In addition to the methods discussed above, there are several other design schemes to realize a double-tuned coil (Bolinger *et al.* 1988, Insko and Leigh 1993, Issac *et al.* 1990, Pascone *et al.* 1993, Rath 1990). Most use a tune circuit, which introduces additional circuit losses. A good review, including an extensive list of references, is given by Fitzsimmons *et al.* (1993).

### 4.7.4 Surface Coils

In the design of transmit/receive RF coils for MRI, one always faces a dilemma: the coil should be as large as possible in order to produce a uniform field, but, by reciprocity, a large coil would receive all of the RF noises generated by the volume it illuminates, while the useful NMR signal would only come from the slice to be imaged. Thus, the SNR of MR images is reduced significantly. Traditionally, this dilemma is solved by employing two separate coils: one for transmitting, which is typically a whole-body birdcage coil, and the other for receiving, which is typically a surface coil because of its small field of view (FOV). A surface coil is particularly useful to obtain images and spectra from tissues close to the surface. A detailed discussion on the surface coil technology is given by Bendall (1988). Recent efforts have focused on the design of surface coils for quadrature detection, as pointed out earlier.

### 4.7.5 Phased Arrays

Surface coils provide a higher SNR than whole-body coils because of their smaller sensitive region, which decreases the amount of noise that is received from the sample. Unfortunately, the usable FOV is also limited to the size of the sensitive region. In clinical imaging, it is desirable to have a large FOV because the region of interest is often not known prior to the first scan. One simple solution is to use a large coil, which has a lower SNR, or to reposition a smaller coil and repeat the study, which is time consuming. Another solution is to use multiple coils or a coil array to provide a large region of sensitivity. Each coil is connected to an independent preamplifier and receiver channel. The outputs from the receiver channels are combined in an optimum manner with a phase correction dependent on the point in space from which the signal originated. In this way, one can obtain the high SNR of surface coils and a large FOV usually associated with large coils, without any penalty in imaging time. Such a coil array is named the NMR phased array and is treated in detail in the classical paper by Roemer *et al.* (1990). Technical issues discussed include how to eliminate the interactions (mutual coupling) between coils with overlapping FOVs (by overlapping adjacent coils and connecting all coils to preamplifiers with a low input impedance) and how to combine the data from the phased array elements to yield an image with optimum SNR. A four element array having a FOV of 48 cm was constructed for spine imaging. This technique was then extended for volume imaging by Hayes *et al.* (1991). The noise correlation in the data simultaneously acquired from multiple coils is studied by Hayes and Roemer (1990) and by Redpath (1992). The major disadvantage of a phased array is the high cost of the additional receiver channels. This is avoided in the designs proposed by Wright *et al.* (1991, 1992) and Porter *et al.* (1994), which either use multiple coils with selectable sensitive regions or employ RF time-multiplexing to enable the use of multiple array elements with one receiver channel.

### 4.7.6 Unicoil Concept and Design

When separate transmit and receive coils are used for MRI, the two coils must be well decoupled. One way to achieve such a decoupling is to place

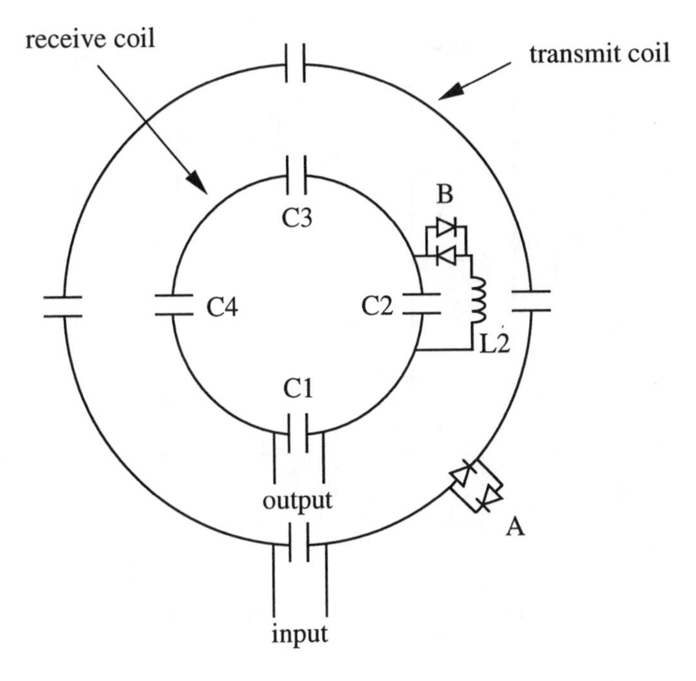


**Figure 4.38.** Concentric transmit and receive coils using crossed diodes for decoupling.

the two coils so that their $B_1$ fields are orthogonal to each other; however, this design is difficult to implement. Another way is to use crossed diodes, as proposed by Bendall (1983) and subsequently employed by Styles *et al.* (1985), Edelstein *et al.* (1986), Bendall *et al.* (1986), Froncisz *et al.* (1986), and Hyde *et al.* (1990). This method is practically convenient and very effective. To illustrate the basic principle of this method, consider the configuration sketched in Fig. 4.38, where a small receive coil is placed inside a large transmit coil. The receive coil is designed so that when the crossed diodes B are open, it resonates at the desired operating frequency. The transmit coil is designed so that when the crossed diodes A are shorted, it resonates at the desired frequency. Therefore, when this system is used in MRI, during transmission, the currents in the two coils are sufficiently strong that both crossed diodes A and B are short-circuited. Because of the effect of $L_2$ in the receive coil, the receive coil's resonant frequency is shifted away from the operating frequency and the mutual coupling is reduced. Furthermore, the high impedance of the $C_2$-$L_2$ circuit prevents significant current flow in the receive coil. Thus, the $B_1$ field produced

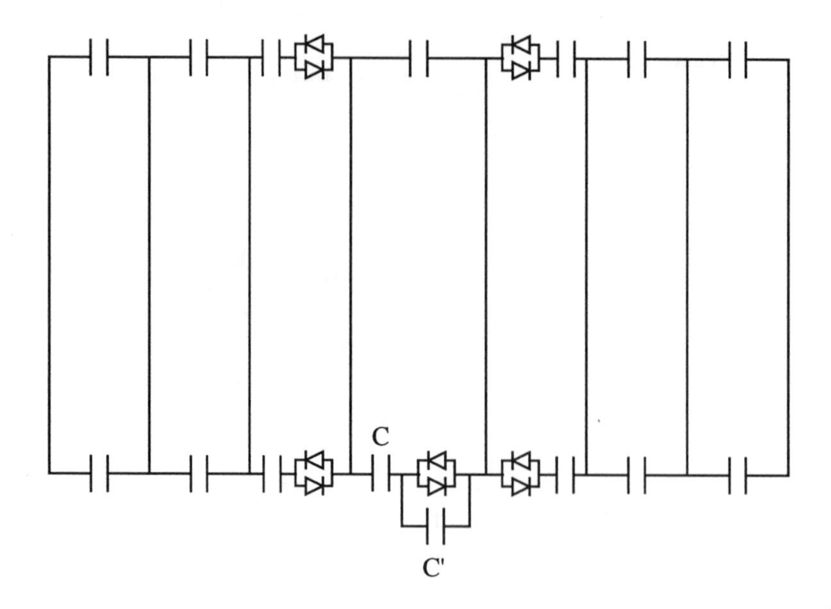


**Figure 4.39.** Schematic sketch of a unicoil.

by the transmit coil is unaffected. During reception, the currents in the two coils are very weak and both crossed diodes A and B are open. The transmit coil becomes an open circuit and the noise picked up by this coil will not be coupled to the receive coil, which now has a resonant frequency the same as the operating frequency.

Note that in the design discussed above, the receive and transmit coils are two separate coils. Another design, proposed by Jin and Perkins (1994), integrates both transmit and receive coils into a single coil: the smaller receive coil is part of the large transmit coil. For this reason, the resulting coil is referred to as a unicoil.

The basic principle of a unicoil can be understood by examining the simple configuration illustrated in Fig. 4.39, which is basically a segment of a highpass ladder network. During the transmission period, the electric currents in the coil are strong so all of the crossed diodes become short-circuited. Therefore, the equivalent circuit during this period becomes the one shown in Fig. 4.40(a). This large coil can produce a relatively uniform $B_1$ field to excite the volume to be imaged. On the other hand, during the reception period, the electric currents in the coil are very small so all of the diodes are basically open. The equivalent circuit during this period has three unconnected sections, as illustrated in Fig. 4.40(b). Since the two

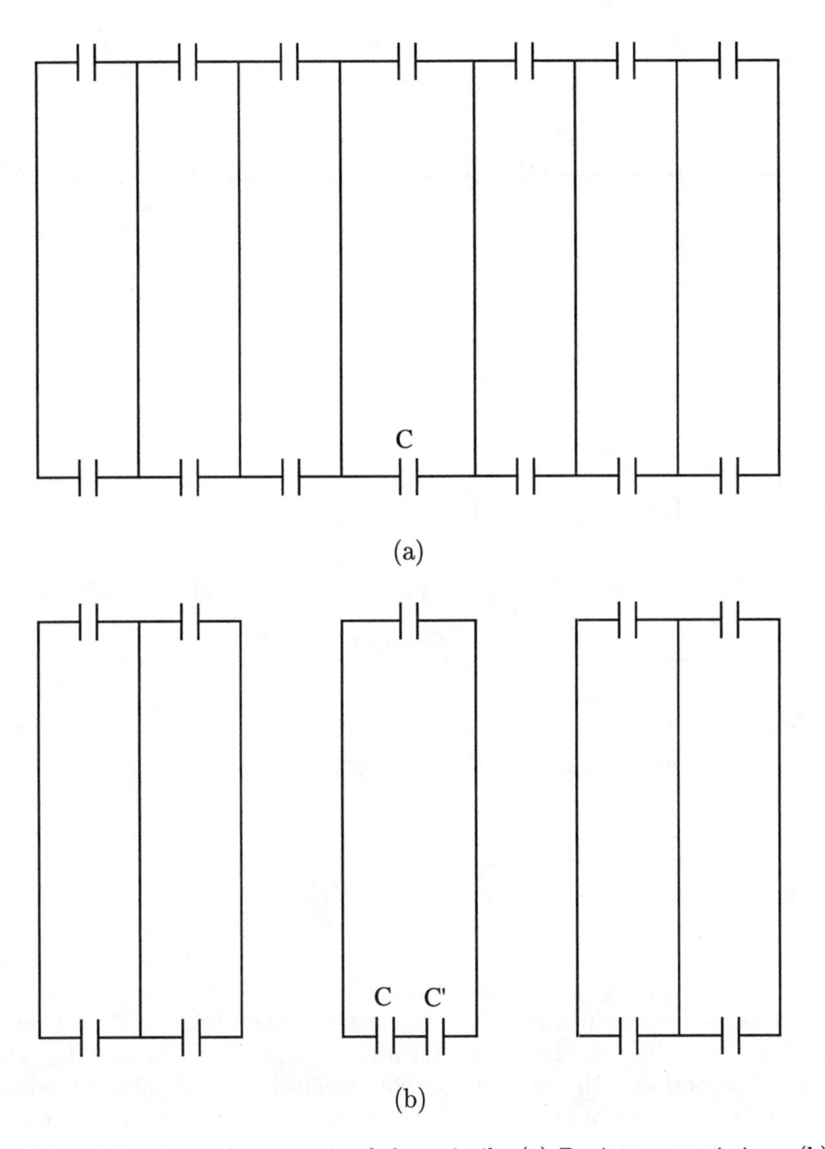


**Figure 4.40.** Equivalent circuit of the unicoil. (a) During transmission. (b) During reception.

sections on the left- and right-hand sides are part of the transmit coil that operates at 63.85 MHz (for 1.5 T MRI systems), the resonant frequencies of these two circuits are much lower than 63.85 MHz. This, however, is

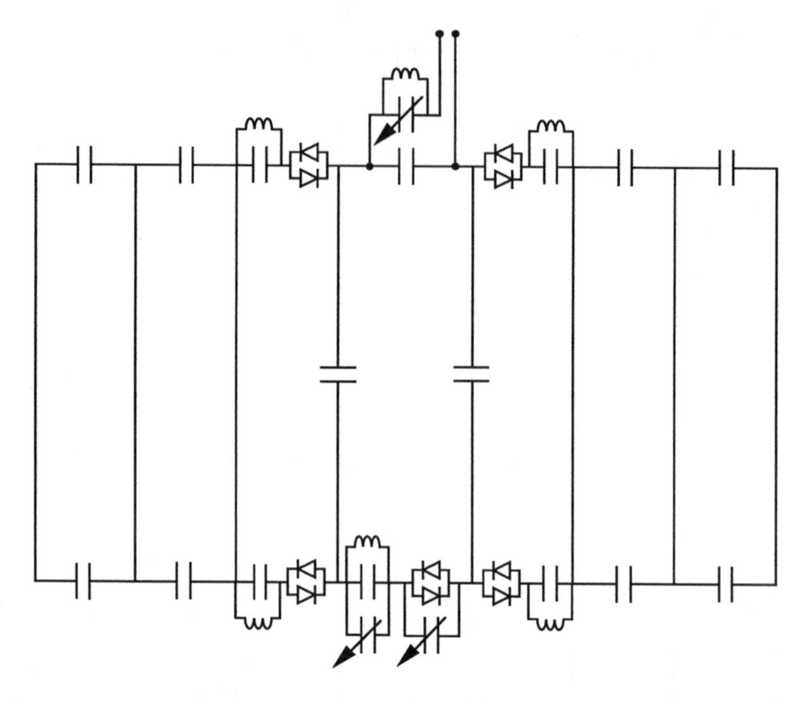

**Figure 4.41.** Practical design of a unicoil with tune and match capacitors. The inductors are added to facilitate the tuning process.

not true for the section in the middle because of capacitor $C'$, which can bring the resonant frequency up to 63.85 MHz. As a result, the circuit in the middle can be used as a receive coil, and, since it is relatively small, it receives noise only from its nearby volume. A practical design of a unicoil is illustrated in Fig. 4.41, which also shows the drive, tune, and match schemes. Several inductors are used to facilitate the tuning of the transmit and receive coils. Experiments (Jin and Perkins 1994) showed that the unicoil outperforms the conventional coil (when the entire coil was used for reception) in terms of SNR by a factor of two on phantoms and a factor of over 1.7 on patients.

## Problems

4.1 Consider the $RLC$ circuit in Fig. 4.3 with $L = 0.025$ $\mu$H and $C = 10$ pF. Plot the current as a function of frequency from 0 to 100 MHz for $R = 0.01$ $\Omega$ and $R = 1$ $\Omega$.

4.2 Because of radiation and conduction losses, an RF coil has a resistance which can be denoted as $r_{\text{coil}}$. When the coil is loaded with a sample, the sample introduces an additional resistance denoted as $r_{\text{sample}}$. Given a coil whose quality factor is $Q_{\text{empty}}$ when it is empty and $Q_{\text{loaded}}$ when it is loaded with the sample, find the ratio between $r_{\text{coil}}$ and $r_{\text{sample}}$.

4.3 A highpass birdcage made of capacitors having the value of 100 pF has the resonant frequency of 55 MHz. Find the desired capacitance so that the resonant frequency becomes 64 MHz.

4.4 Consider two problems illustrated below. In problem (a), a magnetization (**M**) in an object induces a voltage ($V_1$) in an RF coil. In problem (b), a current ($I_2$) produces a magnetic field ($\mathbf{B}_2$) inside the object through the RF coil. Starting from Maxwell's equations for these two problems, derive Eq. (4.20).

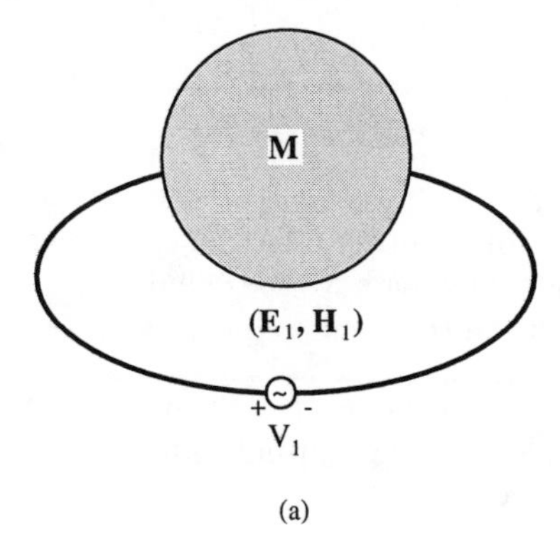


(a)

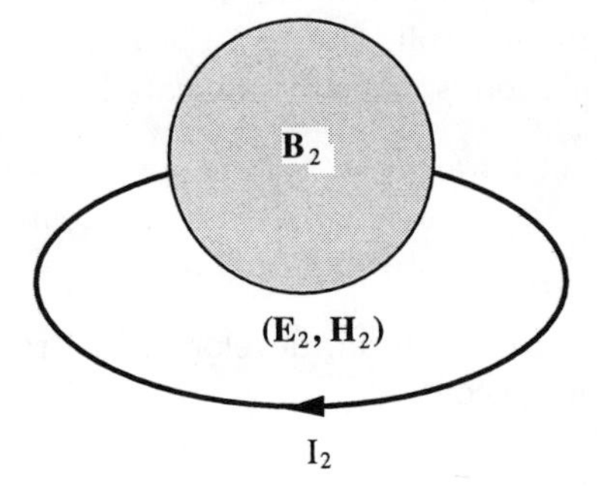


(b)

4.5 Consider a surface coil whose equivalent circuit is shown below. This coil can be used as a quadrature receiver. (a) Find all resonant frequencies of this coil. (b) Sketch the current in the coil for each resonant mode. Indicate the direction of the magnetic field of each mode above the coil. (c) Find the value of $C'$ so that the two resonant modes have the same resonant frequencies.

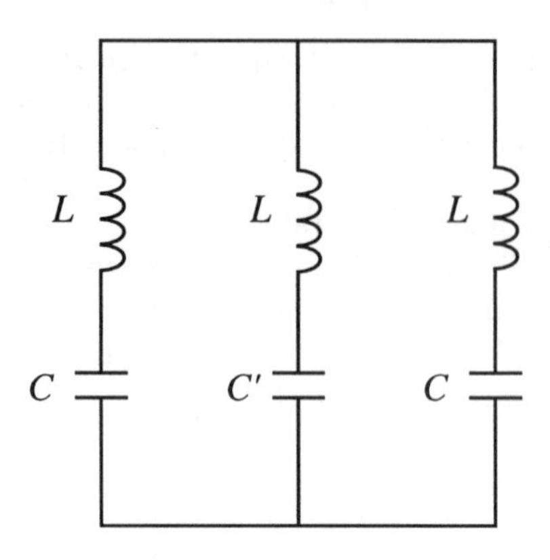


4.6 Consider a highpass birdcage coil whose two end-rings have different capacitors. The capacitors in one end-ring have the value of $C^u$ and those in the other end-ring have the value of $C^l$. Neglect all the mutual inductance. Find the resonant frequencies of the coil.

4.7 Consider an open coil made of a segment of hybrid ladder network (Fig. 4.10). Neglect all the mutual inductance and find the resonant frequencies of the coil.

4.8 Based on the formulation given in Eqs. (4.32) to (4.38), write a computer program to calculate the resonant frequencies and currents of a highpass birdcage coil. (Neglect the $L_{j,k}$ when $j \neq k$ and all $\tilde{L}_{j,k}$ since their calculation is rather complicated.)

4.9 Based on the Biot-Savart law, write a computer program to calculate the $B_1$ field in the axial plane across the center of a birdcage coil. Integrate this program into the program developed in Problem 4.8.

4.10 Modify the computer program developed in Problem 4.8 for lowpass and hybrid birdcage coils.

4.11 Modify the computer program developed in Problem 4.8 for an open highpass coil.

4.12 Include the effect of an RF shield in the computer programs developed in Problems 4.8 to 4.11.

4.13 Consider a circular loop placed in front of a large conducting plane in a parallel manner. Use the image method to find the magnetic field along the axis of the coil.

4.14 Based on the formulation in Section 4.7, write a method of moments program to analyze the surface coil in Fig. 4.5. Compare the numerical result to the approximate result given in Eq. (4.25). (The reader can choose appropriate values for the coil size and the capacitor.)

4.15 Apply the method of moments program developed in Problem 4.14 to the surface coil shown below. Compare the numerical result to the approximate solution obtained using the equivalent circuit method in Problem 4.5.

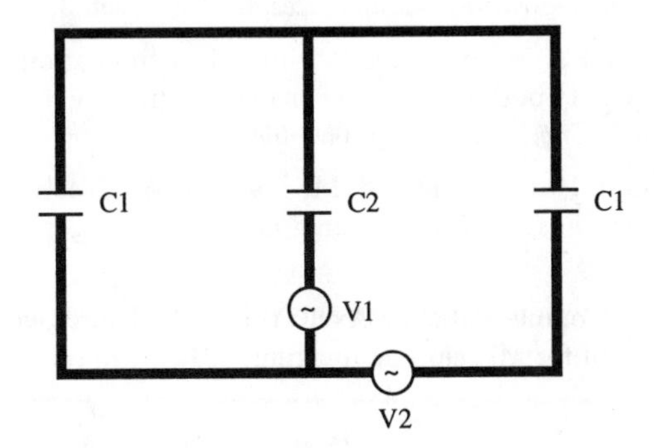


4.16 Consider two circular coils placed in the same plane. Find the overlapping area so that there is no mutual coupling between the coils.

## References

Many papers have been written on the design of RF coils for MRI applications. The following list is not exhaustive; many good papers may have been neglected.

D. Ballon, M. C. Graham, S. Miodownik, and J. A. Koutcher (1990), "A 64 MHz half-birdcage resonator for clinical imaging," *J. Magn. Reson.*, vol. 90, pp. 131–140.

M. R. Bendall (1983), "Portable NMR sample localization method using inhomogeneous RF irradiation coils," *Chem. Phys. Lett.*, vol. 99, pp. 310–315.

M. R. Bendall, A. Connelly, and J. M. McKendry (1986), "Elimination of coupling between cylindrical transmit coils and surface receive coils for invivo NMR," *Magn. Reson. Med.*, vol. 3, pp. 157–163.

M. R. Bendall (1988), "Surface coil technology," in *Magnetic Resonance Imaging*, Vol II. C. L. Partain *et al.* Eds. Philadelphia: W. B. Saunders Company.

L. Bolinger, M. G. Prammer, and J. S. Leigh (1988), "A multiple-frequency coil with a highly uniform $B_1$ field," *J. Magn. Reson.*, vol. 81, pp. 162–166.

E. Boskamp, J. S. Hyde, and M. Wolski (1992), "A new approach to planar quadrature coils," *Works in Progress, 11th Annu. Sci. Mtg. Soc. Magn. Reson. Med.*, p. 4006.

C.-N. Chen, D. I. Hoult, and V. J. Sank (1983), "Quadrature detection coils—A further improvement in sensitivity," *J. Magn. Reson.*, vol. 54, pp. 324–327.

C.-N. Chen, V. J. Sank, S. M. Cohen, and D. I. Hoult (1986), "The field dependence of NMR imaging. I. Laboratory assessment of signal-to-noise ratio and power deposition," *Magn. Reson. Med.*, vol. 3, pp. 722–729.

J. Chen, Z. Feng, and J. M. Jin (1998), "Numerical simulation of SAR and $B_1$-field inhomogeneity of shielded RF coils loaded with the human head," *IEEE Trans. Biomed. Eng.*, vol. 45, pp. 650–659.

W. A. Edelstein, C. J. Hardy, and O. M. Mueller (1986), "Electronic decoupling of surface-coil receivers for NMR imaging and spectroscopy," *J. Magn. Reson.*, vol. 67, pp. 156–161.

Z. A. Fayad, T. J. Connick, and L. Axel (1995), "An improved quadrature or phased-array coil for MR cardiac imaging," *Magn. Reson. Med.*, vol. 34, pp. 186–193.

J. R. Fitzsimmons and B. L. Beck (1992), "The application of quadrature technology to quasi-volume geometries," *Works in Progress, 11th Annu. Sci. Mtg. Soc. Magn. Reson. Med.*, p. 4043.

J. R. Fitzsimmons, B. L. Beck, and H. R. Brooker (1993), "Double resonant quadrature birdcage," *Magn. Reson. Med.*, vol. 30, pp. 107–114.

W. Froncisz, A. Jesmanowicz, J. Kneeland, and J. S. Hyde (1986), "Counter rotating current local coils for high resolution magnetic resonance imaging," *Magn. Reson. Med.*, vol. 3, pp. 590–603.

G. H. Glover, C. E. Hayes, N. J. Pelc, W. A. Edelstein, O. M. Muller, H. R. Hart, C. J. Hardy, M. O'Donnell, and W. D. Barber (1985), "Comparison of linear and circular polarization for magnetic resonance imaging," *J. Magn. Reson.*, vol. 64, pp. 255–270.

R. F. Harrington (1961), *Time-Harmonic Electromagnetic Fields.* New York: McGraw-Hill.

R. F. Harrington (1993), *Field Computation by Moment Methods.* New York: IEEE Press.

C. E. Hayes (1986), "An end-cap birdcage resonator for quadrature head imaging," *Works in Progress, 5th Annu. Sci. Mtg. Soc. Magn. Reson. Med.*, pp. 39–40.

C. E. Hayes and M. G. Eash (1987), "Shield for decoupling RF and gradient coils in an NMR apparatus," U.S. patent: 4,642,569.

C. E. Hayes, W. A. Edelstein, and J. F. Schenck (1986), "Radio frequency coils," in *NMR in Medicine*, S. R. Thomas and R. L. Dixon, Eds. New York: American Association Physicists Med., pp. 142–165.

C. E. Hayes, W. A. Edelstein, J. F. Schenck, O. M. Mueller, and M. Eash (1985), "An efficient, highly homogeneous radiofrequency coil for whole-body NMR imaging at 1.5 T," *J. Magn. Reson.*, vol. 63, pp. 622–628.

C. E. Hayes, N. Hattes, and P. B. Roemer (1991), "Volume imaging with MR phased arrays," *Magn. Reson. Med.*, vol. 18, pp. 309–319.

C. E. Hayes and P. B. Roemer (1990), "Noise correlations in data simultaneously acquired from multiple surface coil arrays," *Magn. Reson. Med.*, vol. 16, pp. 181–191.

D. I. Hoult and R. E. Richards (1976), "The signal-to-noise ratio of the nuclear magnetic resonance experiment," *J. Magn. Reson.*, vol. 24, pp. 71–85.

J. S. Hyde, A. Jesmanowicz, T. M. Grist, W. Froncisz, and J. B. Kneeland (1987), "Quadrature detection surface coil," *Magn. Reson. Med.*, vol. 4, pp. 179–184.

J. S. Hyde, R. J. Rilling, and A. Jesmanowicz (1990), "Passive decoupling of surface coils by pole insertion," *J. Magn. Reson.*, vol. 89, pp. 485–495.

E. K. Insko and J. S. Leigh (1993), "A double discrete cosine quadrature coil design," *J. Magn. Reson. Series A*, vol. 104, pp. 78–82.

G. Isaac, M. D. Schnall, R. T. Lenkinski, and K. Vogele (1990), "A design for double-tuned birdcage coil for use in an integrated MRI/MRS examination," *J. Magn. Reson.*, vol. 89, pp. 41–50.

J. M. Jin, G. Shen, and T. Perkins (1993), "Analysis of open coils including shielding effects for MRI applications," *Proc. 12th Annu. Mtg. Soc. Magn. Reson. Med.*, p. 1354.

J. M. Jin and T. Perkins (1994), "An innovative design of combined transmit/receive RF coils for MR imaging," *Proc. 2nd Mtg. Soc. Magn. Reson.*, p. 1116.

J. M. Jin, G. Shen, and T. Perkins (1994), "On the field inhomogeneity of birdcage coils," *Magn. Reson. Med.*, vol. 32, pp. 418–422.

J. M. Jin, R. L. Magin, G. Shen, and T. Perkins (1995), "A simple method to incorporate the effects of an RF shield into RF resonator analysis for MRI applications," *IEEE Trans. Biomed. Eng.*, vol. 42, pp. 840–843.

P. M. Joseph and D. Lu (1989), "A technique for double resonant operation of birdcage imaging coils," *IEEE Trans. Med. Imaging*, vol. 8, pp. 286–294.

W. P. Kuan and C. J. Leu (1992), "A comparison between quadrature and optimized linear surface coil," *Book of Abstracts, 11th Annu. Sci. Mtg. Soc. Magn. Reson. Med.*, p. 280.

C. T. Lee, R. Pavlovich, and E. Boskamp (1990), "3D anatomically shaped quadrature surface coils," *Book of Abstracts, 9th Annu. Sci. Mtg. Soc. Magn. Reson. Med.*, p. 524.

D. Lu and P. M. Joseph (1991), "A technique of double-resonant operation of $^{19}$F and $^{1}$H quadrature birdcage coils," *Magn. Reson. Med.*, vol. 19, pp. 180–185.

K. I. Marro, C. E. Hayes, and T. L. Richards (1992), "An inductively driven 200 MHz bird-cage resonator with built-in variable tuning capacitors," *Works in Progress, 11th Annu. Sci. Mtg. Soc. Magn. Reson. Med.*, p. 4001.

H. Ochi, E. Yamamoto, K. Sawaya, and S. Adachi (1994), "Analysis of magnetic resonance imaging antenna inside an RF shield," *Electron. Comm. Japan*, Part 1, vol. 77, pp. 37–44.

R. J. Pascone, B. J. Garcia, T. M. Fitzgerald, T. Vullo, R. Zipagan, and P. T. Cahill (1991), "Generalized electrical analysis of low-pass and high-pass birdcage resonators," *Magn. Reson. Imaging*, vol. 9, pp. 395–408.

R. Pascone, T. Vullo, J. Farrelly, R. Mancuso, and P. T. Cahill, (1993), "Use of transmission line analysis for multi-tuning of birdcage resonators," *Magn. Reson. Imaging*, vol. 11, pp. 705–715.

P. Pimmel and A. Briguet (1992), "A hybrid bird cage resonator for sodium observation at 4.7 T," *Magn. Reson. Med.*, vol. 24, pp. 158–162.

J. R. Porter, S. M. Wright, and N. Famili (1994), "A four channel time domain multiplexer: A cost-effective alternative to multiple receivers," *Magn. Reson. Med.*, vol. 32, pp. 499–504.

S. M. Rao, D. R. Wilton, and A. W. Glisson (1982), "Electromagnetic scattering by surfaces of arbitrary shape," *IEEE Trans. Antennas Propagat.*, vol. 30, pp. 409–418.

A. R. Rath (1990), "Design and performance of double-tuned bird-cage coil," *J. Magn. Reson.*, vol. 86, pp. 488–495.

T. W. Redpath (1992), "Noise correlation in multicoil receiver systems," *Magn. Reson. Med.*, vol. 24, pp. 85–89.

P. B. Roemer, W. A. Edelstein, C. E. Hayes, S. P. Souza, and O. M. Muller (1990), "The NMR phased array," *Magn. Reson. Med.*, vol. 16, pp. 192–225.

G. Shen (1992), "Doubled-sided stripline RF shield," *Works in Progress, 11th Annu. Sci. Mtg. Soc. Magn. Reson. Med.*, p. 4048.

P. Styles, M. B. Smith, R. W. Briggs, and G. K. Radda (1985), "A concentric surface-coil probe for the production of homogeneous $B_1$ fields," *J. Magn. Reson.*, vol. 62, pp. 397–405.

J. Tropp (1989), "The theory of the bird-cage resonator," *J. Magn. Reson.*, vol. 82, pp. 51–62.

J. Tropp (1992), "The hybrid bird cage resonator," *Works in Progress, 11th Annu. Sci. Mtg. Soc. Magn. Reson. Med.*, p. 4009.

J. T. Vaughan, H. P. Hetherington, J. G. Harrison, J. O. Otu, J. W. Pan, P. J. Noa, and G. M. Pohost (1993), "High frequency coils for clinical nuclear magnetic resonance imaging and spectroscopy," *Phys. Med.*, vol. IX, pp. 147–153.

J. T. Vaughan, H. P. Hetherington, J. O. Otu, J. W. Pan, and G. M. Pohost (1994), "High frequency volume coils for clinical NMR imaging and spectroscopy," *Magn. Reson. Med.*, vol. 32, pp. 206–218.

T. Vullo, R. T. Zipagan, R. Pascone, J. P. Whalen, and P. T. Cahill (1992), "Experimental and fabrication of birdcage resonators for magnetic resonance imaging," *Magn. Reson. Med.*, vol. 24, pp. 243–252.

J. C. Watkins and E. Fukushima (1988), "High-pass bird-cage coil for nuclear magnetic resonance," *Rev. Sci. Instrum.*, vol. 59, pp. 926–929.

E. C. Wong, E. Boskamp, and J. S. Hyde (1992), "A volume optimized quadrature elliptical end-cap birdcage brain coil," *Works in Progress, 11th Annu. Sci. Mtg. Soc. Magn. Reson. Med.*, p. 4015.

S. M. Wright, R. L. Magin, and J. R. Kelton (1991), "Arrays of mutually coupled receiver coils: Theory and application," *Magn. Reson. Med.*, vol. 17, pp. 252–268.

S. M. Wright and J. R. Porter (1992), "Parallel acquisition of MR images using time multiplexed coils," *Electron. Lett.*, vol. 28, pp. 71–72.

# Chapter 5

# RF Fields in Biological Objects

## 5.1 Introduction

As discussed earlier, in magnetic resonance imaging (MRI) the nuclei are excited by the radiofrequency (RF) magnetic field known as the $B_1$ field. For MRI systems that use a low (less than 0.5 T) static magnetic field known as the $B_0$ field, the Larmor frequency and, hence, the frequency of the $B_1$ field, is very low and the dimension of the human body is only a small fraction of the wavelength. In this case, the interaction between the $B_1$ field and the human body can be neglected and the $B_1$ field can be evaluated in the absence of the human body. Also, the electric field associated with the $B_1$ field is negligible and so is the specific energy absorption rate (SAR).[1]

However, because of the limitation of the signal-to-noise ratio (SNR) associated with low frequencies, low $B_0$-field MRI systems cannot produce SNR high enough for some advanced studies such as functional MRI. To enhance the SNR, MRI systems using a high $B_0$ field have been developed. Systems with 1.5 T have been commercially available for several years, and many research institutions are developing systems with the $B_0$ field as high as 8 T. However, as the strength of the $B_0$ field increases, the frequency of the $B_1$ field increases linearly. For example, the frequency of the $B_1$ field for the 4 T system is 171 MHz for proton imaging. At such a high frequency, the interaction between the $B_1$ field and the human body can no longer

[1] The specific absorption rate (SAR) is a measure of power dissipated in a biological sample. It is defined as

$$\text{SAR} = \frac{\text{total RF energy dissipated in sample (Joules)}}{\text{exposure time (Seconds)} \cdot \text{sample weight (Kg)}} \quad \text{(Watts/Kg)}.$$

The United Sates Food and Drug Administration (USFDA) recommends that the SAR be limited. The SAR must be less than 0.4 W/Kg for the whole body and 3.2 W/Kg for the head. For any one gram of tissue, it must be less than 8.0 W/Kg (Leigh 1990).

be neglected. This interaction is caused by dielectric resonance since the effective wavelength of the $B_1$ field is now comparable to or even smaller than the dimension of the human body (Glover *et al.* 1985, Roeschmann 1987). Such a strong interaction not only degrades substantially the $B_1$ field homogeneity and thus the imaging quality, but can also cause concern about the safety, because the electric field associated with the $B_1$ field increases with the inhomogeneity of the $B_1$ field. Some parts of the body, such as the brain and eyes, can be sensitive to a change of temperature caused by the increased SAR.

The electromagnetic interaction with the human body associated with MRI has been studied by a number of researchers. Early work was based on a simple model that approximates the human body with an infinitely long circular cylinder or the head with a homogeneous sphere (Bottomley and Andrew 1978, Mansfield and Morris 1982, Glover *et al.* 1985, Bottomley *et al.* 1985, Foo *et al.* 1991, Keltner *et al.* 1991). The analytical solution for such a problem showed, indeed, that as the frequency increases, the interaction between electromagnetic fields and the biological object becomes stronger. Recognizing the basic limitations of analytical methods, recent work has concentrated on numerical methods. Most of these, however, focused on the two-dimensional (2D) approximation and few dealt with three-dimensional (3D) analysis. For example, Yang *et al.* (1993) employed a 2D finite element method (FEM) and studied the effect of dielectric resonance. Han and Wright (1993) used the finite-difference time-domain (FDTD) method and studied RF penetration effects caused by surface coils. Ochi *et al.* (1992, 1995) developed a moment method for the analysis of MRI coils based on an integral equation. Jin and Chen (1996) developed a fast 2D FEM to study the $B_1$-field inhomogeneity and SAR of both linear and quadrature, shielded and unshielded birdcage coils loaded with the human head or human trunk. Furthermore, Yang *et al.* (1994), Harrison and Vaughan (1996), and Simunic *et al.* (1996) applied the 3D FEM to model head coils loaded with a simple model of the human head. Jin *et al.* (1996) and Chen *et al.* (1998) developed two efficient and accurate numerical methods to investigate the electromagnetic field interaction with the human head using an anatomically accurate 3D model. One method uses the biconjugate gradient algorithm in combination with the fast Fourier transform to solve a matrix equation resulting from the discretization of an integrodifferential equation representing the original physical problem. The method is applicable only to open coils. The other method employs the FDTD method in conjunction with perfectly matched layers to solve Maxwell's equations in time domain directly and is capable of dealing with both open and shielded coils. Both methods can compute the electric field, the SAR, and the $B_1$ field excited by any MRI coils. While the literature

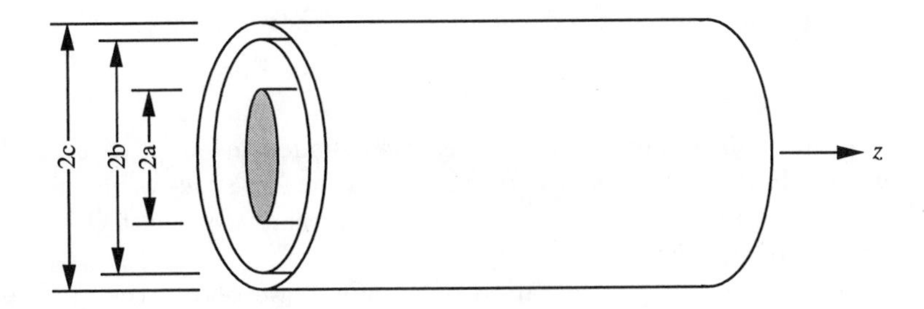


**Figure 5.1.** A lossy dielectric cylinder placed inside a cylindrical surface current enclosed in a conducting shell.

on the numerical simulation of electromagnetic fields for MRI applications is limited, there have been many articles on electromagnetic simulations for other applications such as RF and microwave hyperthermia, mostly using the FEM and the FDTD method (Grandolfo *et al.* 1990, Chen and Gandhi 1991, Gandhi *et al.* 1992, Sullivan 1992, Paulsen *et al.* 1993).

In this chapter, we describe both analytical and numerical methods to study the RF field in biological objects related to MRI applications. The analytical method is for simple models, which can be used to validate numerical methods. The numerical methods include the finite difference, finite element, finite-difference time-domain, and moment methods.

## 5.2 Analytical Methods

In this section, we consider two examples to illustrate the basic procedures of analytical methods for analyzing RF fields in dielectric objects. One is a two-dimensional example and the other is a three-dimensional example.

### 5.2.1 Two-Dimensional Example

Consider the problem illustrated in Fig. 5.1, where a lossy dielectric cylinder of radius $a$, representing the body, is placed inside a surface cylindrical current of radius $b$, approximating an RF coil, which is, in turn, enclosed by an RF shield of radius $c$. The current in the coil has only a $z$-component, which is given by

$$J_z(\phi) = J_0 \cos\phi \tag{5.1}$$

where $J_0$ is a constant. Such a current will excite an electric field that has only a $z$-component. From Eq. (2.114), we obtain the differential equation

$$\nabla^2 E_z + k_0^2 \epsilon_c E_z = 0 \tag{5.2}$$

for the electric field inside the dielectric cylinder ($\rho < a$) and

$$\nabla^2 E_z + k_0^2 E_z = 0 \tag{5.3}$$

for the electric field outside the dielectric cylinder ($a < \rho < b$) and ($b < \rho < c$). In the above, $k_0 = \omega\sqrt{\mu_0\epsilon_0}$ denotes the free-space wavenumber and $\epsilon_c = \epsilon_r + i\sigma/\omega\epsilon_0$, with $\epsilon_r$ and $\sigma$ being the relative permittivity and conductivity of the dielectric cylinder.

Using the method of separation of variables, we obtain the general solutions of Eqs. (5.2) and (5.3) as

$$E_z(\rho,\phi) = \sum_{m=-\infty}^{\infty} A_m J_m(k_d\rho)e^{im\phi} \qquad (\rho < a) \tag{5.4}$$

$$E_z(\rho,\phi) = \sum_{m=-\infty}^{\infty} \left[B_m J_m(k_0\rho) + C_m Y_m(k_0\rho)\right] e^{im\phi} \qquad (a < \rho < b) \tag{5.5}$$

$$E_z(\rho,\phi) = \sum_{m=-\infty}^{\infty} \left[D_m J_m(k_0\rho) + E_m Y_m(k_0\rho)\right] e^{im\phi} \qquad (b < \rho < c) \tag{5.6}$$

where $k_d = k_0\sqrt{\epsilon_c}$, $A_m$, $B_m$, $C_m$, $D_m$, and $E_m$ are the unknown expansion coefficients to be determined later, $J_m$ and $Y_m$ denote the $m$th-order Bessel functions of the first and second kinds, which are discussed in detail in Appendix 5.A. Note that $Y_m$ is not included in Eq. (5.4) because it is singular when $\rho = 0$. Since $E_z$ must be continuous across the interfaces at $\rho = a$ and $\rho = b$ and vanish at $\rho = c$, we have

$$A_m J_m(k_d a) = B_m J_m(k_0 a) + C_m Y_m(k_0 a) \tag{5.7}$$

$$B_m J_m(k_0 b) + C_m Y_m(k_0 b) = D_m J_m(k_0 b) + E_m Y_m(k_0 b) \tag{5.8}$$

$$D_m J_m(k_0 c) + E_m Y_m(k_0 c) = 0. \tag{5.9}$$

To arrive at these, we employed the orthogonality relations of the exponential functions given in Eq. (3.56). To solve for $A_m$, $B_m$, $C_m$, $D_m$, and $E_m$, we need another two equations, which can be obtained from the boundary conditions for the magnetic field. From Maxwell's equations, we obtain the $\phi$-component of the magnetic field

$$H_\phi(\rho,\phi) = \frac{ik_d}{\omega\mu_0} \sum_{m=-\infty}^{\infty} A_m J_m'(k_d\rho)e^{im\phi} \qquad (\rho < a) \tag{5.10}$$

$$H_\phi(\rho,\phi) = \frac{ik_0}{\omega\mu_0} \sum_{m=-\infty}^{\infty} \left[B_m J_m'(k_0\rho) + C_m Y_m'(k_0\rho)\right] e^{im\phi} \qquad (a < \rho < b) \tag{5.11}$$

$$H_\phi(\rho,\phi) = \frac{ik_0}{\omega\mu_0} \sum_{m=-\infty}^{\infty} \left[D_m J'_m(k_0\rho) + E_m Y'_m(k_0\rho)\right] e^{im\phi} \qquad (b < \rho < c). \tag{5.12}$$

Since $H_\phi$ must be continuous across the interface at $\rho = a$, we have

$$A_m k_d J'_m(k_d a) = k_0 \left[B_m J'_m(k_0 a) + C_m Y'_m(k_0 a)\right] \tag{5.13}$$

and, since $H_\phi$ at $\rho = b$ must satisfy the boundary condition in Eq. (2.107), we obtain

$$\sum_{m=-\infty}^{\infty} [D_m J'_m(k_0 b) + E_m Y'_m(k_0 b)] e^{im\phi} - \sum_{m=-\infty}^{\infty} [B_m J'_m(k_0 b) + C_m Y'_m(k_0 b)] e^{im\phi} = \frac{\omega\mu_0}{ik_0} J_0 \cos\phi. \tag{5.14}$$

Solving Eqs. (5.7)–(5.9), (5.13), and (5.14) for the unknown coefficients and substituting them into Eqs. (5.4) and (5.10), we finally obtain the fields inside the dielectric cylinder as

$$E_z(\rho,\phi) = A J_1(k_d\rho)\cos\phi \tag{5.15}$$

$$H_\phi(\rho,\phi) = A \frac{ik_d}{\omega\mu_0} J'_1(k_d\rho)\cos\phi \tag{5.16}$$

$$H_\rho(\rho,\phi) = A \frac{i}{\omega\mu_0\rho} J_1(k_d\rho)\sin\phi \tag{5.17}$$

where

$$A = \frac{b}{a} \frac{J_1(k_0 b) Y_1(k_0 c) - J_1(k_0 c) Y_1(k_0 b)}{k_d J'_1(k_d a) F(k_0,a,c) - k_0 J_1(k_d a) G(k_0,a,c)} \tag{5.18}$$

in which

$$F(k_0,a,c) = J_1(k_0 a) Y_1(k_0 c) - J_1(k_0 c) Y_1(k_0 a)$$
$$G(k_0,a,c) = J'_1(k_0 a) Y_1(k_0 c) - J_1(k_0 c) Y'_1(k_0 a).$$

With the formulation described above and the subroutine given in Appendix 5.A, one can easily write a computer program to calculate the SAR and $B_1$ field. This capability permits one to study various effects on the SAR and $B_1$ field, such as those caused by the shield and the frequency. The solution can also be used to validate the numerical methods discussed in the next section.

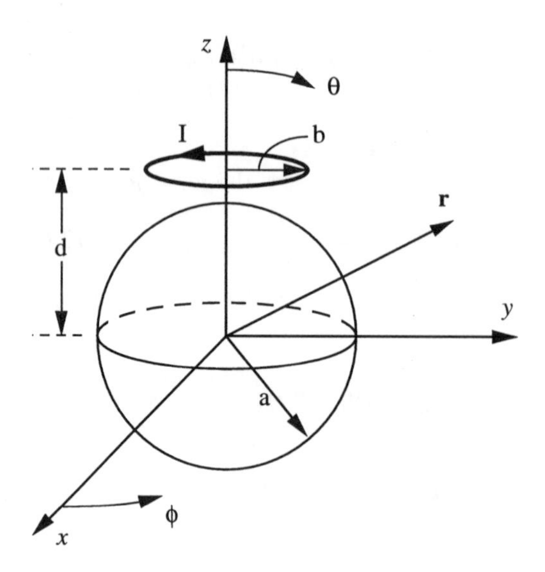


**Figure 5.2.** A surface coil is placed adjacent to a lossy dielectric sphere.

### 5.2.2 Three-Dimensional Example

Consider the problem illustrated in Fig. 5.2, where a loop (representing a surface coil) of radius $b$ carrying uniform current $I$ is placed adjacent to a lossy dielectric sphere of radius $a$. We wish to calculate the electric and magnetic fields induced inside the sphere. For convenience, we chose a spherical coordinate system, whose origin is located at the center of the sphere and whose $z$-axis coincides with the axis of the current loop. Because of the axisymmetric arrangement of the geometry, the fields produced by the current will not have any $\phi$-variation. Furthermore, because the current has only a $\phi$-component, the electric field $\mathbf{E}$ will not have a radial component, that is, $E_r = 0$. Such a field is known as a transverse electric (TE) field, which can be expressed in terms of the Debye potential $\pi_m$ (Chew 1995):

$$\mathbf{E} = \nabla \times (\mathbf{r}\pi_m) \tag{5.19}$$

and the magnetic field is then

$$\mathbf{H} = \frac{1}{i\omega\mu}\nabla \times \mathbf{E} = \frac{1}{i\omega\mu}\nabla \times \nabla \times (\mathbf{r}\pi_m). \tag{5.20}$$

By substituting the above into the source-free Maxwell's equations, we obtain

$$(\nabla^2 + k^2)\pi_m = 0 \tag{5.21}$$

where $k = \omega\sqrt{\mu\epsilon}$. Using the method of separation of variables, we obtain the general solution of Eq. (5.21) as

$$\pi_m = \sum_{n=0}^{\infty} \sum_{m=-n}^{n} \begin{Bmatrix} j_n(kr) \\ h_n^{(1)}(kr) \end{Bmatrix} P_n^m(\cos\theta) \begin{Bmatrix} \cos m\phi \\ \sin m\phi \end{Bmatrix} \tag{5.22}$$

where the brackets imply "linear combination of." In the above, $j_n(kr)$ is the $n$th-order spherical Bessel function of the first kind and $h_n^{(1)}(kr)$ is the $n$th-order spherical Hankel function of the first kind, both of which are discussed in Appendix 5.B. Also, $P_n^m(\cos\theta)$ is the associated Legendre polynomial, discussed in Appendix 2.B.

Although we can start from Eq. (5.22) to derive the general expressions for the electric and magnetic fields, the resulting expressions are lengthy and complicated. Therefore, let us first simplify Eq. (5.22) for our problem. Because of the axisymmetry, $\pi_m$ does not vary with $\phi$. Hence, $\pi_m$ can be simplified as

$$\pi_m = \sum_{n=0}^{\infty} \begin{Bmatrix} j_n(kr) \\ h_n^{(1)}(kr) \end{Bmatrix} P_n(\cos\theta) \tag{5.23}$$

where $P_n(\cos\theta)$ denotes the Legendre polynomial. Substituting Eq. (5.23) into Eqs. (5.19) and (5.20), we obtain the field expressions:

$$E_r = E_\theta = H_\phi = 0 \tag{5.24}$$

$$E_\phi = -\frac{\partial \pi_m}{\partial \theta} \tag{5.25}$$

$$H_r = \frac{1}{i\omega\mu}\left(\frac{\partial^2}{\partial r^2} + k^2\right)(r\pi_m) \tag{5.26}$$

$$H_\theta = \frac{1}{i\omega\mu}\frac{\partial^2(r\pi_m)}{r\partial r\partial\theta}. \tag{5.27}$$

With the solution given above, we now consider the fields in each specific region and then relate them to the excitation. For the field inside the dielectric sphere ($r < a$), we should exclude $h_n^{(1)}(kr)$ because of its singularity at the origin. Therefore, we have

$$E_\phi^{\text{in}} = -\sum_{n=1}^{\infty} a_n j_n(k_d r)\frac{\partial P_n(\cos\theta)}{\partial\theta} \tag{5.28}$$

$$H_r^{\text{in}} = \frac{1}{i\omega\mu_0}\frac{1}{r}\sum_{n=1}^{\infty} a_n n(n+1) j_n(k_d r) P_n(\cos\theta) \tag{5.29}$$

$$H_\theta^{\text{in}} = \frac{1}{i\omega\mu_0}\frac{1}{r}\sum_{n=1}^{\infty} a_n \frac{\partial[r j_n(k_d r)]}{\partial r}\frac{\partial P_n(\cos\theta)}{\partial\theta} \tag{5.30}$$

where $k_d = k_0\sqrt{\epsilon_c}$, $k_0 = \omega\sqrt{\mu_0\epsilon_0}$, and $\epsilon_c = \epsilon_r + i\sigma/\omega\epsilon_0$. In the middle region between the dielectric sphere and the spherical surface that contains the surface coil ($a < r < c$ where $c = \sqrt{b^2 + d^2}$), we have

$$E_\phi^{\text{mid}} = -\sum_{n=0}^{\infty}\left[b_n j_n(k_0 r) + c_n h_n^{(1)}(k_0 r)\right]\frac{\partial P_n(\cos\theta)}{\partial\theta} \tag{5.31}$$

$$H_r^{\text{mid}} = \frac{1}{i\omega\mu_0}\frac{1}{r}\sum_{n=0}^{\infty} n(n+1)\left[b_n j_n(k_0 r) + c_n h_n^{(1)}(k_0 r)\right]P_n(\cos\theta) \tag{5.32}$$

$$H_\theta^{\text{mid}} = \frac{1}{i\omega\mu_0}\frac{1}{r}\sum_{n=0}^{\infty}\left[b_n\frac{\partial[r j_n(k_0 r)]}{\partial r} + c_n\frac{\partial[r h_n^{(1)}(k_0 r)]}{\partial r}\right]\frac{\partial P_n(\cos\theta)}{\partial\theta}. \tag{5.33}$$

Finally, in the outer region ($r > c$), since the field should propagate away from the source, its expression should contain only $h_n^{(1)}(k_0 r)$. Therefore,

$$E_\phi^{\text{out}} = -\sum_{n=0}^{\infty} d_n h_n^{(1)}(k_0 r)\frac{\partial P_n(\cos\theta)}{\partial\theta} \tag{5.34}$$

$$H_r^{\text{out}} = \frac{1}{i\omega\mu_0}\frac{1}{r}\sum_{n=0}^{\infty} d_n n(n+1) h_n^{(1)}(k_0 r)P_n(\cos\theta) \tag{5.35}$$

$$H_\theta^{\text{out}} = \frac{1}{i\omega\mu_0}\frac{1}{r}\sum_{n=0}^{\infty} d_n\frac{\partial[r h_n^{(1)}(k_0 r)]}{\partial r}\frac{\partial P_n(\cos\theta)}{\partial\theta}. \tag{5.36}$$

It then remains to determine the expansion coefficients $a_n$, $b_n$, $c_n$, and $d_n$. For this, we apply the boundary conditions at the spherical surfaces $r = a$ and $r = c$. Since both the tangential electric and magnetic fields are continuous across the spherical surface $r = a$, we have

$$E_\phi^{\text{in}} = E_\phi^{\text{mid}}, \quad H_\theta^{\text{in}} = H_\theta^{\text{mid}} \quad \text{at } r = a \tag{5.37}$$

from which we obtain

$$a_n j_n(k_d a) = b_n j_n(k_0 a) + c_n h_n^{(1)}(k_0 a) \tag{5.38}$$

$$a_n k_d j_n'(k_d a) = b_n k_0 j_n'(k_0 a) + c_n k_0 h_n'^{(1)}(k_0 a). \tag{5.39}$$

In arriving at these, we applied the orthogonal relation

$$\int_0^\pi \frac{\partial P_n(\cos\theta)}{\partial\theta}\frac{\partial P_{n'}(\cos\theta)}{\partial\theta}\sin\theta d\theta = \begin{cases} 0 & n \neq n' \\ \dfrac{2n(n+1)}{2n+1} & n = n' \end{cases}. \tag{5.40}$$

Similarly, since the tangential electric field is continuous, but the tangential magnetic field is discontinuous across the spherical surface $r = c$, we have

$$E_\phi^{\text{out}} = E_\phi^{\text{mid}}, \quad H_\theta^{\text{out}} - H_\theta^{\text{mid}} = J_\phi \qquad \text{at } r = c \tag{5.41}$$

where $J_\phi = I\delta(\theta - \theta_0)/c$ denotes the surface current density of the current loop and $\theta_0 = \sin^{-1}(b/c)$ denotes the position of the loop. From Eq. (5.41), we obtain

$$b_n j_n(k_0 c) + c_n h_n^{(1)}(k_0 c) = d_n h_n^{(1)}(k_0 c) \tag{5.42}$$

$$d_n h_n^{\prime(1)}(k_0 c) - b_n j_n'(k_0 c) - c_n h_n^{\prime(1)}(k_0 c) = \frac{iZ_0 I}{c} \times \frac{2n+1}{2n(n+1)} \sin\theta_0 \left. \frac{\partial P_n(\cos\theta)}{\partial \theta} \right|_{\theta=\theta_0} \tag{5.43}$$

where $Z_0$ is the free-space wave impedance given by $Z_0 = \sqrt{\mu_0/\epsilon_0}$. Again, in arriving at these, we applied Eq. (5.40). Solving Eqs. (5.38), (5.39), (5.42), and (5.43), we obtain

$$a_n = \frac{ik_0 Z_0 I b^2}{a^2 c} \frac{2n+1}{2n(n+1)} \frac{h_n^{(1)}(k_0 c) P_n'(\cos\theta_0)}{k_d j_n'(k_d a) h_n^{(1)}(k_0 a) - k_0 j_n(k_d a) h_n^{\prime(1)}(k_0 a)}. \tag{5.44}$$

This result is the same as derived by Keltner *et al.* (1991). Substituting Eq. (5.44) into Eqs. (5.28)–(5.30), we obtain the expressions for the field inside the dielectric sphere. Given the fields everywhere, one can calculate the power dissipated in the sphere and the power radiated into free space (Keltner *et. al.* 1991).

## 5.3 Two-Dimensional Numerical Analysis

The problems considered in the preceding section are two of very few problems that can be solved analytically. When the dielectric cylinder/sphere, the surface current/loop current, or the RF shield has an arbitrary cross section, or when the dielectric cylinder/sphere is inhomogeneous, the problems can be solved only by using a numerical method. In this section, we describe the finite difference and finite element methods for solving such a problem.

### 5.3.1 Finite Difference Method

Consider the differential equation

$$\nabla^2 E_z + k_0^2 \epsilon_c E_z = -i\omega\mu_0 J_z \tag{5.45}$$

where $\epsilon_c$ may be a function of position. This equation can be written more explicitly in Cartesian coordinates as

$$\frac{\partial^2 E_z}{\partial x^2} + \frac{\partial^2 E_z}{\partial y^2} + k_0^2 \epsilon_c E_z = -i\omega\mu_0 J_z. \tag{5.46}$$

To solve this equation in the region of interest, we first enclose the region in a rectangular area and then divide the rectangular area uniformly into many small rectangular grids, as illustrated in Fig. 5.3. Further, we use two integers $(m, n)$ to denote the position of each node or, in other words, the coordinates of each node can be expressed as $x = m\Delta x$ and $y = n\Delta y$. In accordance with the finite difference method, the derivatives in Eq. (5.46) can be approximated as

$$\frac{\partial^2 E_z}{\partial x^2} = \frac{E_z(m+1,n) - 2E_z(m,n) + E_z(m-1,n)}{(\Delta x)^2} \tag{5.47}$$

$$\frac{\partial^2 E_z}{\partial y^2} = \frac{E_z(m,n+1) - 2E_z(m,n) + E_z(m,n-1)}{(\Delta y)^2}. \tag{5.48}$$

Substituting these into Eq. (5.46), we obtain

$$\begin{aligned} E_z(m,n) = & \left[\frac{2}{(\Delta x)^2} + \frac{2}{(\Delta y)^2} + k_0^2 \epsilon_c(m,n)\right]^{-1} \\ & \times \left\{ \frac{1}{(\Delta x)^2} [E_z(m+1,n) + E_z(m-1,n)] \right. \\ & \left. + \frac{1}{(\Delta y)^2} [E_z(m,n+1) + E_z(m,n-1)] + i\omega\mu_0 J_z(m,n) \right\}. \end{aligned} \tag{5.49}$$

Equation (5.49) defines a set of linear equations, which can be solved easily using an iterative method such as the Gauss-Seidel method. In this method, we first set all $E_z(m,n)$ to zero, that is, $E_z^0(m,n) = 0$. Here, we use the superscript to denote the iteration number. Then, we calculate a new set of values for $E_z(m,n)$ using Eq. (5.49) or, more specifically,

$$\begin{aligned} E_z^l(m,n) = & \left[\frac{2}{(\Delta x)^2} + \frac{2}{(\Delta y)^2} + k_0^2 \epsilon_c(m,n)\right]^{-1} \\ & \times \left\{ \frac{1}{(\Delta x)^2} \left[E_z^{l-1}(m+1,n) + E_z^{l-1}(m-1,n)\right] \right. \\ & \left. + \frac{1}{(\Delta y)^2} \left[E_z^{l-1}(m,n+1) + E_z^{l-1}(m,n-1)\right] + i\omega\mu_0 J_z(m,n) \right\} \end{aligned} \tag{5.50}$$

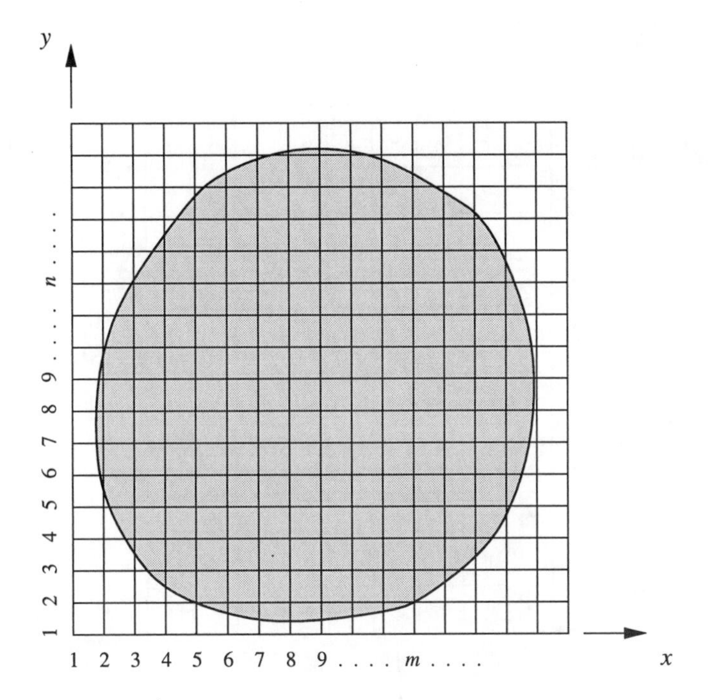


**Figure 5.3.** The finite difference mesh.

for $l = 1$. This process is repeated until a convergence is achieved, that is, the values of $E_z(m,n)$ do not change significantly. Once the electric field is obtained, the magnetic field at the center of each grid can be calculated using the central differencing as

$$B_x(m+\tfrac{1}{2}, n+\tfrac{1}{2}) = \frac{E_z(m+1,n+1) + E_z(m,n+1) - E_z(m+1,n) - E_z(m,n)}{2i\omega\Delta y} \tag{5.51}$$

$$B_y(m+\tfrac{1}{2}, n+\tfrac{1}{2}) = -\frac{E_z(m+1,n+1) + E_z(m+1,n) - E_z(m,n+1) - E_z(m,n)}{2i\omega\Delta x}. \tag{5.52}$$

The finite difference method can also be applied in time domain to solve Maxwell's equations for both electric and magnetic fields. The resulting formulation is called the finite-difference time-domain (FDTD) method (Yee 1966, Kunz and Luebbers 1994, Taflove 1995). Again, consider a

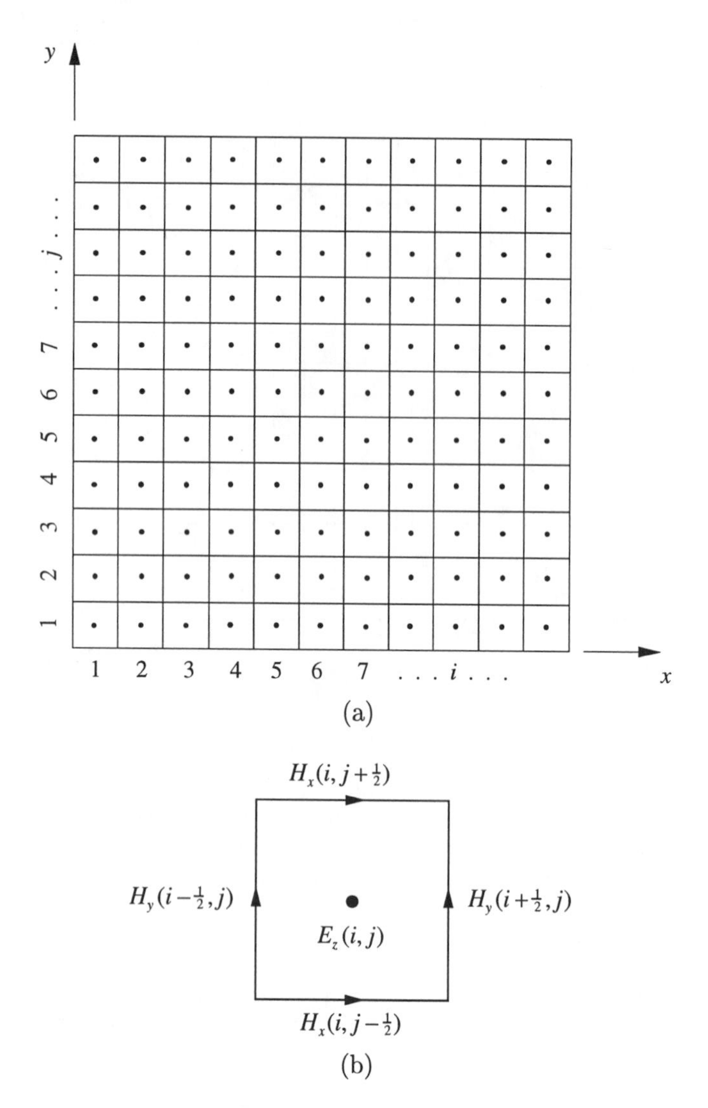


**Figure 5.4.** (a) The two-dimensional FDTD cells. (b) A single FDTD cell.

two-dimensional problem with a source $\mathbf{J} = \hat{z}J_z$. Maxwell's equations for this problem can be reduced to

$$\frac{\partial E_z}{\partial y} = -\mu_0 \frac{\partial H_x}{\partial t} \tag{5.53}$$

$$\frac{\partial E_z}{\partial x} = \mu_0 \frac{\partial H_y}{\partial t} \tag{5.54}$$

$$\frac{\partial H_y}{\partial x} - \frac{\partial H_x}{\partial y} = \epsilon \frac{\partial E_z}{\partial t} + \sigma E_z + J_z. \tag{5.55}$$

To solve for $(E_z, H_x, H_y)$, we again enclose the region in a rectangular area and then divide the rectangular area uniformly into many small rectangular cells, as illustrated in Fig. 5.4(a). The center of each cell is denoted by two integers $(i, j)$. As shown in Fig. 5.4(b), we assign the unknown $E_z$ at the centers of the cells, the unknown $H_x$ at the horizontal sides of the cells, and the unknown $H_y$ at the vertical sides of the cells. By using the central differencing, Eq. (5.53) can be written as

$$\frac{E_z^n(i,j+1) - E_z^n(i,j)}{\Delta y} = -\mu_0 \frac{H_x^{n+\frac{1}{2}}(i,j+\frac{1}{2}) - H_x^{n-\frac{1}{2}}(i,j+\frac{1}{2})}{\Delta t} \tag{5.56}$$

from which we obtain

$$H_x^{n+\frac{1}{2}}(i,j+\tfrac{1}{2}) = H_x^{n-\frac{1}{2}}(i,j+\tfrac{1}{2}) - \frac{\Delta t}{\mu_0 \Delta y}\left[E_z^n(i,j+1) - E_z^n(i,j)\right] \tag{5.57}$$

where $\Delta t$ denotes the time step and the superscript denotes the time. For example, the superscript $n$ indicates that the associated quantity is at $t = n\Delta t$. Similarly, from Eqs. (5.54) and (5.55), we obtain

$$H_y^{n+\frac{1}{2}}(i+\tfrac{1}{2},j) = H_y^{n-\frac{1}{2}}(i+\tfrac{1}{2},j) + \frac{\Delta t}{\mu_0 \Delta x}\left[E_z^n(i+1,j) - E_z^n(i,j)\right] \tag{5.58}$$

and

$$\begin{aligned} E_z^{n+1}(i,j) = {} & \frac{1}{\beta(i,j)} \\ & \times \left\{ \alpha(i,j) E_z^n(i,j) + \frac{\Delta t}{\Delta x}\left[H_y^{n+\frac{1}{2}}(i+\tfrac{1}{2},j) - H_z^{n+\frac{1}{2}}(i-\tfrac{1}{2},j)\right] \right. \\ & \left. - \frac{\Delta t}{\Delta y}\left[H_x^{n+\frac{1}{2}}(i,j+\tfrac{1}{2}) - H_y^{n-\frac{1}{2}}(i,j-\tfrac{1}{2})\right] - J_z^{n+\frac{1}{2}}(i,j) \right\} \end{aligned} \tag{5.59}$$

where

$$\alpha = \frac{\epsilon}{\Delta t} - \frac{\sigma}{2}, \qquad \beta = \frac{\epsilon}{\Delta t} + \frac{\sigma}{2}. \tag{5.60}$$

It can be proven that the discretization above is of second order in accuracy in terms of the cell size and, for a stable time marching, the time step has to satisfy the Courant-Friedrichs-Lewy stability criterion (Chew 1995)

$$\Delta t < \frac{1}{c_{\max}\sqrt{(1/\Delta x)^2 + (1/\Delta y)^2}} \tag{5.61}$$

where $c_{\max}$ is the maximum propagation speed of the electromagnetic waves in the simulation region.

### 5.3.2 Finite Element Method

The finite difference method described above is simple and easy to implement. However, since it divides the region of interest into rectangular cells, it cannot accurately model arbitrary geometries. This disadvantage can be alleviated by the finite element method (Jin 1993), which divides the region of interest into irregular triangular cells. Since the shape of the triangular cells can be arbitrary, the finite element method can accurately model arbitrary geometries. This section describes the basic procedure of the finite element method, as applied to Eq. (5.45), which is rewritten as

$$\nabla^2\phi + k_0^2\epsilon_c\phi = f \tag{5.62}$$

where $\phi = E_z$ and $f = -i\omega\mu_0 J_z$.

In the finite element method, instead of solving Eq. (5.62) directly, we seek a solution to the weighted integral of Eq. (5.62), which is obtained by multiplying Eq. (5.62) by a weighting function $w(x,y)$ and integrating the resultant equation over the region of interest:

$$\iint_\Omega w(x,y)\left[\nabla^2\phi(x,y) + k_0^2\epsilon_c\phi(x,y)\right] dxdy = \iint_\Omega w(x,y) f(x,y)\, dxdy. \tag{5.63}$$

Using the first scalar Green's theorem[2]

$$\iint_\Omega (w\nabla^2\phi + \nabla w\cdot\nabla\phi)\, dxdy = \oint_C w\frac{\partial\phi}{\partial n}\, dl, \tag{5.64}$$

[2] This Green's theorem can be obtained from the two-dimensional version of Gauss's theorem given in Eq. (2.2), which can be written as

$$\iint_\Omega \nabla\cdot\mathbf{A}\, dxdy = \oint_C \mathbf{A}\cdot\hat{n}\, dl$$

by letting $\mathbf{A} = w\nabla\phi$ and using vector identity $\nabla\cdot(w\nabla\phi) = w\nabla^2\phi + \nabla w\cdot\nabla\phi$.

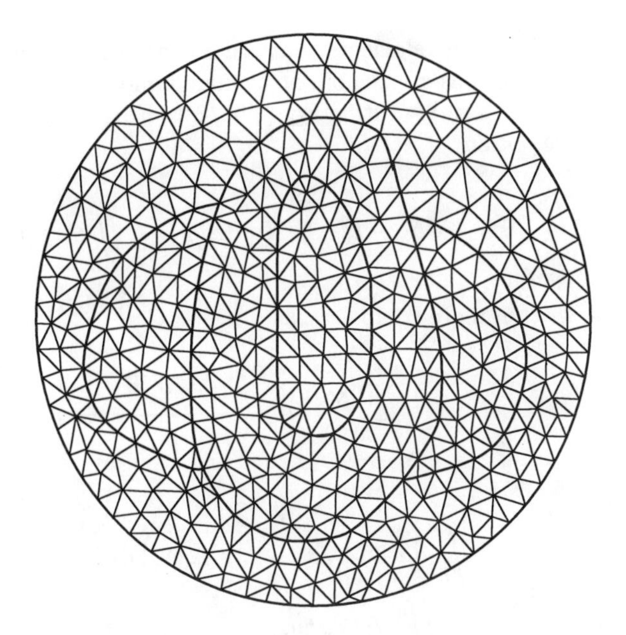

**Figure 5.5.** A finite element mesh.

Eq. (5.63) can be written as

$$\iint_\Omega \left[\nabla w \cdot \nabla\phi - k_0^2\epsilon_c w\phi\right] dxdy = \oint_C w\frac{\partial\phi}{\partial n}\, dl - \iint_\Omega wf\, dxdy. \quad (5.65)$$

As mentioned above, the first step of the finite element method is to subdivide the region of interest into small triangular cells, which are called elements (Fig. 5.5). Assume that at the boundary of the region of interest, the electric field vanishes, as is the case for a shielded coil. Therefore, we have to solve only for the electric field inside the region of interest. Assign a value of the electric field at each internal node as $\phi_i$ where $i$ denotes the nodal number. Furthermore, assume that the field within each element is a linear interpolation of the fields at the three nodes of that element. Then, the field in the entire region of interest can be expressed as

$$\phi(x, y) = \sum_{i=1}^{N} N_i(x, y)\phi_i \quad (5.66)$$

where $N$ denotes the total number of internal nodes and $N_i(x, y)$ is called the expansion function or the basis function associated with node $i$. For linear elements, $N_i(x, y)$ is illustrated in Fig. 5.6, where we see that $N_i(x, y)$

is nonzero only within the elements that are directly connected to node $i$. Furthermore, $N_i(x,y)$ has a value of one at node $i$ and decreases to zero at the neighboring nodes. Substituting Eq. (5.66) into Eq. (5.65) and choosing $w = N_i(x,y)$, we obtain

$$\sum_{j=1}^{N} \phi_j \iint_\Omega \left[\nabla N_i \cdot \nabla N_j - k_0^2 \epsilon_c N_i N_j\right] dxdy = -\iint_\Omega N_i f \, dxdy \quad (5.67)$$

which can be written more compactly as

$$\sum_{j=1}^{N} K_{ij} \phi_j = b_i \quad (5.68)$$

where

$$K_{ij} = \iint_\Omega \left[\nabla N_i \cdot \nabla N_j - k_0^2 \epsilon_c N_i N_j\right] dxdy \quad (5.69)$$

$$b_i = -\iint_\Omega N_i f \, dxdy. \quad (5.70)$$

Equation (5.68) defines a set of linear equations, which can be solved using one of many standard algorithms. Its solution provides the value of $E_z$ at each node, from which the magnetic field can be calculated using Maxwell's equations.

### 5.3.3 Numerical Simulations

In this section, we present numerical results obtained using the finite element method to demonstrate the electric field, magnetic field, and SAR generated by both linear and quadrature birdcage coils at four different frequencies. The electric currents used for simulation are calculated using the equivalent circuit method described in the preceding chapter. This is followed by a detailed comparison of the SAR and $B_1$-field inhomogeneity for different coils at different frequencies. The SAR is calculated from the electric field using

$$\text{SAR} = \frac{\sigma |\mathbf{E}|^2}{2\rho} \quad (5.71)$$

where $\rho$ denotes the density of the tissue. For the results given in this chapter, we assume that the total exposure time to the RF field is 4.7 seconds and the SAR is averaged over 6 minutes.

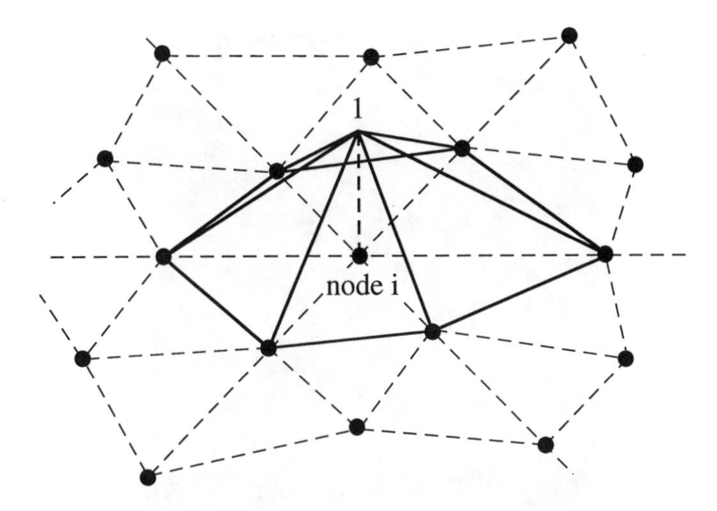


**Figure 5.6.** Illustration of the basis function for node $i$.

To study the electromagnetic interaction with the human head, we need an electromagnetic model of the head. This model can be constructed by segmenting MRI images into voxels in the shape of cubes. Each voxel is then given a tag which identifies its tissue type. The electromagnetic model used in this study is shown in Fig. 5.7 (see color insert following page 240), and is provided by National Radiological Protection Board of U.K. (Dimbylow and Mann 1994). The tissues are skin, muscle, bone, brain, cerebrospinal fluid (CSF), air (sinuses), lens, vitreous humour, and cartilage. Their material properties $\rho$, $\epsilon_r = \epsilon/\epsilon_0$, and $\sigma$ are given in Table 5.1, which are derived by using the Cole-Cole dispersion relation (Gabriel *et al.* 1996b). These data are a little different from those used in our calculation, which are obtained by inter- and extrapolation of the data given by Stuchly and Stuchly (1980) and Simunic *et al.* (1996). A recent survey on the dielectric properties of biological tissues is given by Gabriel *et al.* (1996a). The interested reader is referred to this article which contains an extensive list of references.[3]

The birdcage coil considered has a diameter of 26 cm, a length of 26 cm, and it consists of 16 elements. The coil is enclosed by a cylindrical shield having a diameter of 30 cm. Therefore, the shield is 2 cm away from the coil's elements, which are about 3.6 cm away from the head. The maximum electric current in the coil is assumed to be 1 A. The four frequencies considered are 64 MHz, 128 MHz, 171 MHz, and 256 MHz,

[3] The following web site provides the capability of computing tissue parameters (permittivity and conductivity) at a given frequency: *http://www.fcc.gov/fcc-bin/dielec.sh*.

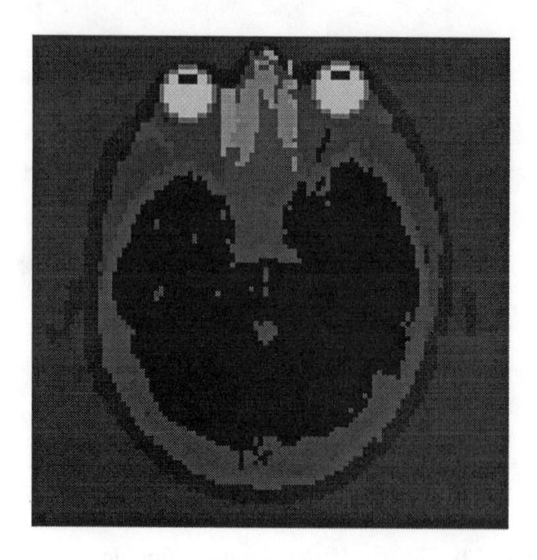

**Figure 5.7.** Axial slice through the eyes of the head model. Reproduced from Jin and Chen (1997).

**Table 5.1.** Tissue Properties.

| Tissue type | $\rho$ (g/cm$^3$) | 64 MHz | | 128 MHz | | 171 MHz | | 256 MHz | |
|---|---|---|---|---|---|---|---|---|---|
| | | $\epsilon_r$ | $\sigma$ (S/m) | $\epsilon_r$ | $\sigma$ (S/m) | $\epsilon_r$ | $\sigma$ (S/m) | $\epsilon_r$ | $\sigma$ (S/m) |
| CSF | 1.06 | 97 | 2.07 | 84 | 2.14 | 79 | 2.17 | 74 | 2.21 |
| air | | 1 | 0 | 1 | 0 | 1 | 0 | 1 | 0 |
| muscle | 1.04 | 72 | 0.71 | 64 | 0.74 | 62 | 0.76 | 60 | 0.78 |
| bone | 1.85 | 17 | 0.06 | 15 | 0.07 | 14 | 0.07 | 14 | 0.08 |
| skin | 1.10 | 77 | 0.49 | 62 | 0.54 | 57 | 0.57 | 53 | 0.61 |
| lens | 1.05 | 50 | 0.29 | 43 | 0.31 | 41 | 0.32 | 39 | 0.34 |
| humor | 1.01 | 69 | 1.50 | 69 | 1.51 | 69 | 1.51 | 69 | 1.51 |
| brain | 1.03 | 83 | 0.40 | 63 | 0.46 | 58 | 0.49 | 53 | 0.53 |
| cartilage | 1.10 | 63 | 0.45 | 53 | 0.49 | 50 | 0.51 | 48 | 0.54 |

corresponding to the frequency of the $B_1$ field in 1.5 T, 3 T, 4 T, and 6 T MRI systems, respectively. These are chosen because of current interest in developing 3 T, 4 T, and 6 T systems for advanced MRI studies. The 1.5 T systems are commercially available and have been widely used in clinical applications.

#### 5.3.3.1 Linear Excitation

When a birdcage coil is fed at a single point, it generates a linearly polarized $B_1$ field. Such an excitation is often referred to as linear excitation. The electric and magnetic fields generated by an empty birdcage coil with linear excitation are shown in Figs. 5.8 and 5.9 (see color insert). It is clear that the electric field, polarized in the direction parallel to the coil's axis, varies linearly along the vertical direction and remains constant in the horizontal direction. This results in a uniform magnetic field polarized in the horizontal direction. Note that both electric and magnetic field distributions are basically the same at the four different frequencies. The $B_1$ field remains uniform in the empty coil even at 256 MHz. This is, however, not true when the coil is loaded with the human head. Figures 5.10 and 5.11 (see color insert) display the SAR and $B_1$ field distributions in the loaded coil. It is observed that the SAR is low in a horizontal strip-shaped region across the center of the head because of the weak electric field, and is very high in the top and bottom regions due to the strong electric field. At low frequencies, the high SAR occurs in the superficial region; however, at 256 MHz the high SAR moves into the deeper region due to dielectric resonance or standing wave phenomena.

The results presented above are pertinent to the horizontally polarized $B_1$ field. By rotating the feed point or the coil 90°, we can obtain the $B_1$ field polarized in the vertical direction. In that case, the electric field is strong in both sides of the head and weak in a vertical strip-shaped region across the center of the head. This reduces significantly the SAR in the eyes. The results are shown in Figs. 5.12 and 5.13 (see color insert).

We note that the magnetic field displayed in Figs. 5.9, 5.11, and 5.13 is the total magnetic field. As explained in Chapter 1, a linearly polarized $B_1$ field can be decomposed into two counter rotating or circularly polarized components. Only the component that rotates in the same sense as the spins precess excites the transverse magnetization and the other component is wasted. Figures 5.14 and 5.15 display this useful circularly polarized component for the horizontally and vertically polarized loaded birdcage coils, respectively. It is observed that even though the total magnetic field is quite uniform at 64 MHz, its circularly polarized component exhibits the diagonal pattern of intensity non-uniformity. This non-uniformity was described by Glover *et al.* (1985) as a "quadrapole" artifact.

#### 5.3.3.2 Quadrature Excitation

When a birdcage coil is fed at two points 90° apart with a phase difference of 90°, it generates a circularly polarized $B_1$ field. Such an excitation is

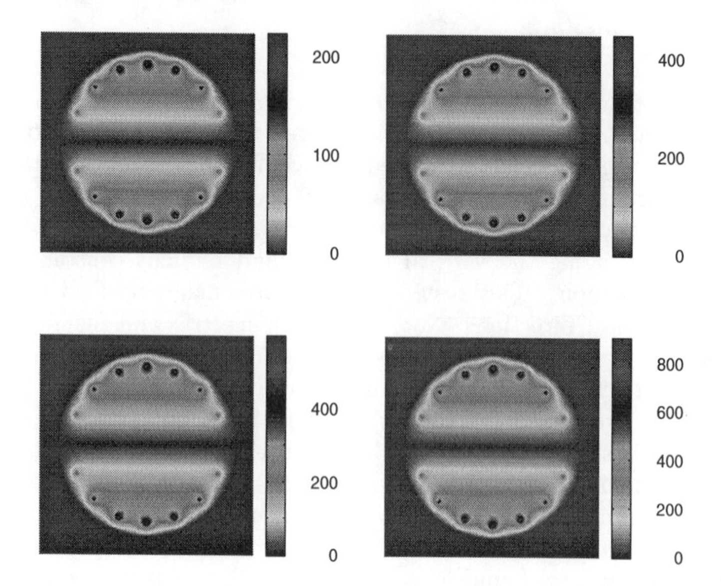


**Figure 5.8.** Electric field (V/m) of an unloaded linear, horizontally polarized birdcage coil. Top-left: 64 MHz. Top-right: 128 MHz. Bottom-left: 171 MHz. Bottom-right: 256 MHz. Reproduced from Jin and Chen (1997).

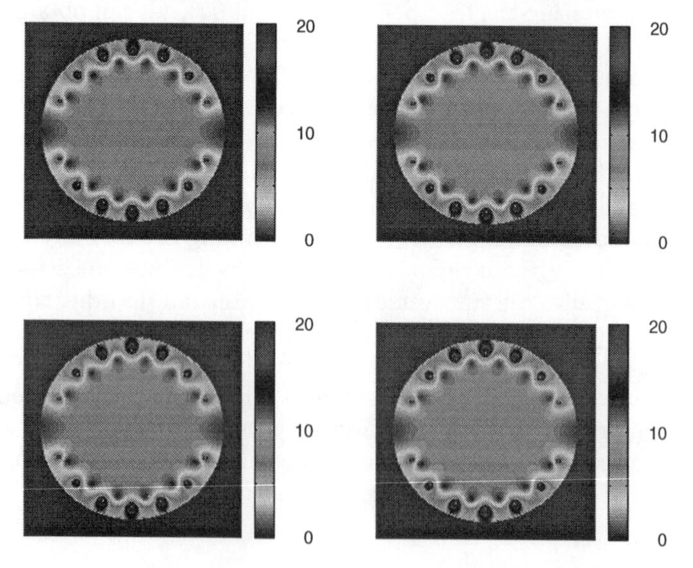


**Figure 5.9.** Magnetic field (A/m) of an unloaded linear, horizontally polarized birdcage coil. Top-left: 64 MHz. Top-right: 128 MHz. Bottom-left: 171 MHz. Bottom-right: 256 MHz. Reproduced from Jin and Chen (1997).

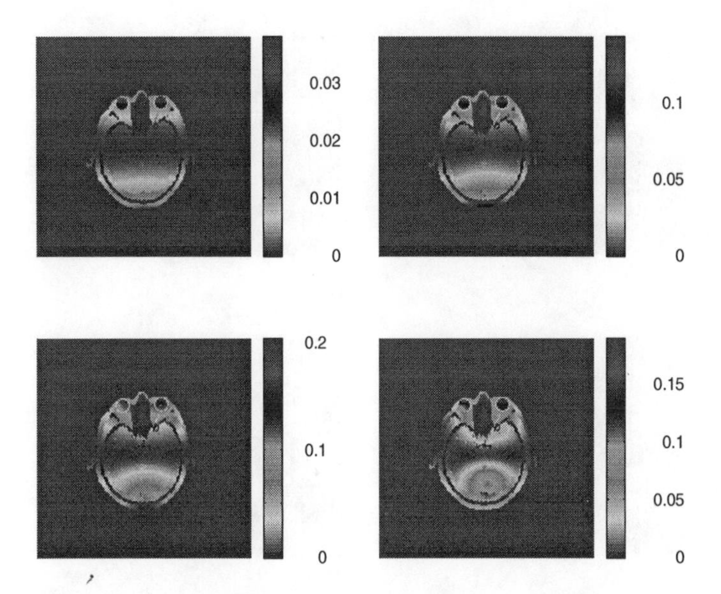


**Figure 5.10.** SAR (W/Kg) of a loaded linear, horizontally polarized birdcage coil. Top-left: 64 MHz. Top-right: 128 MHz. Bottom-left: 171 MHz. Bottom-right: 256 MHz. Reproduced from Jin and Chen (1997).

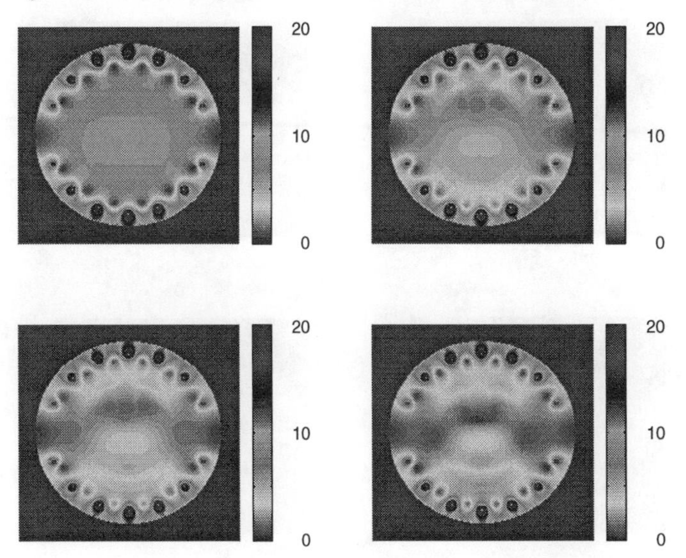


**Figure 5.11.** Magnetic field (A/m) of a loaded linear, horizontally polarized birdcage coil. Top-left: 64 MHz. Top-right: 128 MHz. Bottom-left: 171 MHz. Bottom-right: 256 MHz. Reproduced from Jin and Chen (1997).

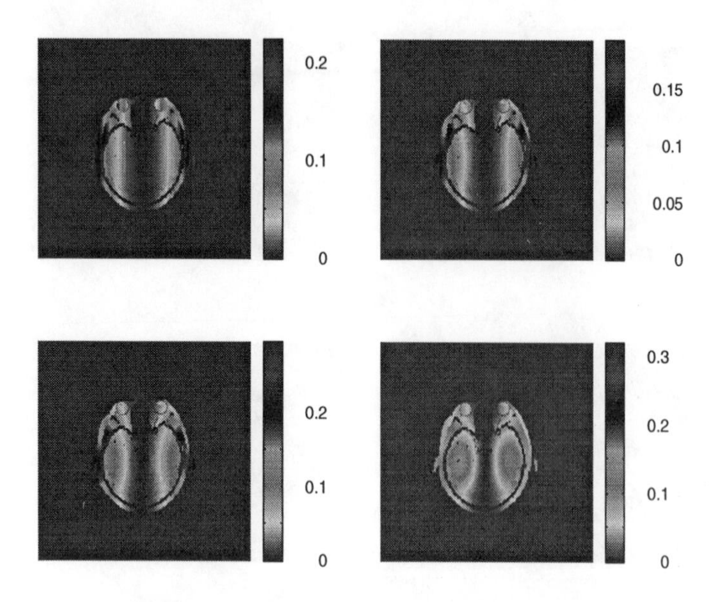


**Figure 5.12.** SAR (W/Kg) of a loaded linear, vertically polarized birdcage coil. Top-left: 64 MHz. Top-right: 128 MHz. Bottom-left: 171 MHz. Bottom-right: 256 MHz.

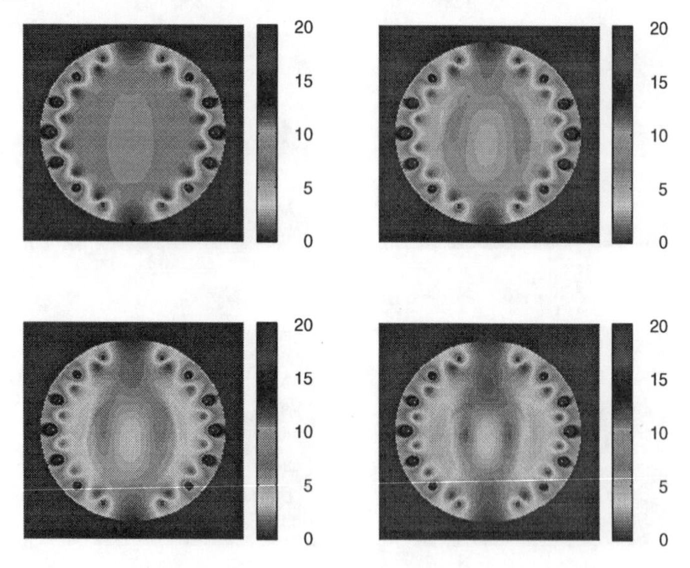


**Figure 5.13.** Magnetic field (A/m) of a loaded linear, vertically polarized birdcage coil. Top-left: 64 MHz. Top-right: 128 MHz. Bottom-left: 171 MHz. Bottom-right: 256 MHz.

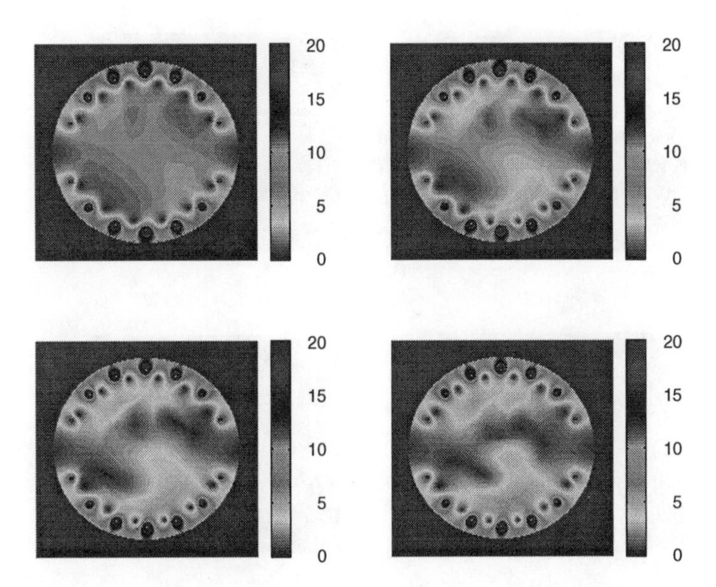


**Figure 5.14.** The circularly polarized component of the magnetic field (A/m) of a loaded linear, horizontally polarized birdcage coil. Top-left: 64 MHz. Top-right: 128 MHz. Bottom-left: 171 MHz. Bottom-right: 256 MHz.

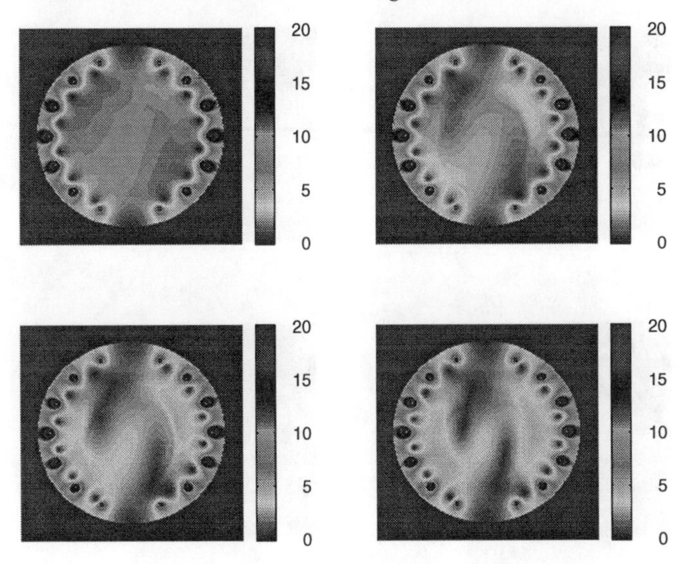


**Figure 5.15.** The circularly polarized component of the magnetic field (A/m) of a loaded linear, vertically polarized birdcage coil. Top-left: 64 MHz. Top-right: 128 MHz. Bottom-left: 171 MHz. Bottom-right: 256 MHz.

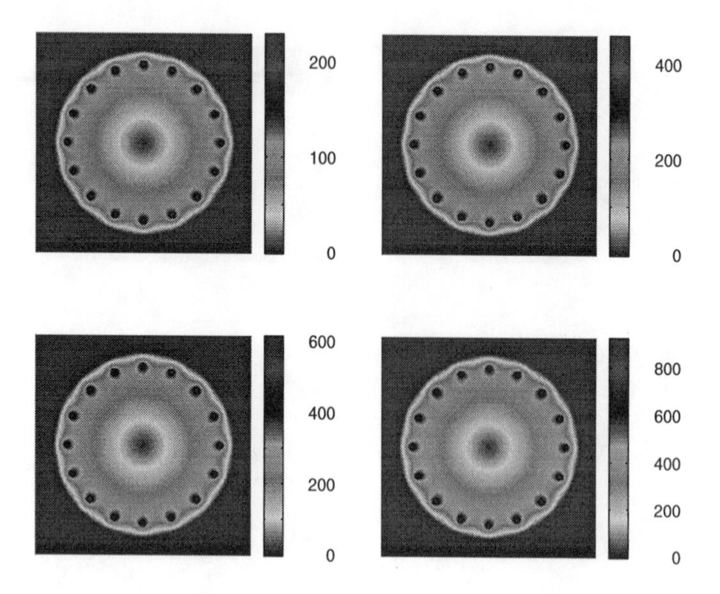


**Figure 5.16.** Electric field (V/m) of an unloaded quadrature birdcage coil. Top-left: 64 MHz. Top-right: 128 MHz. Bottom-left: 171 MHz. Bottom-right: 256 MHz. Reproduced from Jin and Chen (1997).

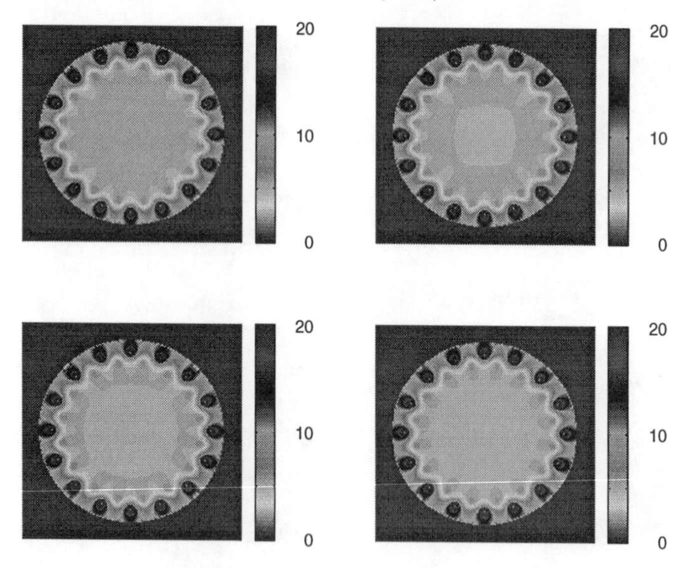


**Figure 5.17.** Magnetic field (A/m) of an unloaded quadrature birdcage coil. Top-left: 64 MHz. Top-right: 128 MHz. Bottom-left: 171 MHz. Bottom-right: 256 MHz. Reproduced from Jin and Chen (1997).

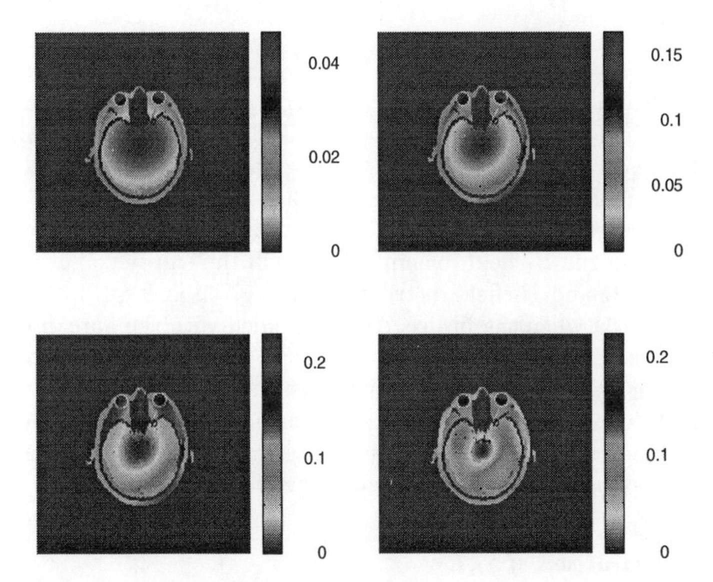


**Figure 5.18.** SAR (W/Kg) of a loaded quadrature birdcage coil. Top-left: 64 MHz. Top-right: 128 MHz. Bottom-left: 171 MHz. Bottom-right: 256 MHz. Reproduced from Jin and Chen (1997).

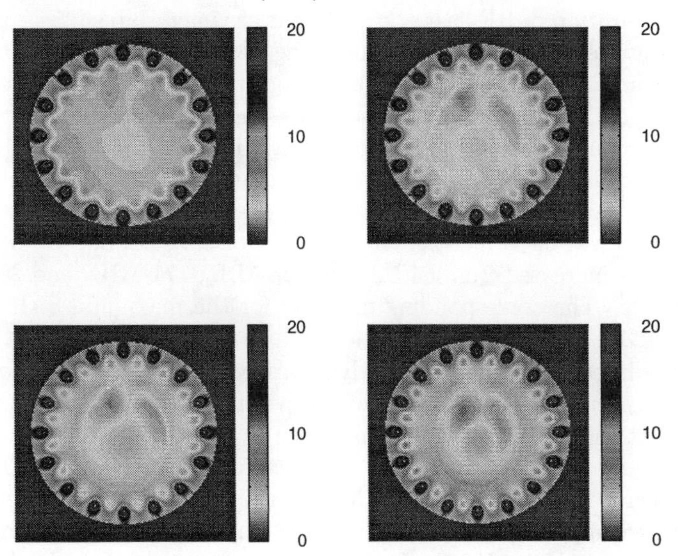


**Figure 5.19.** Magnetic field (A/m) of a loaded quadrature birdcage coil. Top-left: 64 MHz. Top-right: 128 MHz. Bottom-left: 171 MHz. Bottom-right: 256 MHz. Reproduced from Jin and Chen (1997).

often referred to as quadrature excitation. The electric and magnetic fields generated by an empty birdcage coil with quadrature excitation are shown in Figs. 5.16 and 5.17 (see color insert). In contrast to the linear excitation, the electric field varies linearly in the radial direction with a minimum at the center and remains constant in the angular direction. This results in a uniform magnetic field with a circular polarization. Again, both electric and magnetic field distributions are basically the same at the four different frequencies and the $B_1$ field remains uniform in the empty coil even at 256 MHz. The SAR and $B_1$ field distributions are given in Figs. 5.18 and 5.19 (see color insert) when the birdcage coil is loaded with the human head. It is observed that the SAR is low in the center of the head because of the weak electric field, and is very high in the outer region. The size of the region with low SAR decreases as the frequency increases and, moreover, at high frequencies the high SAR penetrates into the deeper region of the head due to dielectric resonance or standing wave phenomena.

#### *5.3.3.3 Comparison of SAR*

To examine in detail the SAR in the human head, we assume that the current in the birdcage coil produces a value of the linearly polarized magnetic field of 21.49 A/m (27 $\mu$T) in the center of the coil. Further, the total duration of RF energy exposure is assumed to be 4.7 seconds and the SAR is averaged over six minutes. The SAR generated by the birdcage coil with linear excitation under such conditions is given in Table 5.2 for eight different tissues at four different frequencies. For each tissue, both the average and maximum SAR are given. The last row of the table gives the SAR in the entire region. It is seen that as the frequency increases, the highest maximum SAR occurs in the muscle. Also, the average SAR in the entire region is increased by a factor of 4.2, 5.8, and 6.9 when the frequency is increased from 64 MHz to 128 MHz, 171 MHz, and 256 MHz, respectively. The corresponding numbers for the maximum SAR are 3.0, 4.1, and 4.4.

As pointed out earlier, a linearly polarized $B_1$ field can be decomposed into two counter rotating or circularly polarized components. Only the component that rotates in the same sense as the spins precess excites the transverse magnetization and the other component is wasted. Therefore, for a linearly polarized $B_1$ field having the strength of 21.49 A/m (27 $\mu$T), its decomposed circularly polarized components have the strength of $21.49/2 = 10.75$ A/m (13.5 $\mu$T). The SAR generated by the birdcage coil with quadrature excitation, that produces a value of the circularly polarized magnetic field of 10.75 A/m (13.5 $\mu$T) in the center of the coil, is given in Table 5.3. The average SAR in the entire region is increased by a factor of

**Table 5.2.** Maximum and Average SAR (W/Kg) for Horizontally Polarized, Linear Birdcage Coil (Jin and Chen 1997).

| Tissue | 64 MHz | | 128 MHz | | 171 MHz | | 256 MHz | |
|---|---|---|---|---|---|---|---|---|
| type | Avg | Max | Avg | Max | Avg | Max | Avg | Max |
| lens | 0.68 | 0.89 | 2.3 | 2.8 | 3.1 | 3.7 | 3.3 | 4.7 |
| humor | 2.9 | 3.8 | 8.9 | 10.8 | 9.2 | 10.7 | 11.7 | 16.6 |
| cartilage | 0.05 | 0.08 | 0.22 | 0.33 | 0.3 | 0.4 | 0.38 | 0.66 |
| bone | 0.02 | 0.06 | 0.08 | 0.26 | 0.13 | 0.33 | 0.17 | 0.4 |
| brain | 0.24 | 1.24 | 1.1 | 5.0 | 1.8 | 6.9 | 2.8 | 9.2 |
| skin | 0.83 | 2.2 | 3.1 | 7.8 | 3.8 | 8.9 | 3.2 | 9.2 |
| CSF | 0.8 | 1.6 | 3.1 | 6.1 | 4.4 | 8.5 | 5.2 | 10.7 |
| muscle | 0.56 | 2.3 | 3.3 | 11.5 | 5.1 | 15.4 | 4.5 | 16.9 |
| overall | 0.45 | 3.8 | 1.9 | 11.5 | 2.6 | 15.4 | 3.1 | 16.9 |

**Table 5.3.** Maximum and Average SAR (W/Kg) for Quadrature Birdcage Coil (Jin and Chen 1997).

| Tissue | 64 MHz | | 128 MHz | | 171 MHz | | 256 MHz | |
|---|---|---|---|---|---|---|---|---|
| type | Avg | Max | Avg | Max | Avg | Max | Avg | Max |
| lens | 0.23 | 0.29 | 0.65 | 0.75 | 0.85 | 0.95 | 1.0 | 1.4 |
| humor | 0.95 | 1.2 | 2.6 | 2.9 | 2.5 | 2.8 | 3.6 | 4.7 |
| cartilage | 0.02 | 0.02 | 0.06 | 0.07 | 0.08 | 0.09 | 0.09 | 0.16 |
| bone | 0.01 | 0.02 | 0.04 | 0.07 | 0.05 | 0.08 | 0.07 | 0.11 |
| brain | 0.1 | 0.3 | 0.5 | 1.2 | 0.85 | 1.7 | 1.5 | 2.6 |
| skin | 0.42 | 0.6 | 1.4 | 1.9 | 1.8 | 2.4 | 1.5 | 3.3 |
| CSF | 0.27 | 0.42 | 0.95 | 1.5 | 1.4 | 2.1 | 1.85 | 2.9 |
| muscle | 0.33 | 0.65 | 1.7 | 2.8 | 2.3 | 3.8 | 2.1 | 4.0 |
| overall | 0.21 | 1.2 | 0.8 | 2.9 | 1.1 | 3.7 | 1.4 | 4.7 |

3.8, 5.2, and 6.7 when the frequency is increased from 64 MHz to 128 MHz, 171 MHz, and 256 MHz, respectively. The corresponding numbers for the maximum SAR are 2.4, 3.2, and 3.9. These numbers are similar to those in the case of linear excitation, although they are slightly smaller.

Compared to the case of linear excitation, the average SAR in the case of quadrature excitation is reduced by a factor of between 2.1 to 2.4, and the maximum SAR is reduced by a factor of between 3.2 to 4.1. This reduction is due to the reduced current in the coil and the more uniform

**Table 5.4.** Comparison of Maximum and Average SAR (W/Kg) for Different Coils (Jin and Chen 1997).

| Coil type | 64 MHz | | 128 MHz | | 171 MHz | | 256 MHz | |
|---|---|---|---|---|---|---|---|---|
| | Avg | Max | Avg | Max | Avg | Max | Avg | Max |
| Coil 1 | 0.45 | 3.8 | 1.9 | 11.5 | 2.6 | 15.4 | 3.1 | 16.9 |
| Coil 2 | 0.22 | 1.2 | 0.8 | 2.9 | 1.1 | 3.8 | 1.4 | 4.7 |
| Coil 3 | 0.21 | 1.3 | 0.75 | 2.9 | 1.1 | 3.7 | 1.3 | 4.9 |
| Coil 4 | 0.30 | 1.3 | 0.5 | 1.8 | 0.6 | 2.0 | 0.5 | 2.2 |
| Coil 5 | 0.20 | 1.3 | 0.75 | 2.9 | 1.1 | 3.5 | 1.4 | 4.7 |

Coil 1: 16 elements, $d = 2$ cm, linear polarization.
Coil 2: 16 elements, $d = 2$ cm, circular polarization.
Coil 3: 16 elements, $d = 5$ cm, circular polarization.
Coil 4: 16 elements, $d = \infty$ (open), circular polarization.
Coil 5: 8 elements, $d = 2$ cm, circular polarization.

distribution of the SAR in the head in the case of quadrature excitation.

Since the two-dimensional simulation method is very efficient, it can be conveniently used to study a variety of coil configurations. In Table 5.4, we give the average and maximum SARs in the entire head region for the two coils considered above and for three additional coils. The first one is a quadrature coil with the distance between the coil and shield (denoted as $d$ in the table) increased to 5 cm. The second one is a quadrature coil without the shield (open coil), and the third is a quadrature coil with the number of elements reduced to eight. In addition to the observations made on the linear versus quadrature excitation, three more observations can be made from the examination of Table 5.4. First, a 3-cm difference in the distance of the shield from the coil's elements does not have a significant effect on the SAR. Second, the open coil has a significantly lower SAR when the frequency increases. This is probably due to the increased radiation of the coil at high frequencies. Third, the difference in the SAR generated by an 8-element coil and a 16-element coil is negligible when the distance between the coil's elements and the head is more than 3 cm.

In passing, we would like to make two points. First, although the numbers given in Tables 5.2–5.4 are for a specific excitation, one can easily calculate the corresponding SAR values for other excitations provided that one knows the desired $B_1$ field, the duration of RF energy exposure, and the period over which the SAR is averaged. Second, the results given in Tables 5.2–5.4 assume that the imaging region is at the center of the head. It is clear in Figs. 5.14, 5.15, and 5.19 that the $B_1$ field is highest at the center of

**Table 5.5.** Comparison of Average Variation in $B_1$ Field for Different Coils (Jin and Chen 1997).

| Coil type | 64 MHz | | 128 MHz | | 171 MHz | | 256 MHz | |
|---|---|---|---|---|---|---|---|---|
| | $\tilde{B}_1$ | $\delta_{\text{ave}}$ (%) | $\tilde{B}_1$ | $\delta_{\text{ave}}$ (%) | $\tilde{B}_1$ | $\delta_{\text{ave}}$ (%) | $\tilde{B}_1$ | $\delta_{\text{ave}}$ (%) |
| Coil 1 | 2.1 | 10.0 | 2.3 | 26 | 2.5 | 35 | 2.5 | 44 |
| Coil 2 | 2.9 | 5.3 | 3.3 | 15 | 3.1 | 21 | 3.3 | 27 |
| Coil 3 | 5.1 | 5.5 | 5.3 | 15 | 5.3 | 21 | 5.2 | 26 |
| Coil 4 | 15.4 | 5.5 | 15.5 | 15 | 15.2 | 20 | 12.7 | 25 |
| Coil 5 | 1.4 | 5.5 | 1.6 | 14 | 1.6 | 21 | 1.7 | 27 |

See Table 5.4 for description of the coils.

the head when the frequency increases due to the standing wave effect. As a result, if the imaging region is elsewhere, the SAR would increase more significantly as the frequency increases.

#### *5.3.3.4 Comparison of $B_1$ Field*

To compare the $B_1$ field inhomogeneity, we calculate the average and maximum variation of the $B_1$ field inside a circular region located at the center of the head. This circular region has a diameter of 16 cm, which is slightly smaller than the size of the head. The average variation is defined as

$$\delta_{\text{ave}} = \frac{1}{A\tilde{B}_1} \iint_A \left| B_1 - \tilde{B}_1 \right| dA \tag{5.72}$$

and the maximum variation is defined as

$$\delta_{\text{max}} = \frac{|B_{1\text{max}} - B_{1\text{min}}|}{\tilde{B}_1} \tag{5.73}$$

where $A$ denotes the circular region and $\tilde{B}_1$ denotes the average value of $B_1$ over $A$.

The average and maximum variations in the $B_1$ field are given in Tables 5.5 and 5.6 for the five different coils at four different frequencies. As can be seen, the $B_1$ field inhomogeneity increases significantly with the frequency. The increase is basically independent of the number of elements in the coil and the radius of the shield. However, this increase is more significant in the linear polarization case than in the circular polarization case.

**Table 5.6.** Comparison of Maximum Variation in $B_1$ Field for Different Coils (Jin and Chen 1997).

| Coil type | 64 MHz | | 128 MHz | | 171 MHz | | 256 MHz | |
|---|---|---|---|---|---|---|---|---|
| | $\tilde{B}_1$ | $\delta_{\max}$ (%) | $\tilde{B}_1$ | $\delta_{\max}$ (%) | $\tilde{B}_1$ | $\delta_{\max}$ (%) | $\tilde{B}_1$ | $\delta_{\max}$ (%) |
| Coil 1 | 2.1 | 69 | 2.3 | 171 | 2.5 | 207 | 2.5 | 233 |
| Coil 2 | 2.9 | 33 | 3.3 | 85 | 3.1 | 127 | 3.3 | 180 |
| Coil 3 | 5.1 | 39 | 5.3 | 85 | 5.3 | 127 | 5.2 | 177 |
| Coil 4 | 15.4 | 33 | 15.5 | 82 | 15.2 | 123 | 12.7 | 172 |
| Coil 5 | 1.4 | 39 | 1.6 | 86 | 1.6 | 128 | 1.7 | 180 |

See Table 5.4 for description of the coils.

## 5.4 Three-Dimensional Numerical Analysis

Although a two-dimensional analysis can provide useful information, its solution is approximate and the accuracy of the approximation depends upon specific problems. If the accuracy is not good enough, one has to resort to three-dimensional analysis. In this section, we describe two methods for such analysis. One is the finite-difference time-domain method, which is particularly suitable for the simulation of shielded RF coils, and the other is a numerical method based on an integral equation, which is especially suited for the analysis of unshielded RF coils.

### 5.4.1 Finite-Difference Time-Domain Method

Consider Maxwell's equations in time domain:

$$\nabla \times \mathbf{E} = -\mu_0 \frac{\partial \mathbf{H}}{\partial t} \tag{5.74}$$

$$\nabla \times \mathbf{H} = \epsilon \frac{\partial \mathbf{E}}{\partial t} + \sigma \mathbf{E} + \mathbf{J}. \tag{5.75}$$

These two vector equations can be written as six scalar equations given by

$$\frac{\partial E_z}{\partial y} - \frac{\partial E_y}{\partial z} = -\mu_0 \frac{\partial H_x}{\partial t} \tag{5.76}$$

$$\frac{\partial E_x}{\partial z} - \frac{\partial E_z}{\partial x} = -\mu_0 \frac{\partial H_y}{\partial t} \tag{5.77}$$

$$\frac{\partial E_y}{\partial x} - \frac{\partial E_x}{\partial y} = -\mu_0 \frac{\partial H_z}{\partial t} \tag{5.78}$$

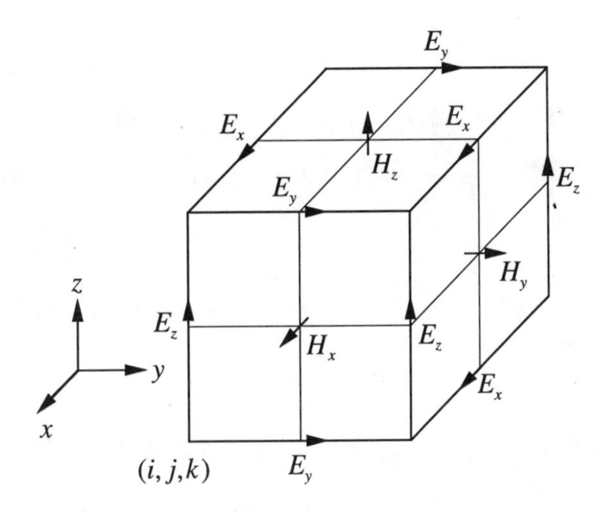


**Figure 5.20.** Illustration of Yee's grid for the FDTD algorithm.

$$\frac{\partial H_z}{\partial y} - \frac{\partial H_y}{\partial z} = \epsilon \frac{\partial E_x}{\partial t} + \sigma E_x + J_x \tag{5.79}$$

$$\frac{\partial H_x}{\partial z} - \frac{\partial H_z}{\partial x} = \epsilon \frac{\partial E_y}{\partial t} + \sigma E_y + J_y \tag{5.80}$$

$$\frac{\partial H_y}{\partial x} - \frac{\partial H_x}{\partial y} = \epsilon \frac{\partial E_z}{\partial t} + \sigma E_z + J_z . \tag{5.81}$$

To solve these equations for the electric and magnetic fields in a volume $V$, we enclose the volume $V$ in a rectangular box and then divide the box into many small rectangular cells. We then assign the electric field components at the center of each edge of the cells and the magnetic field components at the center of each face of the cells, as illustrated in Fig. 5.20. Using the central differencing scheme, Eqs. (5.76)–(5.78) can be written as

$$\begin{aligned} H_x^{n+\frac{1}{2}}(i, j+\tfrac{1}{2}, k+\tfrac{1}{2}) &= H_x^{n-\frac{1}{2}}(i, j+\tfrac{1}{2}, k+\tfrac{1}{2}) \\ &- \frac{\Delta t}{\mu_0 \Delta y}\left[E_z^n(i, j+1, k+\tfrac{1}{2}) - E_z^n(i, j, k+\tfrac{1}{2})\right] \\ &+ \frac{\Delta t}{\mu_0 \Delta z}\left[E_y^n(i, j+\tfrac{1}{2}, k+1) - E_y^n(i, j+\tfrac{1}{2}, k)\right] \end{aligned} \tag{5.82}$$

$$\begin{aligned} H_y^{n+\frac{1}{2}}(i+\tfrac{1}{2}, j, k+\tfrac{1}{2}) &= H_y^{n-\frac{1}{2}}(i+\tfrac{1}{2}, j, k+\tfrac{1}{2}) \\ &- \frac{\Delta t}{\mu_0 \Delta z}\left[E_x^n(i+\tfrac{1}{2}, j, k+1) - E_x^n(i+\tfrac{1}{2}, j, k)\right] \end{aligned}$$

$$+ \frac{\Delta t}{\mu_0 \Delta x} \left[E_z^n(i+1,j,k+\tfrac{1}{2}) - E_z^n(i,j,k+\tfrac{1}{2})\right] \quad (5.83)$$

$$\begin{aligned} H_z^{n+\frac{1}{2}}(i+\tfrac{1}{2},j+\tfrac{1}{2},k) &= H_z^{n-\frac{1}{2}}(i+\tfrac{1}{2},j+\tfrac{1}{2},k) \\ &- \frac{\Delta t}{\mu_0 \Delta x} \left[E_y^n(i+1,j+\tfrac{1}{2},k) - E_y^n(i,j+\tfrac{1}{2},k)\right] \\ &+ \frac{\Delta t}{\mu_0 \Delta y} \left[E_x^n(i+\tfrac{1}{2},j+1,k) - E_x^n(i+\tfrac{1}{2},j,k)\right] \end{aligned} \quad (5.84)$$

where the superscript $n$ denotes the time ($t = n\Delta t$) and $i$, $j$, $k$ stand for the $x$, $y$, $z$ coordinates of a specific cell ($x = i\Delta x$, $y = j\Delta y$, $z = k\Delta z$). Similarly, Eqs. (5.79)–(5.81) can be discretized as

$$\begin{aligned} E_x^n(i+\tfrac{1}{2},j,k) = \frac{1}{\beta(i+\tfrac{1}{2},j,k)} \Big\{ &\alpha(i+\tfrac{1}{2},j,k) E_x^{n-1}(i+\tfrac{1}{2},j,k) \\ &+ \frac{\Delta t}{\Delta y} \left[H_z^{n-\frac{1}{2}}(i+\tfrac{1}{2},j+\tfrac{1}{2},k) - H_z^{n-\frac{1}{2}}(i+\tfrac{1}{2},j-\tfrac{1}{2},k)\right] \\ &- \frac{\Delta t}{\Delta z} \left[H_y^{n-\frac{1}{2}}(i+\tfrac{1}{2},j,k+\tfrac{1}{2}) - H_y^{n-\frac{1}{2}}(i+\tfrac{1}{2},j,k-\tfrac{1}{2})\right] \\ &- J_x^{n-1}(i+\tfrac{1}{2},j,k) \Big\} \end{aligned} \quad (5.85)$$

$$\begin{aligned} E_y^n(i,j+\tfrac{1}{2},k) = \frac{1}{\beta(i,j+\tfrac{1}{2},k)} \Big\{ &\alpha(i,j+\tfrac{1}{2},k) E_y^{n-1}(i,j+\tfrac{1}{2},k) \\ &+ \frac{\Delta t}{\Delta z} \left[H_x^{n-\frac{1}{2}}(i,j+\tfrac{1}{2},k+\tfrac{1}{2}) - H_x^{n-\frac{1}{2}}(i,j+\tfrac{1}{2},k-\tfrac{1}{2})\right] \\ &- \frac{\Delta t}{\Delta x} \left[H_z^{n-\frac{1}{2}}(i+\tfrac{1}{2},j+\tfrac{1}{2},k) - H_z^{n-\frac{1}{2}}(i-\tfrac{1}{2},j+\tfrac{1}{2},k)\right] \\ &- J_y^{n-1}(i,j+\tfrac{1}{2},k) \Big\} \end{aligned} \quad (5.86)$$

$$\begin{aligned} E_z^n(i,j,k+\tfrac{1}{2}) = \frac{1}{\beta(i,j,k+\tfrac{1}{2})} \Big\{ &\alpha(i,j,k+\tfrac{1}{2}) E_z^{n-1}(i,j,k+\tfrac{1}{2}) \\ &+ \frac{\Delta t}{\Delta x} \left[H_y^{n-\frac{1}{2}}(i+\tfrac{1}{2},j,k+\tfrac{1}{2}) - H_z^{n-\frac{1}{2}}(i-\tfrac{1}{2},j,k+\tfrac{1}{2})\right] \\ &- \frac{\Delta t}{\Delta y} \left[H_x^{n-\frac{1}{2}}(i,j+\tfrac{1}{2},k+\tfrac{1}{2}) - H_y^{n-\frac{1}{2}}(i,j-\tfrac{1}{2},k+\tfrac{1}{2})\right] \\ &- J_z^{n-1}(i,j,k+\tfrac{1}{2}) \Big\} \end{aligned} \quad (5.87)$$

where

$$\alpha = \frac{\epsilon}{\Delta t} - \frac{\sigma}{2}, \qquad \beta = \frac{\epsilon}{\Delta t} + \frac{\sigma}{2}. \quad (5.88)$$

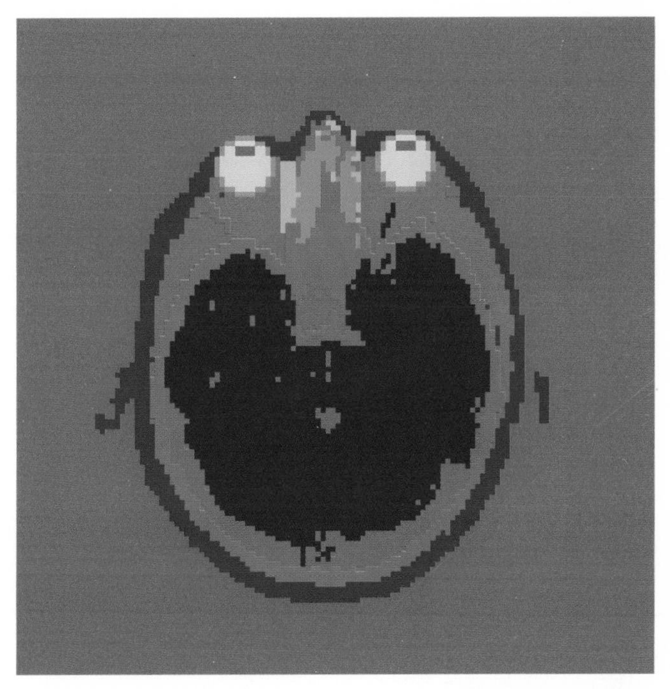

**Figure 5.7.** Axial slice through the eyes of the head model. Reproduced from Jin and Chen (1997).

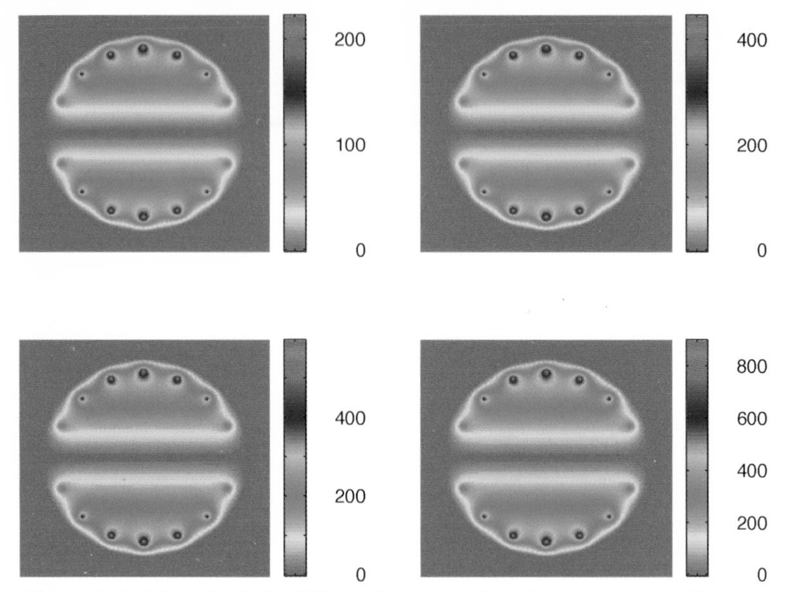


**Figure 5.8.** Electric field (V/m) of an unloaded linear, horizontally polarized birdcage coil. Top-left: 64 MHz. Top-right: 128 MHz. Bottom-left: 171 MHz. Bottom-right: 256 MHz. Reproduced from Jin and Chen (1997).

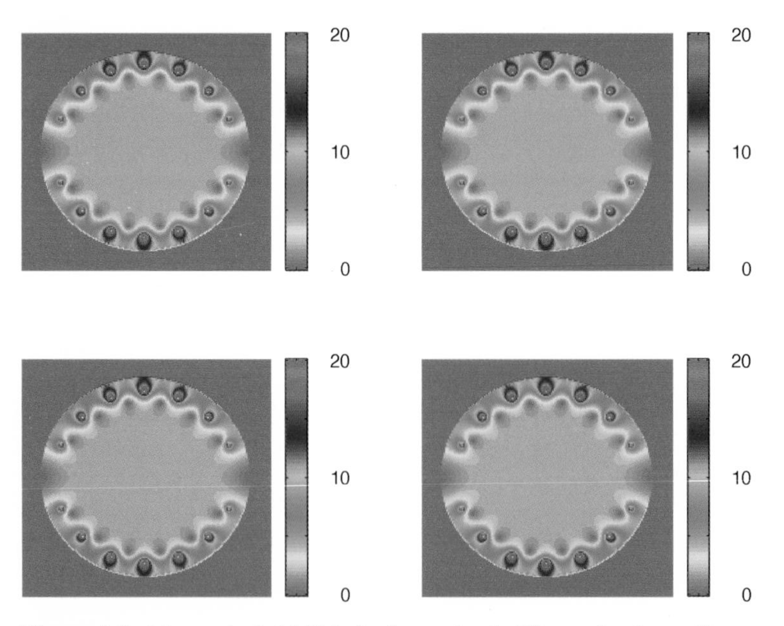


**Figure 5.9.** Magnetic field (A/m) of an unloaded linear, horizontally polarized birdcage coil. Top-left: 64 MHz. Top-right: 128 MHz. Bottom-left: 171 MHz. Bottom-right: 256 MHz. Reproduced from Jin and Chen (1997).

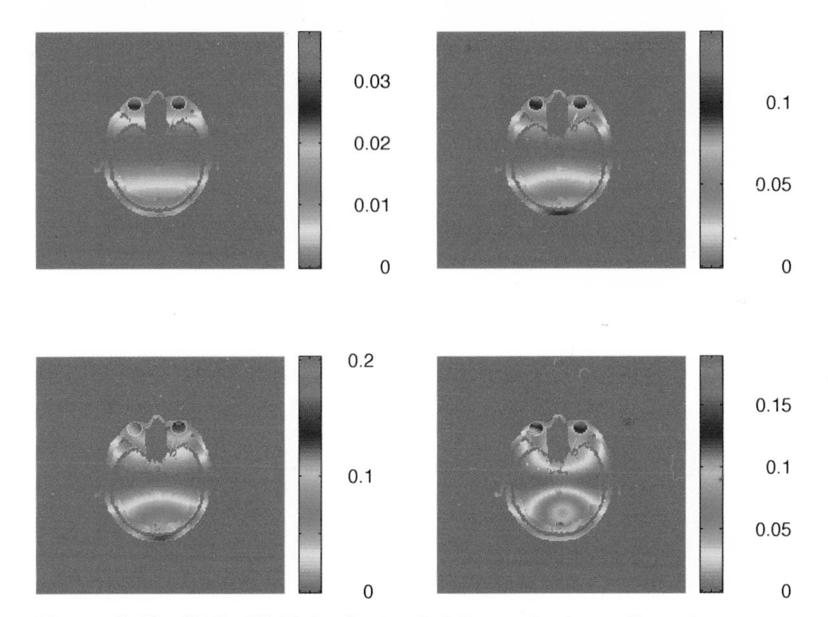


**Figure 5.10.** SAR (W/Kg) of a loaded linear, horizontally polarized birdcage coil. Top-left: 64 MHz. Top-right: 128 MHz. Bottom-left: 171 MHz. Bottom-right: 256 MHz. Reproduced from Jin and Chen (1997).

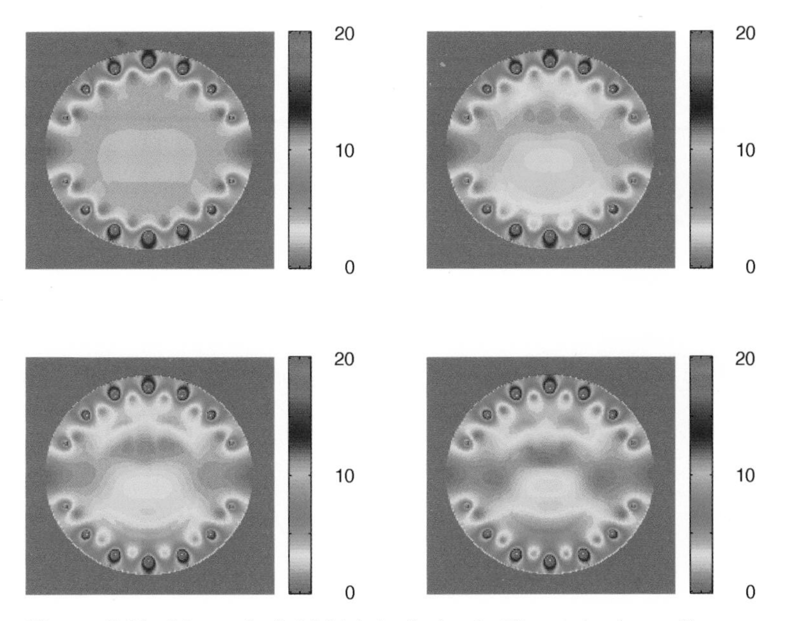


**Figure 5.11.** Magnetic field (A/m) of a loaded linear, horizontally polarized birdcage coil. Top-left: 64 MHz. Top-right: 128 MHz. Bottom-left: 171 MHz. Bottom-right: 256 MHz. Reproduced from Jin and Chen (1997).

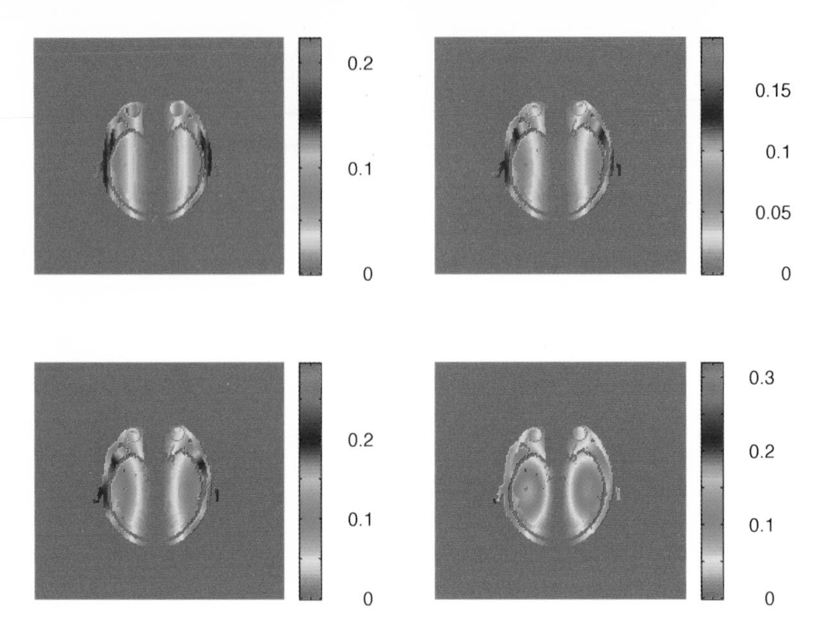


**Figure 5.12.** SAR (W/Kg) of a loaded linear, vertically polarized birdcage coil. Top-left: 64 MHz. Top-right: 128 MHz. Bottom-left: 171 MHz. Bottom-right: 256 MHz.

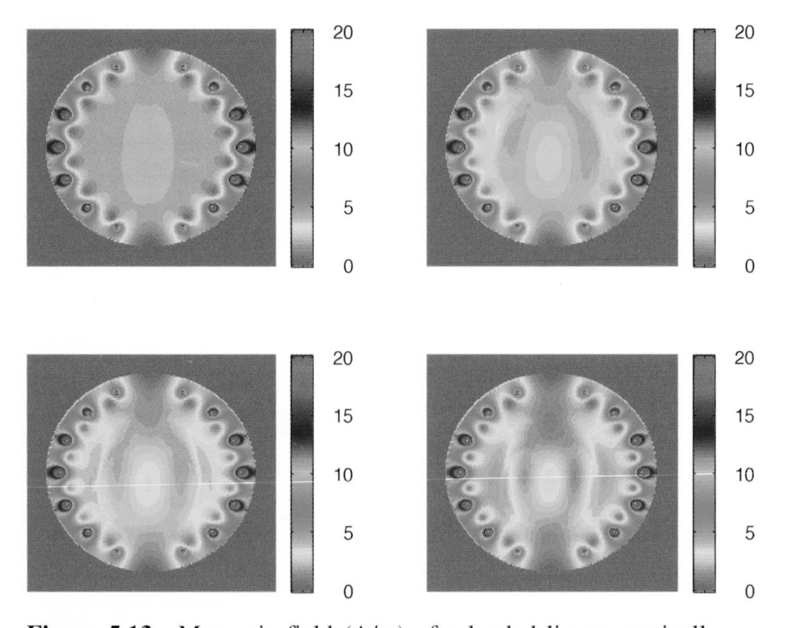


**Figure 5.13.** Magnetic field (A/m) of a loaded linear, vertically polarized birdcage coil. Top-left: 64 MHz. Top-right: 128 MHz. Bottom-left: 171 MHz. Bottom-right: 256 MHz.

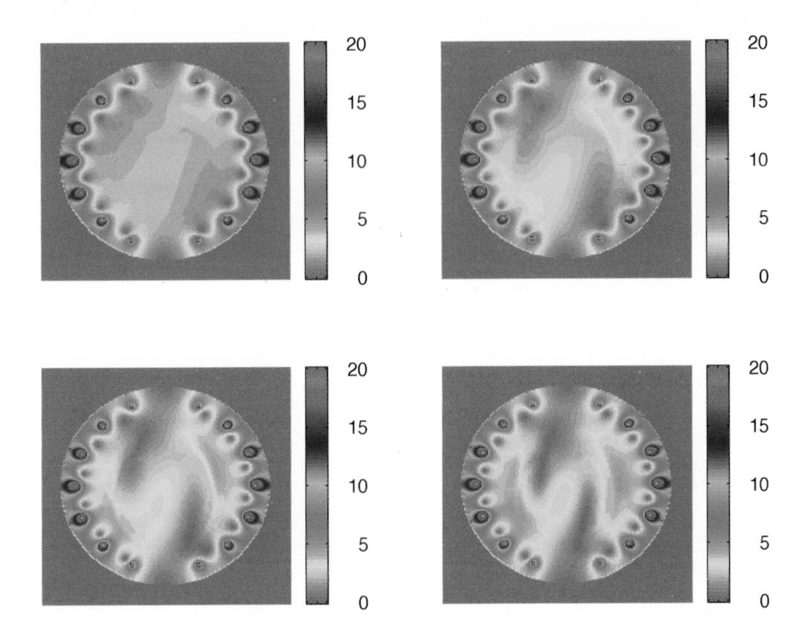


**Figure 5.14.** The circularly polarized component of the magnetic field (A/m) of a loaded linear, horizontally polarized birdcage coil. Top-left: 64 MHz. Top-right: 128 MHz. Bottom-left: 171 MHz. Bottom-right: 256 MHz.

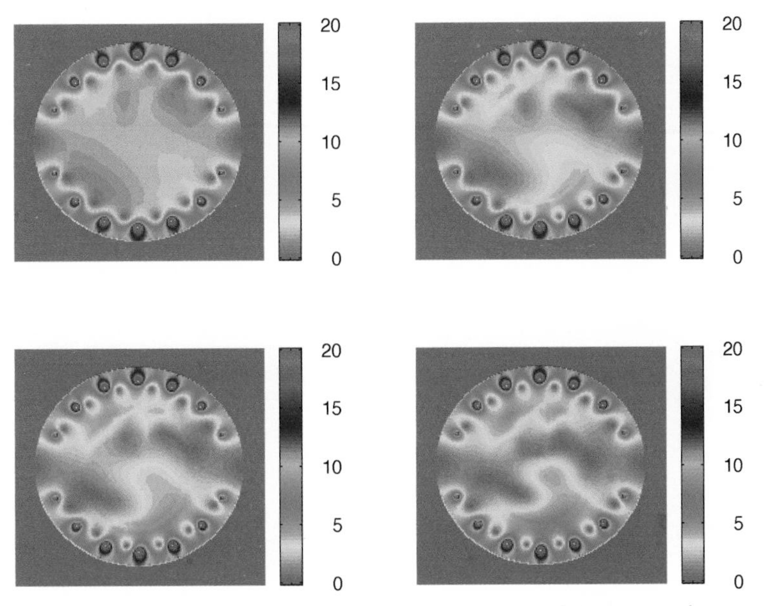


**Figure 5.15.** The circularly polarized component of the magnetic field (A/m) of a loaded linear, vertically polarized birdcage coil. Top-left: 64 MHz. Top-right: 128 MHz. Bottom-left: 171 MHz. Bottom-right: 256 MHz.

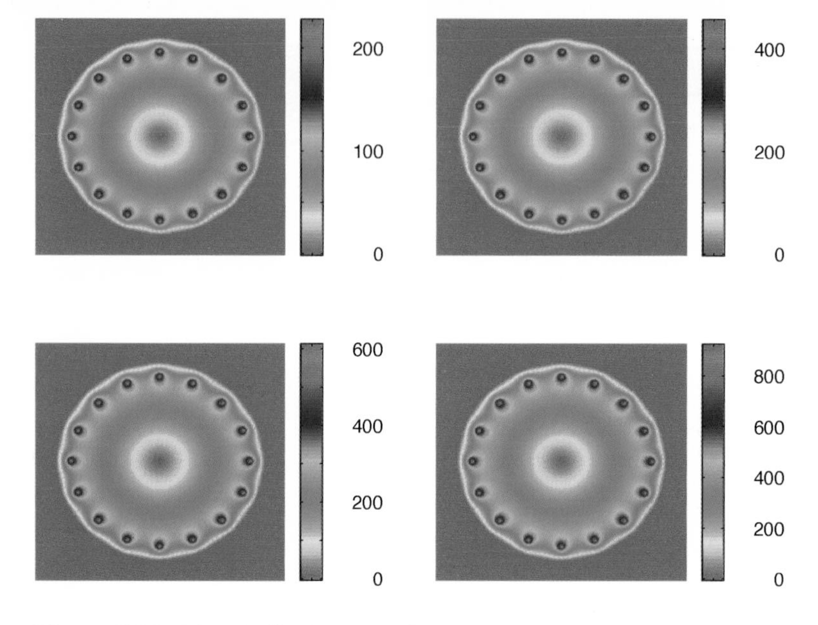


**Figure 5.16.** Electric field (V/m) of an unloaded quadrature birdcage coil. Top-left: 64 MHz. Top-right: 128 MHz. Bottom-left: 171 MHz. Bottom-right: 256 MHz. Reproduced from Jin and Chen (1997).

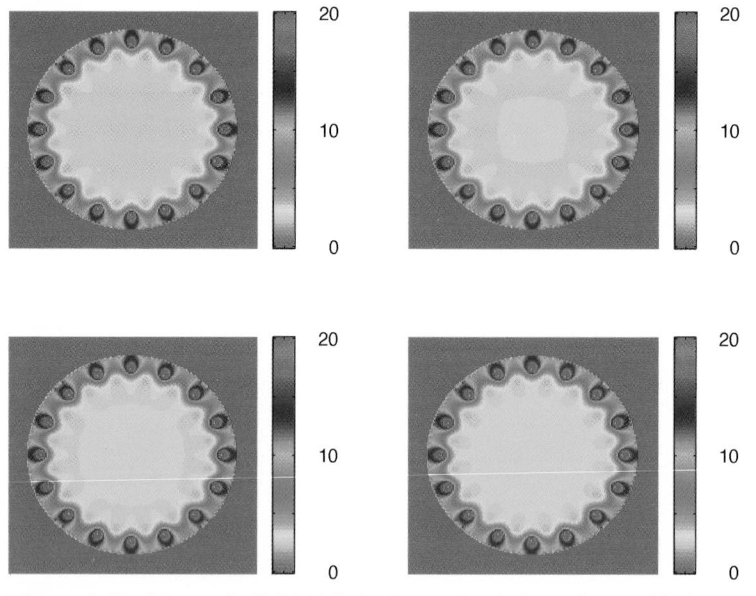


**Figure 5.17.** Magnetic field (A/m) of an unloaded quadrature birdcage coil. Top-left: 64 MHz. Top-right: 128 MHz. Bottom-left: 171 MHz. Bottom-right: 256 MHz. Reproduced from Jin and Chen (1997).

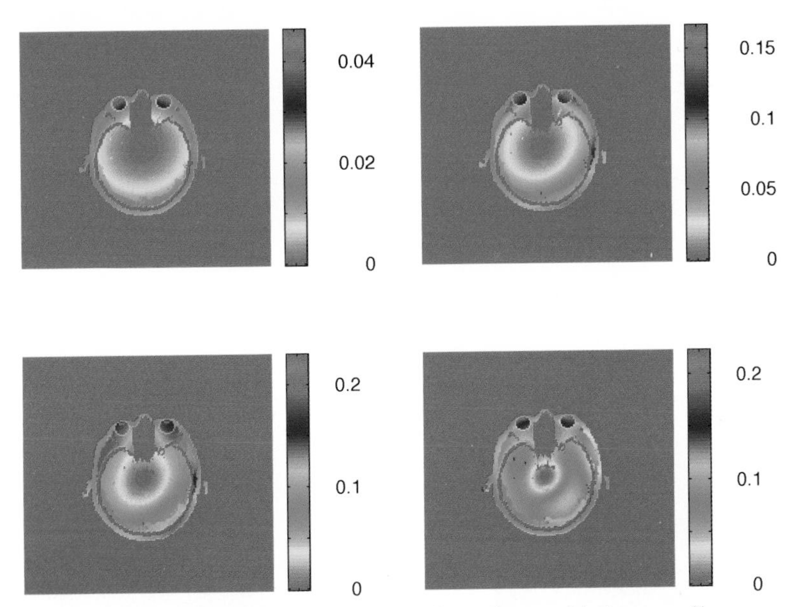


**Figure 5.18.** SAR (W/Kg) of a loaded quadrature birdcage coil. Top-left: 64 MHz. Top-right: 128 MHz. Bottom-left: 171 MHz. Bottom-right: 256 MHz. Reproduced from Jin and Chen (1997).

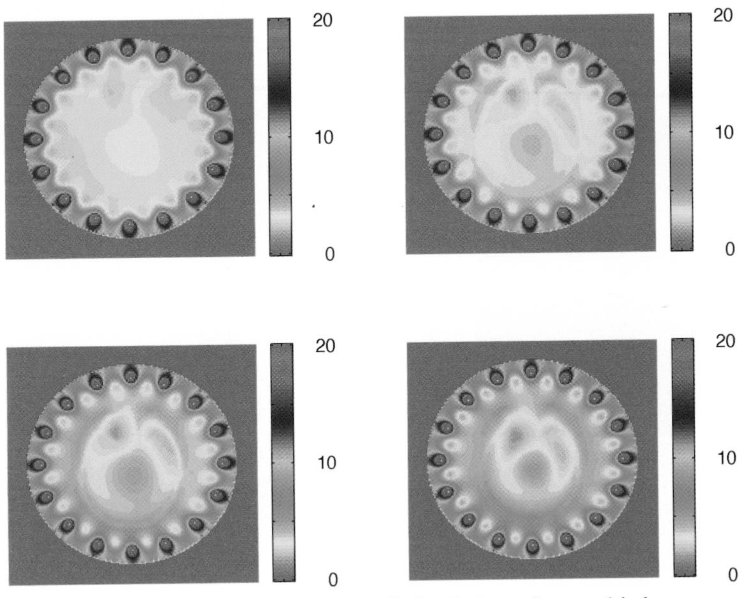


**Figure 5.19.** Magnetic field (A/m) of a loaded quadrature birdcage coil. Top-left: 64 MHz. Top-right: 128 MHz. Bottom-left: 171 MHz. Bottom-right: 256 MHz. Reproduced from Jin and Chen (1997).

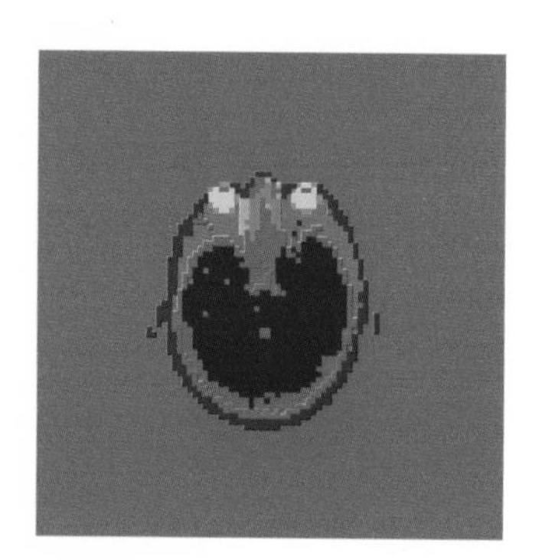

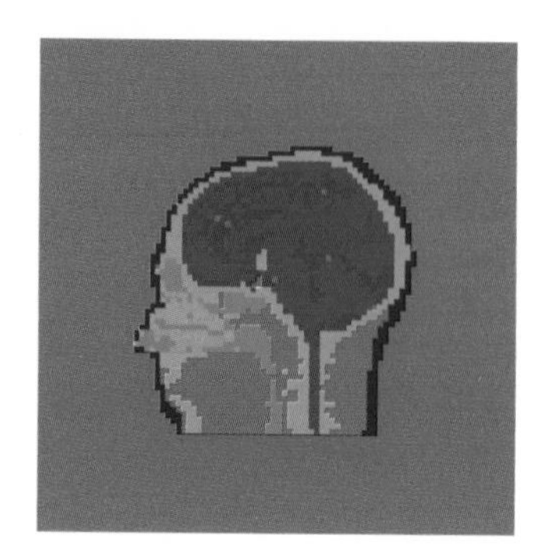

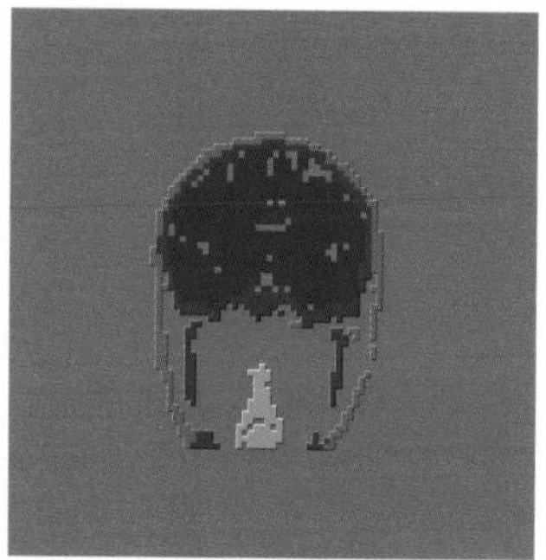

**Figure 5.21.** The axial, sagittal, and coronal slices of the head model. Reproduced from Chen et al. (1998), © 1998 IEEE.

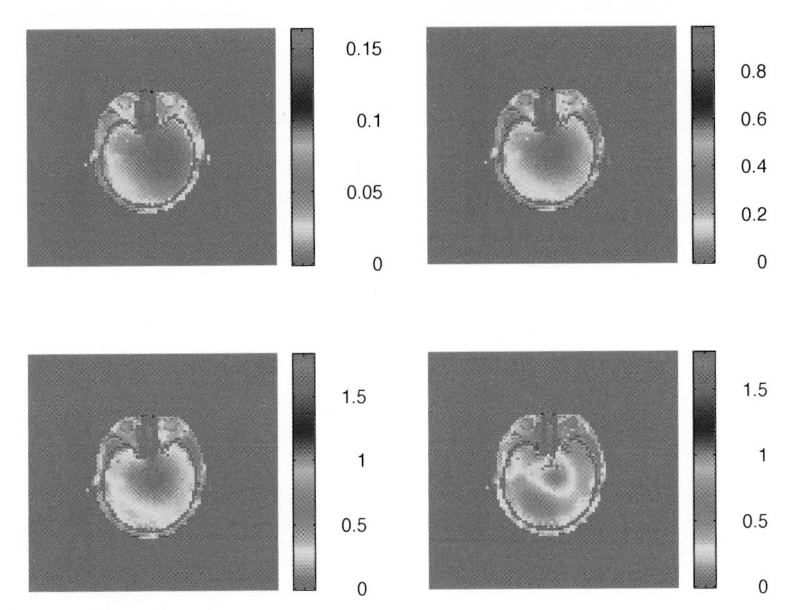


**Figure 5.22.** SAR (W/Kg) distribution in the axial slice for a shielded birdcage coil. Top-left: 64 MHz. Top-right: 128 MHz. Bottom-left: 171 MHz. Bottom-right: 256 MHz. Reproduced from Chen et al. (1998), © 1998 IEEE.

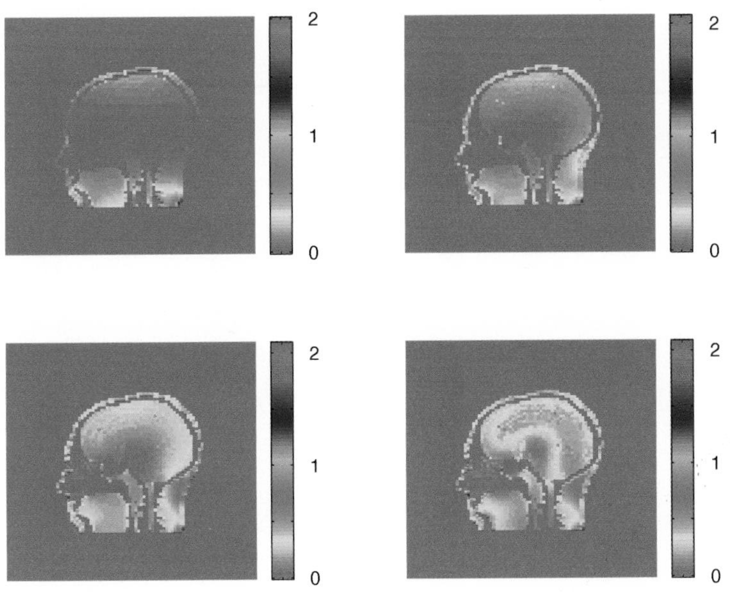


**Figure 5.23.** SAR (W/Kg) distribution in the sagittal slice for a shielded birdcage coil. Top-left: 64 MHz. Top-right: 128 MHz. Bottom-left: 171 MHz. Bottom-right: 256 MHz. Reproduced from Chen et al. (1998), © 1998 IEEE.

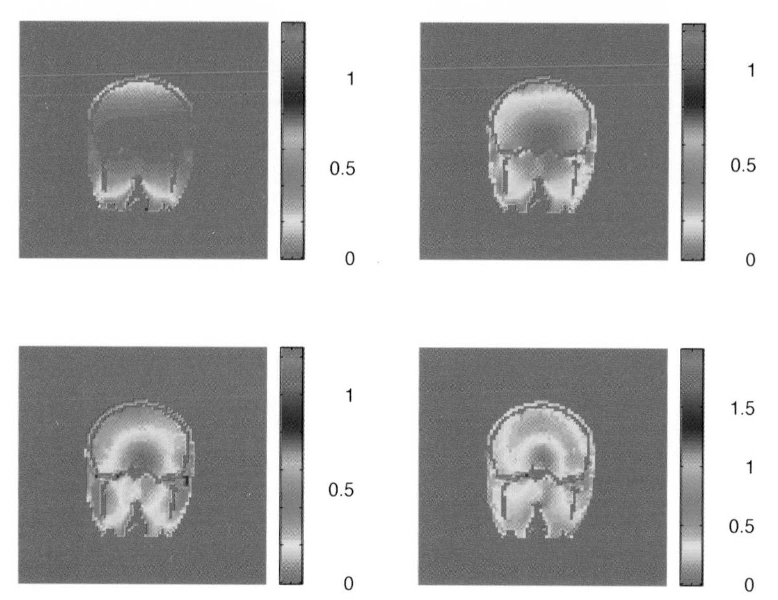


**Figure 5.24.** SAR (W/Kg) distribution in the coronal slice for a shielded birdcage coil. Top-left: 64 MHz. Top-right: 128 MHz. Bottom-left: 171 MHz. Bottom-right: 256 MHz. Reproduced from Chen et al. (1998), © 1998 IEEE.

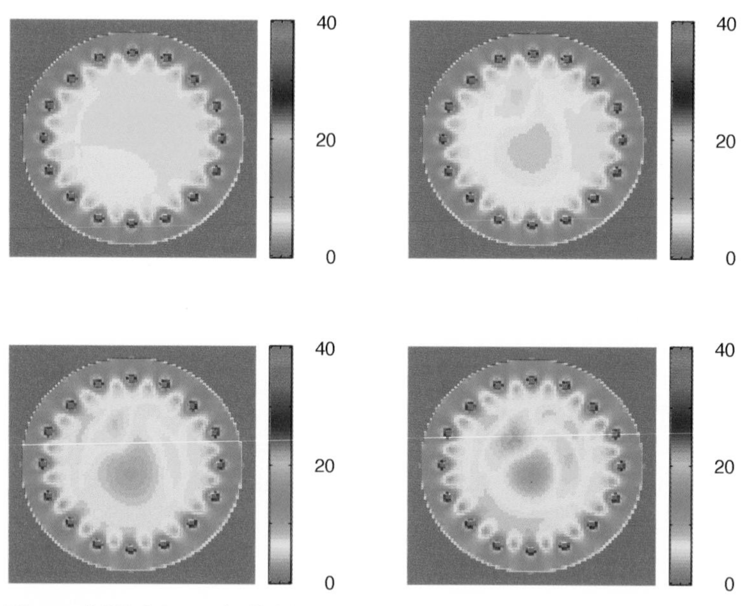


**Figure 5.25.** Magnetic field (A/m) distribution in the axial slice for a shielded birdcage coil. Top-left: 64 MHz. Top-right: 128 MHz. Bottom-left: 171 MHz. Bottom-right: 256 MHz. Reproduced from Chen et al. (1998), © 1998 IEEE.

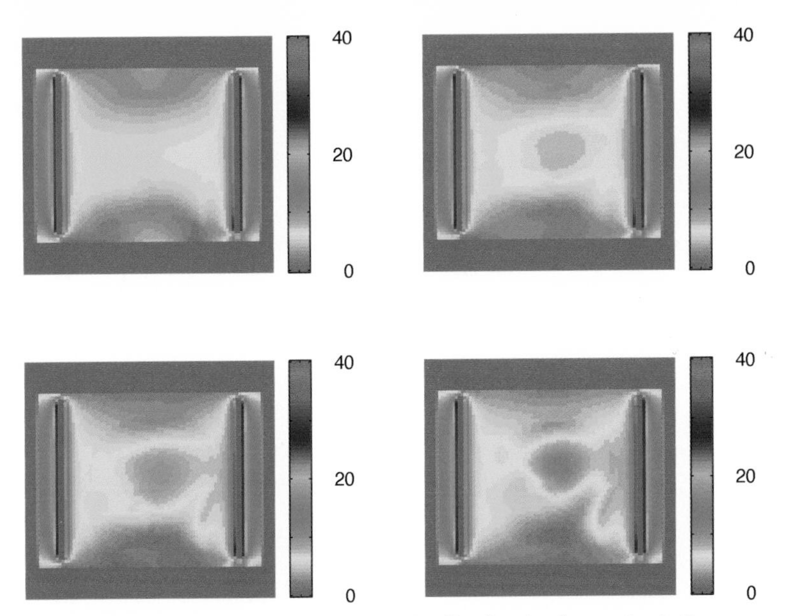


**Figure 5.26.** Magnetic field (A/m) distribution in the sagittal slice for a shielded birdcage coil. Top-left: 64 MHz. Top-right: 128 MHz. Bottom-left: 171 MHz. Bottom-right: 256 MHz. Reproduced from Chen et al. (1998), © 1998 IEEE.

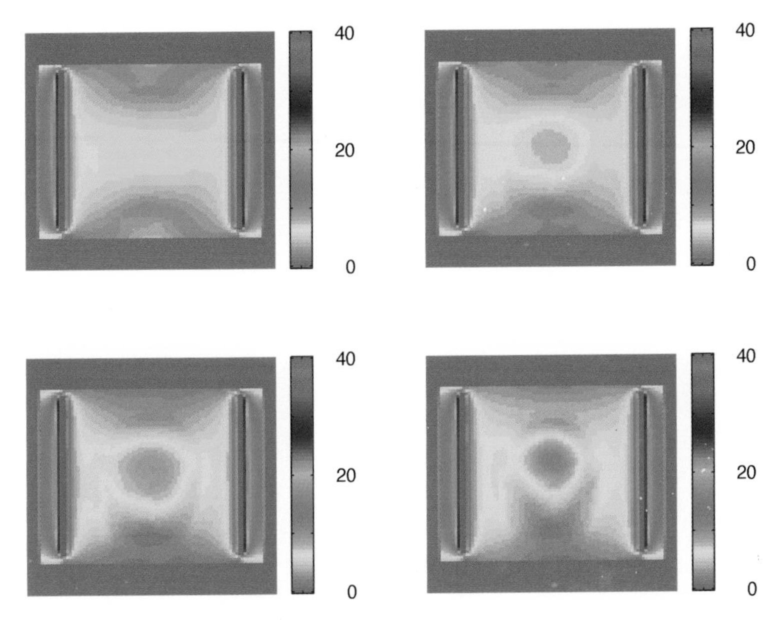


**Figure 5.27.** Magnetic field (A/m) distribution in the coronal slice for a shielded birdcage coil. Top-left: 64 MHz. Top-right: 128 MHz. Bottom-left: 171 MHz. Bottom-right: 256 MHz. Reproduced from Chen et al. (1998), © 1998 IEEE.

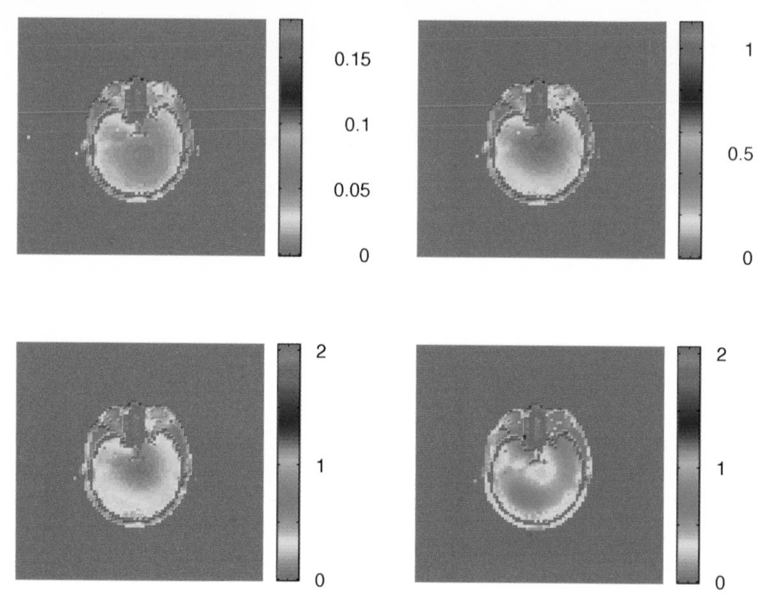


**Figure 5.28.** SAR (W/Kg) distribution in the axial slice for an end-capped shielded birdcage coil. Top-left: 64 MHz. Top-right: 128 MHz. Bottom-left: 171 MHz. Bottom-right: 256 MHz.

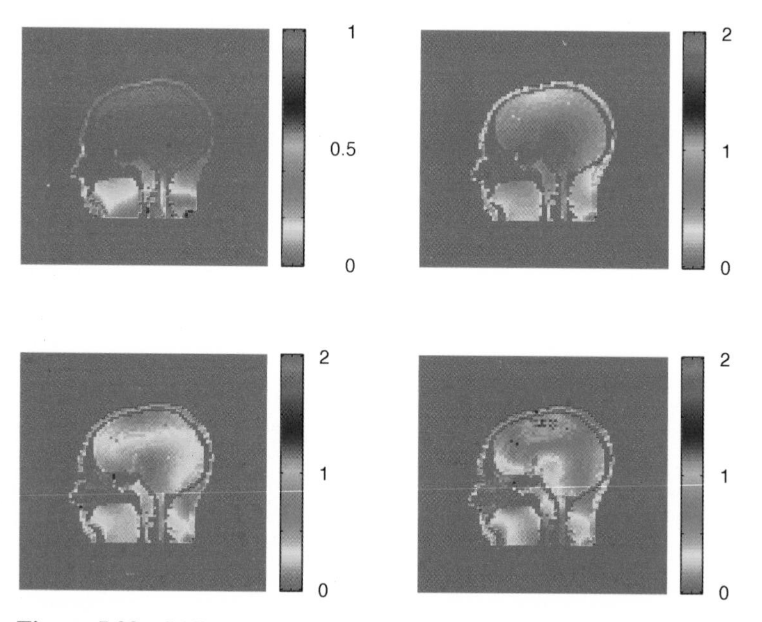


**Figure 5.29.** SAR (W/Kg) distribution in the sagittal slice for an end-capped shielded birdcage coil. Top-left: 64 MHz. Top-right: 128 MHz. Bottom-left: 171 MHz. Bottom-right: 256 MHz.

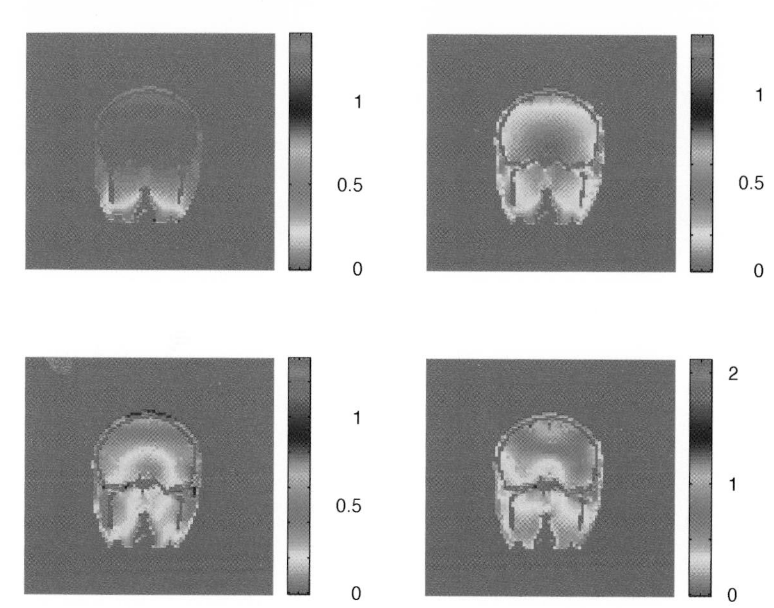


**Figure 5.30.** SAR (W/Kg) distribution in the coronal slice for an end-capped shielded birdcage coil. Top-left: 64 MHz. Top-right: 128 MHz. Bottom-left: 171 MHz. Bottom-right: 256 MHz.

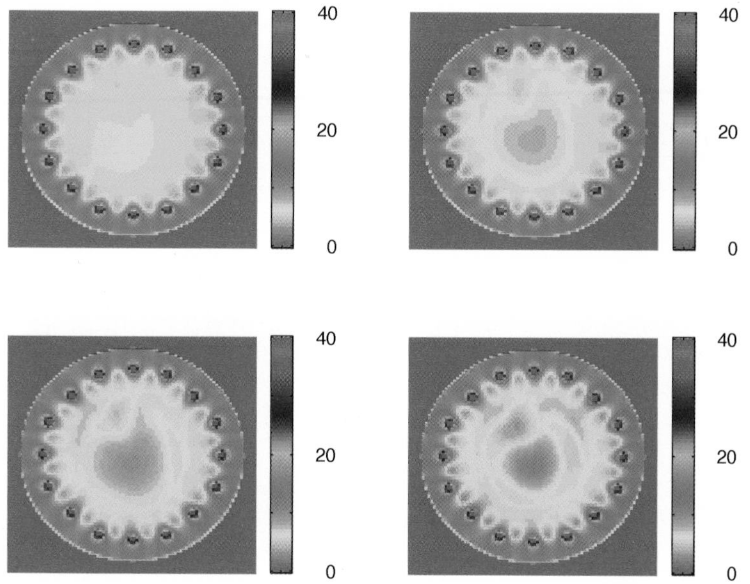


**Figure 5.31.** Magnetic field (A/m) distribution in the axial slice for an end-capped shielded birdcage coil. Top-left: 64 MHz. Top-right: 128 MHz. Bottom-left: 171 MHz. Bottom-right: 256 MHz.

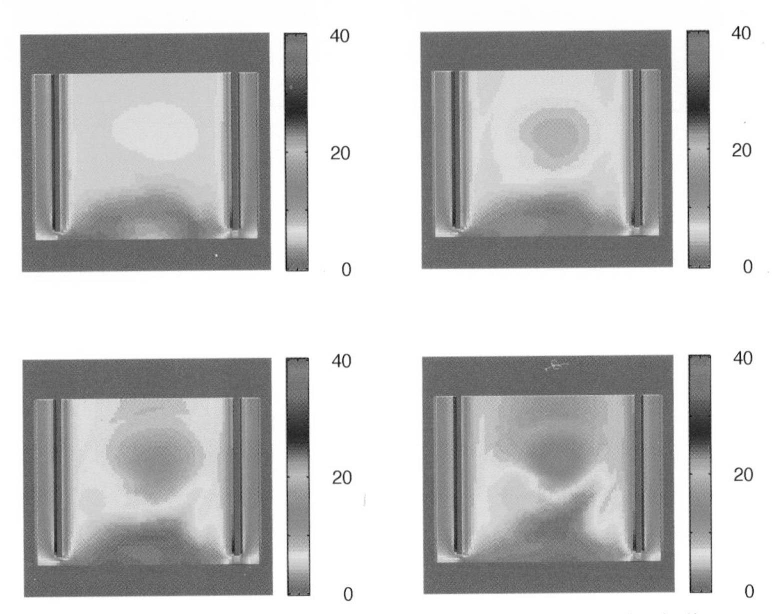


**Figure 5.32.** Magnetic field (A/m) distribution in the sagittal slice for an end-capped shielded birdcage coil. Top-left: 64 MHz. Top-right: 128 MHz. Bottom-left: 171 MHz. Bottom-right: 256 MHz.

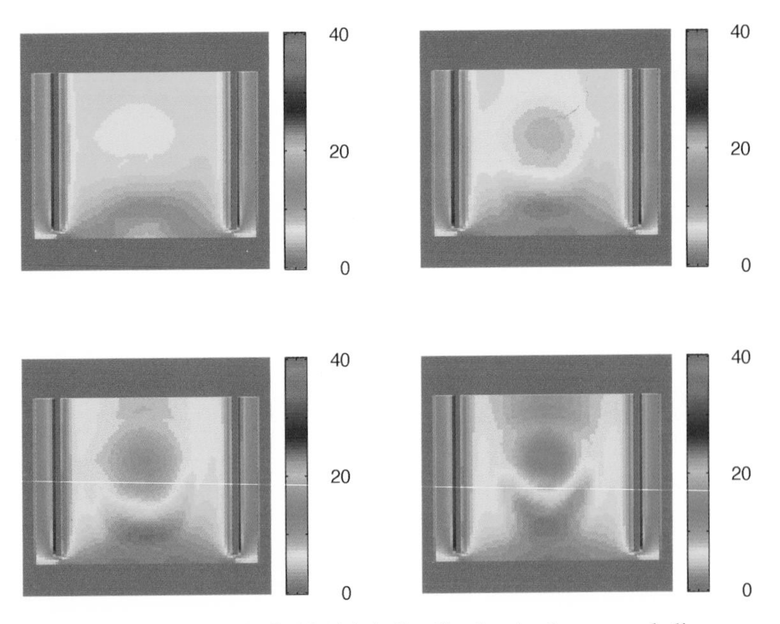


**Figure 5.33.** Magnetic field (A/m) distribution in the coronal slice for an end-capped shielded birdcage coil. Top-left: 64 MHz. Top-right: 128 MHz. Bottom-left: 171 MHz. Bottom-right: 256 MHz.

Clearly, given the excitation and initial values for the electric and magnetic fields, we can use Eqs. (5.82)–(5.84) to calculate the magnetic field and Eqs. (5.85)–(5.87) to calculate the electric field at a new time step. It can be proven that the discretization above is of second order in accuracy in terms of the cell size, and for a stable time marching, the time step has to satisfy the Courant-Friedrichs-Lewy stability criterion (Chew 1995)

$$\Delta t < \frac{1}{c_{\max}\sqrt{(1/\Delta x)^2 + (1/\Delta y)^2 + (1/\Delta z)^2}} \tag{5.89}$$

where $c_{\max}$ is the maximum propagation speed of the electromagnetic waves in the simulation region.

Since all RF coils (even the shielded ones) are basically open structures, the field generated by the coil radiates into a large space. However, the numerical simulation described above can be performed only inside a finite space. Therefore, we must first truncate the simulation space by using a conducting box to enclose the solution volume. Unfortunately, the conducting box will reflect the outgoing field back into the solution volume, rendering a totally useless solution. One remedy is to apply an absorbing boundary condition (ABC) on the inner surface of the box to reduce the artificial reflection produced by the box (Kunz and Luebbers 1994, Taflove 1995). An alternative is to place a layer of artificial absorbing material on the inner surface of the box to achieve the same purpose. The best artificial absorbing material developed so far is called the perfectly matched layer (PML) introduced by Berenger (1994) and extended by Chew and Weedon (1994). This PML is equivalent to a uniaxial medium with constitutive parameters (Sacks *et al.* 1995)

$$[\epsilon] = \epsilon_0 \begin{bmatrix} a & 0 & 0 \\ 0 & a & 0 \\ 0 & 0 & a^{-1} \end{bmatrix} \tag{5.90}$$

and

$$[\mu] = \mu_0 \begin{bmatrix} a & 0 & 0 \\ 0 & a & 0 \\ 0 & 0 & a^{-1} \end{bmatrix} \tag{5.91}$$

for the layer perpendicular to the $z$-axis. It can be shown that for such a layer, the wave can enter into the layer without reflection from the interface. In Eqs. (5.90) and (5.91), $a$ is chosen such that the wave will be sufficiently attenuated in the layer. The usual choice is

$$a = 1 + i\frac{\sigma}{\omega\epsilon_0} \tag{5.92}$$

where $\epsilon_0$ denotes the free-space permittivity and $\sigma$ is the conductivity, large enough to attenuate the wave.

Finally, we note that in order to obtain accurate electric and magnetic fields at a certain frequency, we have to continue the FDTD calculation until it reaches the steady state. This process can be sped up by using a tapered sinusoidal excitation instead of an excitation with a finite jump. For example, if we are interested in the solution at frequency $\omega$, instead of using $\mathbf{J}(\mathbf{r},t) = \mathbf{J}(\mathbf{r})\sin(\omega t)u(t)$ as an excitation, we can use the tapered excitation

$$\mathbf{J}(\mathbf{r},t) = \mathbf{J}(\mathbf{r})\left(1 - e^{-\alpha t}\right)\sin(\omega t)u(t) \tag{5.93}$$

where $\alpha$ is the constant chosen to ensure that the excitation has a smooth transient. Usually, $\alpha$ is chosen to be $\alpha = \omega/5$ so that the current excitation will reach its full strength after three periods of the operating frequency. The data after this time instant can then be used to obtain a spectral domain solution using either peak detection or the fast Fourier transform (FFT) method.

### 5.4.2 Method of Moments

The method of moments (MoM) is one of the popular methods for the computation of electromagnetic fields in arbitrarily-shaped, inhomogeneous dielectric bodies (Livesay and Chen 1974, Schaubert *et al.* 1984). In this method, an integro-differential equation is first formulated in terms of volumetric equivalent current that accounts for the effect of the permittivity and conductivity of an inhomogeneous body. This integro-differential equation is then discretized using Galerkin's procedure. The discretization results in a matrix equation, whose solution provides a numerical solution to the problem.

Consider electromagnetic fields $(\mathbf{E}, \mathbf{H})$ excited by current density $\mathbf{J}^{\text{ex}}$ in the presence of an inhomogeneous dielectric body characterized by permittivity $\epsilon$ and conductivity $\sigma$. From Maxwell's equations, we have

$$\nabla \times \mathbf{E} = i\omega\mu_0\mathbf{H} \tag{5.94}$$

$$\nabla \times \mathbf{H} = -i\omega\epsilon\mathbf{E} + \sigma\mathbf{E} + \mathbf{J}^{\text{ex}}. \tag{5.95}$$

Equation (5.95) can also be written as

$$\begin{aligned}\nabla \times \mathbf{H} &= -i\omega\epsilon_c\epsilon_0\mathbf{E} + \mathbf{J}^{\text{ex}} \\ &= -i\omega\epsilon_0\mathbf{E} + \mathbf{J}^{\text{eq}} + \mathbf{J}^{\text{ex}}\end{aligned} \tag{5.96}$$

where $\epsilon_c\epsilon_0 = \epsilon + i\sigma/\omega$ and

$$\mathbf{J}^{\text{eq}} = -i\omega\epsilon_0(\epsilon_c - 1)\mathbf{E}. \tag{5.97}$$

It is obvious from Eq. (5.96) that $(\mathbf{E}, \mathbf{H})$ can be thought of as the electromagnetic fields generated by $\mathbf{J}^{\text{ex}}$ and $\mathbf{J}^{\text{eq}}$ in free space. In other words, the effect of the inhomogeneous body can be accounted for by a volumetric equivalent current $\mathbf{J}^{\text{eq}}$.

The electric fields generated by $\mathbf{J}^{\text{ex}}$ and $\mathbf{J}^{\text{eq}}$ can be expressed as

$$\mathbf{E}^{\text{ex}}(\mathbf{r}) = (k_0^2 + \nabla\nabla\cdot)\mathbf{A}^{\text{ex}}(\mathbf{r}) \tag{5.98}$$

$$\mathbf{E}^{\text{eq}}(\mathbf{r}) = (k_0^2 + \nabla\nabla\cdot)\mathbf{A}^{\text{eq}}(\mathbf{r}) \tag{5.99}$$

where $k_0 = \omega\sqrt{\mu_0\epsilon_0}$ and

$$\mathbf{A}^{\text{ex}}(\mathbf{r}) = \frac{i}{\omega\epsilon_0}\iiint_V G(\mathbf{r}, \mathbf{r}')\mathbf{J}^{\text{ex}}(\mathbf{r}')\, dV' \tag{5.100}$$

$$\mathbf{A}^{\text{eq}}(\mathbf{r}) = \frac{i}{\omega\epsilon_0}\iiint_V G(\mathbf{r}, \mathbf{r}')\mathbf{J}^{\text{eq}}(\mathbf{r}')\, dV' \tag{5.101}$$

in which $G(\mathbf{r}, \mathbf{r}')$ is the free-space Green's function given by

$$G(\mathbf{r}, \mathbf{r}') = \frac{\exp(ik_0|\mathbf{r} - \mathbf{r}'|)}{4\pi|\mathbf{r} - \mathbf{r}'|}. \tag{5.102}$$

The total electric field is then

$$\mathbf{E} = \mathbf{E}^{\text{ex}} + \mathbf{E}^{\text{eq}}. \tag{5.103}$$

Substituting Eqs. (5.97)–(5.102) into Eq. (5.103), we obtain the integro-differential equation expressed in terms of $\mathbf{D}(\mathbf{r})$ as

$$\frac{\mathbf{D}(\mathbf{r})}{\epsilon_c(\mathbf{r})\epsilon_0} - (k_0^2 + \nabla\nabla\cdot)\mathbf{A}(\mathbf{r}) = \mathbf{E}^{\text{ex}}(\mathbf{r}) \tag{5.104}$$

where

$$\mathbf{A}(\mathbf{r}) = \frac{1}{\epsilon_0}\iiint_V G(\mathbf{r}, \mathbf{r}')\chi(\mathbf{r}')\mathbf{D}(\mathbf{r}')\, dV' \tag{5.105}$$

with

$$\chi(\mathbf{r}) = \frac{\epsilon_c(\mathbf{r}) - 1}{\epsilon_c(\mathbf{r})}. \tag{5.106}$$

To discretize Eq. (5.104), we place the object in a uniform mesh with grid widths of $\Delta x$, $\Delta y$, and $\Delta z$ in the $x$, $y$, and $z$ directions, respectively. Therefore, the object is modeled approximately as a collection of small grids. The center of each grid is denoted as $\mathbf{r}_{M,N,P} = \hat{x}(M - \frac{1}{2})\Delta x +$

$\hat{y}(N - \frac{1}{2})\Delta y + \hat{z}(P - \frac{1}{2})\Delta z$ and within each grid the complex permittivity is assumed to be constant with value $\epsilon_{cM,N,P} = \epsilon_c(\mathbf{r}_{M,N,P})$.

To convert Eq. (5.104) into a matrix equation, we expand the electric flux density and the vector potential as

$$\mathbf{D}(\mathbf{r}) = \epsilon_0 \sum_{q=1}^{3} \sum_{I,J,K} d_{I,J,K}^{(q)} \mathbf{f}_{I,J,K}^{(q)}(\mathbf{r}) \tag{5.107}$$

$$\mathbf{A}(\mathbf{r}) = \sum_{q=1}^{3} \sum_{I,J,K} A_{I,J,K}^{(q)} \mathbf{f}_{I,J,K}^{(q)}(\mathbf{r}) \tag{5.108}$$

where $\mathbf{f}_{I,J,K}^{(1)}$, $\mathbf{f}_{I,J,K}^{(2)}$, and $\mathbf{f}_{I,J,K}^{(3)}$ are vector volumetric rooftop functions in the $x$, $y$, and $z$ directions, respectively. They are defined as

$$\mathbf{f}_{I,J,K}^{(1)} = \hat{x}\Lambda(I)\Pi(J)\Pi(K) \tag{5.109}$$

$$\mathbf{f}_{I,J,K}^{(2)} = \hat{y}\Pi(I)\Lambda(J)\Pi(K) \tag{5.110}$$

$$\mathbf{f}_{I,J,K}^{(3)} = \hat{z}\Pi(I)\Pi(J)\Lambda(K) \tag{5.111}$$

where

$$\Lambda(I) = \begin{cases} 1 - |x - I\Delta x|/\Delta x & |x - I\Delta x| < \Delta x \\ 0 & |x - I\Delta x| > \Delta x \end{cases} \tag{5.112}$$

$$\Pi(I) = \begin{cases} 1 & |x - I\Delta x| < \Delta x/2 \\ 0 & |x - I\Delta x| > \Delta x/2. \end{cases} \tag{5.113}$$

We then apply the Galerkin's testing formulation to Eq. (5.104) [that is, multiply Eq. (5.104) by $\mathbf{f}_{M,N,P}^{(p)}$ and integrate over the volume] and obtain

$$\begin{aligned} \langle \mathbf{f}_{M,N,P}^{(p)}(\mathbf{r}), \frac{\mathbf{D}(\mathbf{r})}{\epsilon_c(\mathbf{r})\epsilon_0} \rangle - k_0^2 \langle \mathbf{f}_{M,N,P}^{(p)}(\mathbf{r}), \mathbf{A}(\mathbf{r}) \rangle + \langle \nabla \cdot \mathbf{f}_{M,N,P}^{(p)}(\mathbf{r}), \nabla \cdot \mathbf{A}(\mathbf{r}) \rangle \\ = \langle \mathbf{f}_{M,N,P}^{(p)}(\mathbf{r}), \mathbf{E}^{\text{ex}}(\mathbf{r}) \rangle \end{aligned} \tag{5.114}$$

for $p = 1, 2, 3$, where $\langle \cdot \rangle$ denotes the inner product of two vector functions defined as

$$\langle \mathbf{f}, \mathbf{g} \rangle = \iiint_V \mathbf{f} \cdot \mathbf{g} \, dV. \tag{5.115}$$

In arriving at Eq. (5.114), we employed the divergence theorem to transfer one del operator from $\mathbf{A}(\mathbf{r})$ to $\mathbf{f}_{M,N,P}^{(p)}(\mathbf{r})$. Substituting Eqs. (5.107) and

(5.108) into Eq. (5.114), we obtain the following weak form of the domain integral equation

$$[u^{(p,q)}_{M,N,P;I,J,K}][d^{(q)}_{I,J,K}] - [k_0^2 v^{(p,q)}_{M,N,P;I,J,K} - w^{(p,q)}_{M,N,P;I,J,K}][A^{(q)}_{I,J,K}] = [e^{\text{ex},(p)}_{M,N,P}] \tag{5.116}$$

where

$$u^{(p,q)}_{M,N,P;I,J,K} = \langle \mathbf{f}^{(p)}_{M,N,P}, \frac{1}{\epsilon_c(\mathbf{r})}\mathbf{f}^{(q)}_{I,J,K}\rangle \tag{5.117}$$

$$v^{(p,q)}_{M,N,P;I,J,K} = \langle \mathbf{f}^{(p)}_{M,N,P}, \mathbf{f}^{(q)}_{I,J,K}\rangle \tag{5.118}$$

$$w^{(p,q)}_{M,N,P;I,J,K} = \langle \nabla\cdot\mathbf{f}^{(p)}_{M,N,P}, \nabla\cdot\mathbf{f}^{(q)}_{I,J,K}\rangle \tag{5.119}$$

$$e^{\text{ex},(p)}_{M,N,P} = \langle \mathbf{f}^{(p)}_{M,N,P}, \mathbf{E}^{\text{ex}}\rangle. \tag{5.120}$$

The relationship between $d^{(q)}_{M,N,P}$ and $A^{(q)}_{M,N,P}$ can be found by substituting Eqs. (5.107) and (5.108) into Eq. (5.105), yielding

$$A^{(q)}_{M,N,P} = \Delta V \sum_{I,J,K} G_{M-I,N-J,P-K}\chi^{(q)}_{I,J,K}d^{(q)}_{I,J,K} \tag{5.121}$$

where $\Delta V = \Delta x \Delta y \Delta z$, and

$$G_{M-I,N-J,P-K} = \frac{1}{\Delta V}\int_{-\Delta x/2}^{\Delta x/2}\int_{-\Delta y/2}^{\Delta y/2}\int_{-\Delta z/2}^{\Delta z/2}\frac{\exp(ik_0R)}{4\pi R}\,dx''dy''dz'' \tag{5.122}$$

with

$$R = \sqrt{[(M-I)\Delta x + x'']^2 + [(N-J)\Delta y + y'']^2 + [(P-K)\Delta z + z'']^2}.$$

Substituting Eq. (5.121) into Eq. (5.116), we obtain a system of linear algebraic equations, which can be symbolically written as

$$\mathbf{Ld} = \mathbf{e}^{\text{ex}}. \tag{5.123}$$

The numerical discretization described above follows that of Zwamborn and van den Berg (1992). Equation (5.123) involves a large number of unknowns and its coefficient matrix **L** is a full matrix. Therefore, its solution using a direct solver, such as Gaussian elimination and $LU$ decomposition method, is basically impractical, because a direct solver has a memory requirement of $O(n^2)$ and computational complexity of $O(n^3)$, where $n$ is the number of unknowns. This difficulty can be circumvented by solving Eq.

(5.123) using an iterative solver. There are many iterative solvers and a good choice for this problem is the transpose-free quasi-minimum residual method (Freund 1993, Saad 1995). Its algorithm for solving Eq. (5.123) with an initial guess $\mathbf{d}_0$ is given as follows:

1. Compute $\mathbf{w}_0 = \mathbf{u}_0 = \mathbf{r}_0 = \mathbf{e}^{\text{ex}} - \mathbf{L}\mathbf{d}_0, \mathbf{v}_0 = \mathbf{L}\mathbf{u}_0, \mathbf{g}_0 = 0$;
2. $\tau_0 = \|\mathbf{r}_0\|, \theta_0 = \eta_0 = 0$;
3. Choose $\mathbf{r}_0^*$ such that $\rho_0 \equiv \langle \mathbf{r}_0^*, \mathbf{r}_0 \rangle \neq 0$.
4. For $m = 0, 1, 2, \ldots$, until convergence Do:
5. If $m$ is even then
6. $\alpha_{m+1} = \alpha_m = \rho_m / \langle \mathbf{v}_m, \mathbf{r}_0^* \rangle$
7. $\mathbf{u}_{m+1} = \mathbf{u}_m - \alpha_m \mathbf{v}_m$
8. Endif
9. $\mathbf{w}_{m+1} = \mathbf{w}_m - \alpha_m \mathbf{L}\mathbf{u}_m$
10. $\mathbf{g}_{m+1} = \mathbf{u}_m + (\theta_m^2/\alpha_m)\eta_m \mathbf{g}_m$
11. $\theta_{m+1} = \|\mathbf{w}_{m+1}\|_2/\tau_m; c_{m+1} = (1 + \theta_{m+1}^2)^{-\frac{1}{2}}$
12. $\tau_{m+1} = \tau_m \theta_{m+1} c_{m+1}; \eta_{m+1} = c_{m+1}^2 \alpha_m$
13. $\mathbf{d}_{m+1} = \mathbf{d}_m + \eta_{m+1} \mathbf{g}_{m+1}$
14. If $m$ is odd then
15. $\rho_{m+1} = \langle \mathbf{w}_{m+1}, \mathbf{r}_0^* \rangle; \beta_{m-1} = \rho_{m+1}/\rho_{m-1}$
16. $\mathbf{u}_{m+1} = \mathbf{w}_{m+1} + \beta_{m-1}\mathbf{u}_m$
17. $\mathbf{v}_{m+1} = \mathbf{L}\mathbf{u}_{m+1} + \beta_{m-1}(\mathbf{L}\mathbf{u}_m + \beta_{m-1}\mathbf{v}_{m-1})$
18. Endif
19. EndDo.

The residual norm of the approximate solution $\mathbf{d}_m$ is given by $\|\mathbf{r}_m\| \leq (m+1)^{\frac{1}{2}}\tau_m$. From the algorithm, it is easy to see that the coefficient matrix $\mathbf{L}$ is involved only in the computation of a matrix-by-vector product. If we generate $\mathbf{L}$ explicitly and carry out this matrix-by-vector product directly, we would need a memory requirement of $O(n^2)$ and computational complexity of $O(n^2)$ for each iteration where $n$ denotes the number of unknowns. However, if we recognize that Eq. (5.121) is a discrete convolution, which can be evaluated using FFT, we can reduce the memory requirement to $O(n)$ and the computational complexity to $O(n \log n)$ for each iteration. To be more specific, the evaluation of the matrix-by-vector product is equivalent to evaluating the left-hand side of Eq. (5.116). This evaluation can be accomplished through two steps. The first step is to calculate $A_{M,N,P}^{(q)}$ from Eq. (5.121), which can be written as

$$A_{M,N,P}^{(q)} = \Delta V \, DFT^{-1}\{DFT\{G_{M,N,P}\} \cdot DFT\{\chi_{M,N,P}^{(q)} d_{M,N,P}^{(q)}\}\}. \tag{5.124}$$

This calculation can be done using FFT with a computational complexity of $O(n \log n)$. The second step is to substitute the calculated $A^{(q)}_{M,N,P}$ into Eq. (5.116). Since the matrices implied in Eq. (5.116) are sparse, their product with a vector can be evaluated with $O(n)$ operations. The $G_{M,N,P}$ in Eq. (5.124) is given by

$$G_{M,N,P} = G_{M-1,N-1,P-1} \tag{5.125}$$

with the right-hand side defined in Eq. (5.122). Using the spherical approximation for $M = N = P = 1$, we obtain

$$G_{1,1,1} = \frac{1}{\Delta V}\left[\left(\frac{1}{k_0^2} - i\frac{r_0}{k_0}\right)e^{ik_0 r_0} - \frac{1}{k_0^2}\right] \tag{5.126}$$

where $r_0 = [3\Delta V/(4\pi)]^{1/3}$. For other cases, we can either use the midpoint approximation to find

$$G_{M,N,P} = \frac{\exp(ik_0 R)}{4\pi R} \tag{5.127}$$

where $R = \sqrt{(M\Delta x)^2 + (N\Delta y)^2 + (P\Delta z)^2}$, or use a slightly more complicated evaluation (Zwamborn and van den Berg 1992) to find

$$G_{M,N,P} = \frac{\exp(ik_0 R)\,[\mathrm{sinc}(ik_0 r_0) - \cos(ik_0 r_0)]}{\frac{1}{3}\pi(k_0 r_0)^2 R} \tag{5.128}$$

which has a better accuracy than Eq. (5.127).

Once the electric field is computed, the magnetic field can be calculated using Eq. (5.94), where the derivatives can be approximated by finite difference. However, because of the finite difference approximation, the result obtained has a very poor accuracy. To calculate the magnetic field accurately, we use the integral expression

$$\mathbf{H}(\mathbf{r}) = \mathbf{H}^{\mathrm{ex}}(\mathbf{r}) + \mathbf{H}^{\mathrm{eq}}(\mathbf{r}) \tag{5.129}$$

where

$$\mathbf{H}^{\mathrm{ex}}(\mathbf{r}) = -i\omega\epsilon_0 \nabla \times \mathbf{A}^{\mathrm{ex}}(\mathbf{r}) \tag{5.130}$$

$$\mathbf{H}^{\mathrm{eq}}(\mathbf{r}) = -i\omega\epsilon_0 \nabla \times \mathbf{A}^{\mathrm{eq}}(\mathbf{r}) \tag{5.131}$$

with $\mathbf{A}^{\mathrm{ex}}(\mathbf{r})$ and $\mathbf{A}^{\mathrm{eq}}(\mathbf{r})$ given in Eqs. (5.100) and (5.101). Using a vector identity, Eq. (5.126) can be written as

$$\mathbf{H}^{\mathrm{eq}}(r) = \iiint_V \chi(\mathbf{r}')\mathbf{D}(\mathbf{r}') \times \nabla G(\mathbf{r}, \mathbf{r}')dV'. \tag{5.132}$$

Since

$$\nabla G(\mathbf{r}, \mathbf{r}') = \frac{\partial G(\mathbf{r}, \mathbf{r}')}{\partial R} \nabla R \tag{5.133}$$

where $R = |\mathbf{R}| = |\mathbf{r} - \mathbf{r}'|$ and

$$\frac{\partial G(\mathbf{r}, \mathbf{r}')}{\partial R} = \left(ik_0 - \frac{1}{R}\right) G(\mathbf{r}, \mathbf{r}'), \quad \nabla R = \frac{\mathbf{R}}{R}, \tag{5.134}$$

we obtain

$$\mathbf{H}^{\mathrm{eq}}(\mathbf{r}) = \iiint_V \chi(\mathbf{r}')\mathbf{D}(\mathbf{r}') \times \frac{\mathbf{R}}{R} \left(ik_0 - \frac{1}{R}\right) G(\mathbf{r}, \mathbf{r}')\, dV' \tag{5.135}$$

which can be evaluated efficiently using the fast Fourier transform.

The numerical approach described above belongs to the $k$-space method introduced by Bojarski (1971). The $k$-space method is also known as the CG-FFT or BCG-FFT method when it employs a conjugate gradient (CG) or a biconjugate gradient (BCG) method as the iterative solver. There is a large body of literature on the CG-FFT and BCG-FFT methods for a variety of electromagnetics problems and it is not our intention to review it here. Instead, we shall mention a few papers on 3D volumetric material problems to give a brief history. The first application of the CG-FFT method to such problems can be found in the analysis of the absorption of electromagnetic power by human bodies (Borup and Gandhi 1984). However, the use of pulse basis functions yielded slow convergence and poor results when dealing with materials with high dielectric contrast. Better formulations were later proposed (Shen *et al.* 1989, Catedra *et al.* 1989, Zwamborn and van den Berg 1992, Gan and Chew 1996), and most of these used mixed-order (linear in one direction and constant in the other two directions) basis functions, as we did in this section. Among these, the methods proposed by Zwamborn and van den Berg (1992) and Gan and Chew (1996) are the most accurate for materials with high dielectric contrast. In particular, the second one has been employed successfully to study RF loaded coils for high-frequency MRI applications (Jin *et al.* 1996). In both methods, one is required to calculate within each iteration the multiplication between the transpose of the system matrix and a vector, in addition to that between the system matrix and a vector, resulting in at least 12 FFTs per iteration. Furthermore, the multiplication between the transpose of the system matrix and a vector is found to be more complicated than that between the system matrix and a vector. These difficulties have been removed in the method described in this section. The use of the transpose-free quasi-minimal residual (TFQMR) algorithm allows

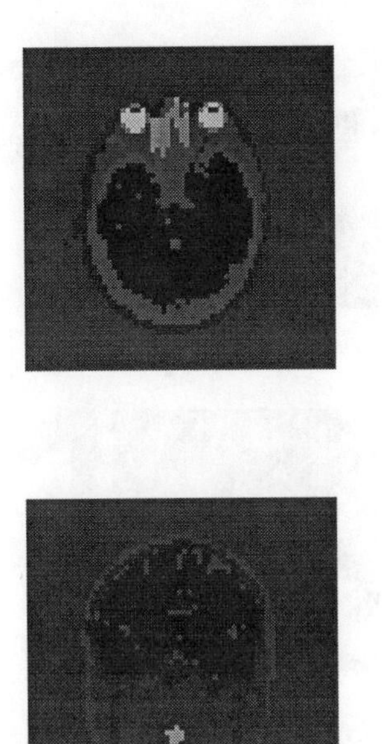

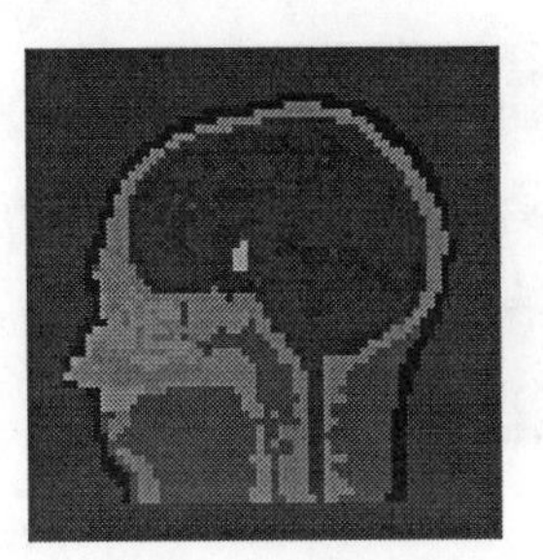

**Figure 5.21.** The axial, sagittal, and coronal slices of the head model. Reproduced from Chen *et al.* (1998), ©1998 IEEE.

us to avoid the complicated multiplication between the transpose of the system matrix and a vector, and reduce the number of FFTs to only six per iteration. Consequently, the resultant method is much simpler and more efficient than other methods (Wang and Jin 1998).

### 5.4.3 Numerical Simulations

The electromagnetic model of the head used in the study is the same one described in Section 5.3.3. Three slices of this model are shown in Fig. 5.21 (see color insert). In this section, we apply the FDTD algorithm to analyze the SAR and $B_1$ field inside the human head generated by a shielded, quadrature birdcage coil. The electric currents in the birdcage coil are calculated using the method of moments described in the preceding chapter and are used as the excitation in the FDTD calculations.

The birdcage coil considered has a diameter of 26 cm, a length of 26 cm, and consists of 16 elements. The coil is enclosed by a cylindrical shield having a diameter of 32 cm and a length of 32 cm. Therefore, the shield is 3 cm away from the coil's elements, which are about 3.6 cm away from the

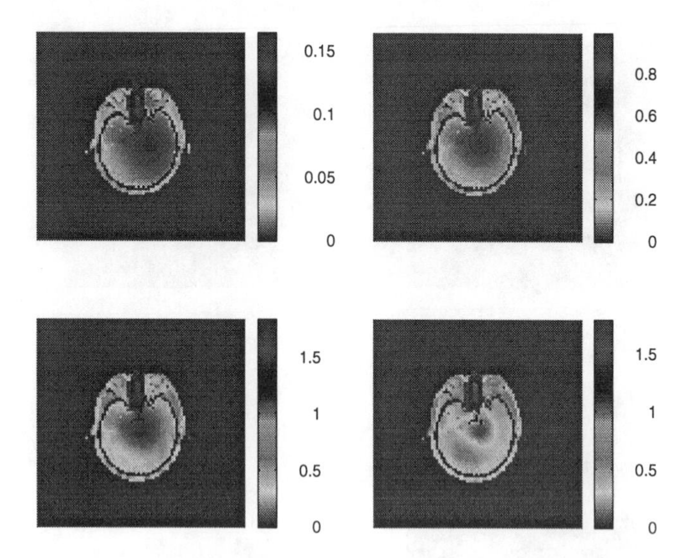


**Figure 5.22.** SAR (W/Kg) distribution in the axial slice for a shielded birdcage coil. Top-left: 64 MHz. Top-right: 128 MHz. Bottom-left: 171 MHz. Bottom-right: 256 MHz. Reproduced from Chen *et al.* (1998), ©1998 IEEE.

head. The maximum electric current in the elements of the coil is assumed to be 1 A. The four frequencies considered are 64 MHz, 128 MHz, 171 MHz, and 256 MHz, corresponding to the frequency of the $B_1$ field in 1.5 T, 3 T, 4 T, and 6 T MRI systems, respectively.

Figures 5.22–5.24 (see color insert) display the SAR distribution in the axial, sagittal, and coronal slices. The corresponding $B_1$ field is given in Figs. 5.25–5.27 (see color insert). As can be seen, at low frequency such as 64 MHz, the high SAR concentrates in the skin region; however, as the frequency increases, the SAR penetrates into the deeper region of the head. It is also observed that at low frequency the $B_1$ field is very homogeneous whereas at high frequency the $B_1$ field exhibits a strong inhomogeneity.

To further demonstrate the capability of the method, we consider the above shielded birdcage coil with its top end capped with a conducting plate. This conducting plate acts as a mirror for the coil and effectively doubles its electrical length. As a result, the homogeneity of the $B_1$ field produced inside the coil, particularly near the end capped with the mirror, can be improved significantly. We have simulated this case and the SAR distribution is shown in Figs. 5.28–5.30 (see color insert) and the corresponding $B_1$ field is given in Figs. 5.31–5.33 (see color insert). It is seen that the end-cap can decrease the SAR at low frequency and increase the SAR at high frequency in the top of the head. It is also seen that at

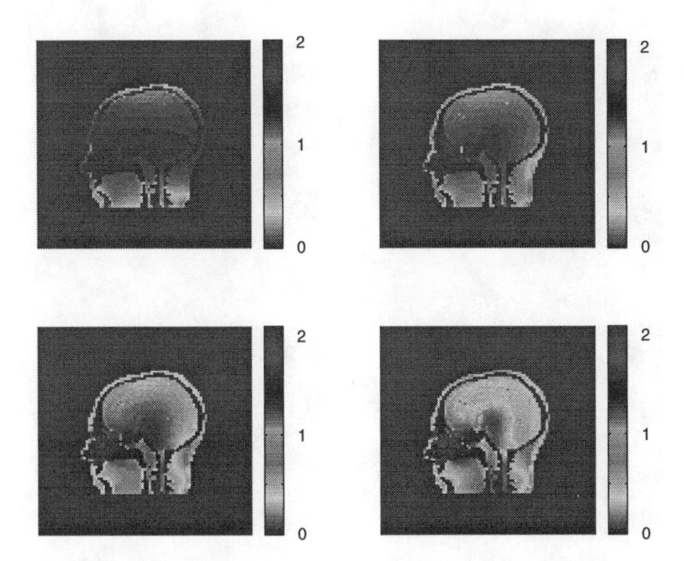


**Figure 5.23.** SAR (W/Kg) distribution in the sagittal slice for a shielded birdcage coil. Top-left: 64 MHz. Top-right: 128 MHz. Bottom-left: 171 MHz. Bottom-right: 256 MHz. Reproduced from Chen *et al.* (1998), ©1998 IEEE.

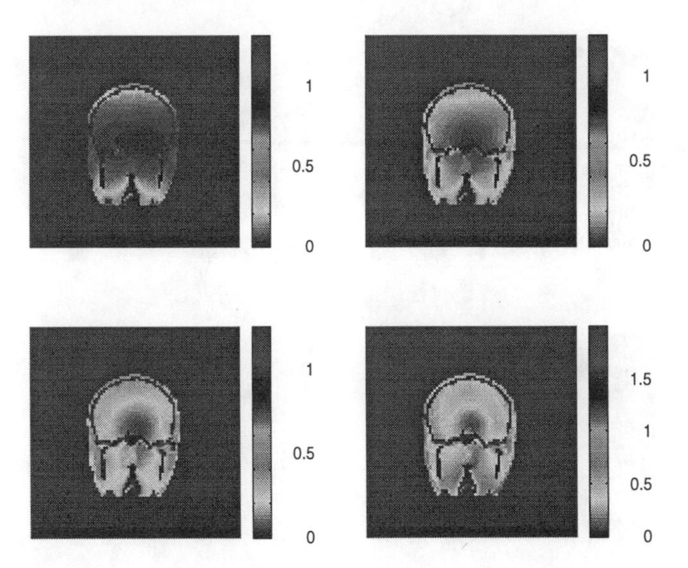


**Figure 5.24.** SAR (W/Kg) distribution in the coronal slice for a shielded birdcage coil. Top-left: 64 MHz. Top-right: 128 MHz. Bottom-left: 171 MHz. Bottom-right: 256 MHz. Reproduced from Chen *et al.* (1998), ©1998 IEEE.

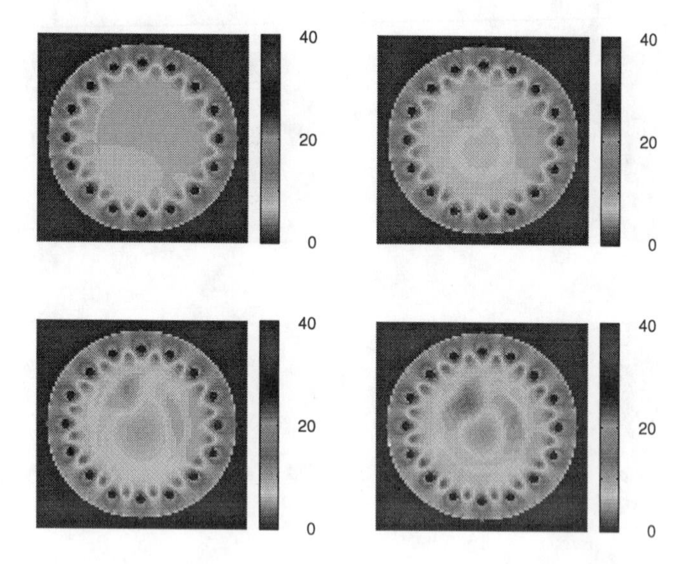


**Figure 5.25.** Magnetic field (A/m) distribution in the axial slice for a shielded birdcage coil. Top-left: 64 MHz. Top-right: 128 MHz. Bottom-left: 171 MHz. Bottom-right: 256 MHz. Reproduced from Chen *et al.* (1998), ©1998 IEEE.

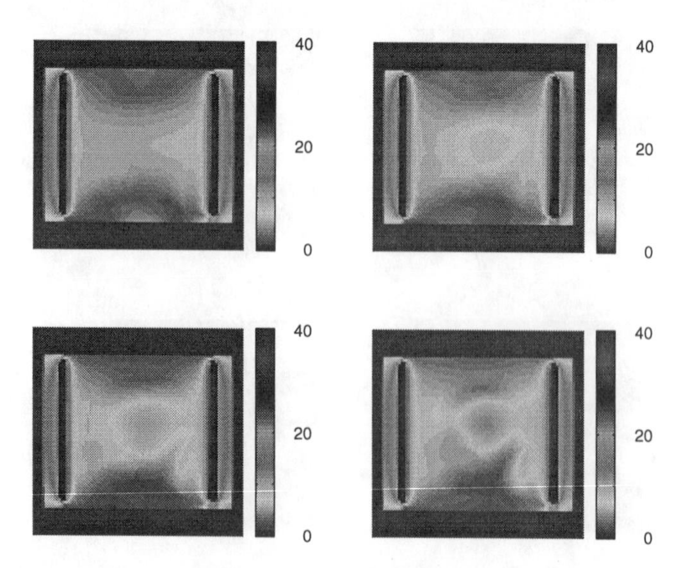


**Figure 5.26.** Magnetic field (A/m) distribution in the sagittal slice for a shielded birdcage coil. Top-left: 64 MHz. Top-right: 128 MHz. Bottom-left: 171 MHz. Bottom-right: 256 MHz. Reproduced from Chen *et al.* (1998), ©1998 IEEE.

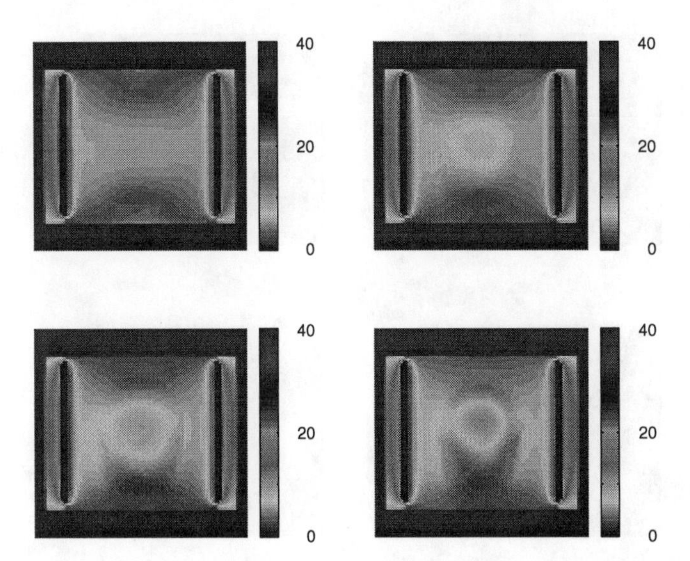


**Figure 5.27.** Magnetic field (A/m) distribution in the coronal slice for a shielded birdcage coil. Top-left: 64 MHz. Top-right: 128 MHz. Bottom-left: 171 MHz. Bottom-right: 256 MHz. Reproduced from Chen *et al.* (1998), ©1998 IEEE.

low frequency, the $B_1$ field homogeneity is indeed improved significantly; however, at high frequency, such improvement becomes rather trivial due to the phase variation or standing wave effect.

In this chapter, we have described several numerical methods to simulate electromagnetic fields inside biological objects. These methods can be used to evaluate the current and new designs of MRI RF coils. Accurate information about the $B_1$ field can be used for MR spectroscopy quantification and for designing new imaging schemes (RF excitation and post acquisition signal processing) that compensate for the field inhomogeneity. It is also useful for a better understanding of the EM-NMR transduction in human anatomy. Accurate information about the SAR can be used to assess more accurately the potential hazards of RF fields on the patient.

## 5.A Bessel Functions

The Bessel functions, denoted by $J_n(z)$ and $Y_n(z)$, are the two linearly independent solutions of the second-order differential equation

$$z^2\frac{d^2y}{dz^2} + z\frac{dy}{dz} + (z^2 - n^2)y = 0 \tag{5.136}$$

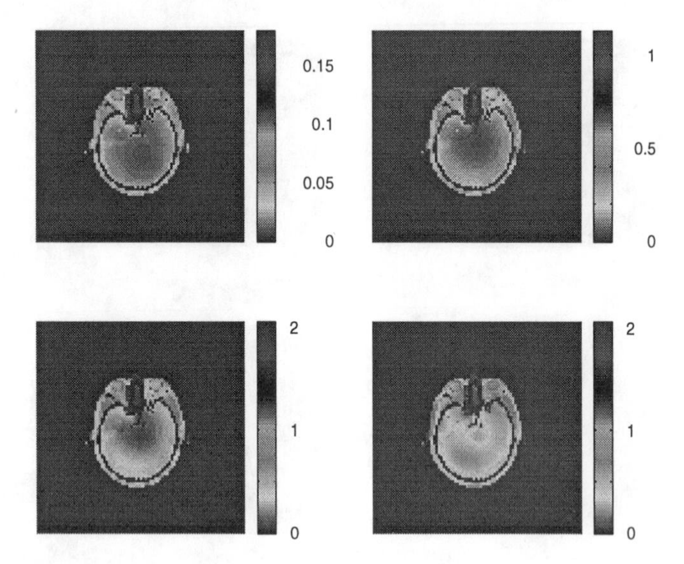


**Figure 5.28.** SAR (W/Kg) distribution in the axial slice for an end-capped shielded birdcage coil. Top-left: 64 MHz. Top-right: 128 MHz. Bottom-left: 171 MHz. Bottom-right: 256 MHz.

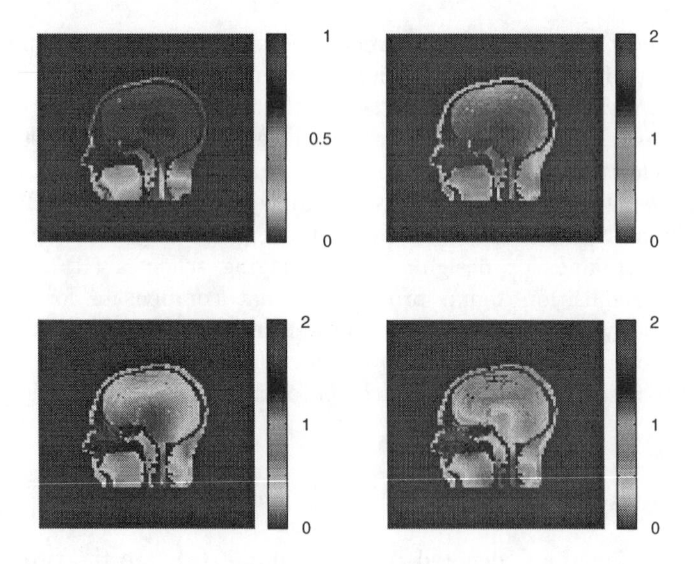


**Figure 5.29.** SAR (W/Kg) distribution in the sagittal slice for an end-capped shielded birdcage coil. Top-left: 64 MHz. Top-right: 128 MHz. Bottom-left: 171 MHz. Bottom-right: 256 MHz.

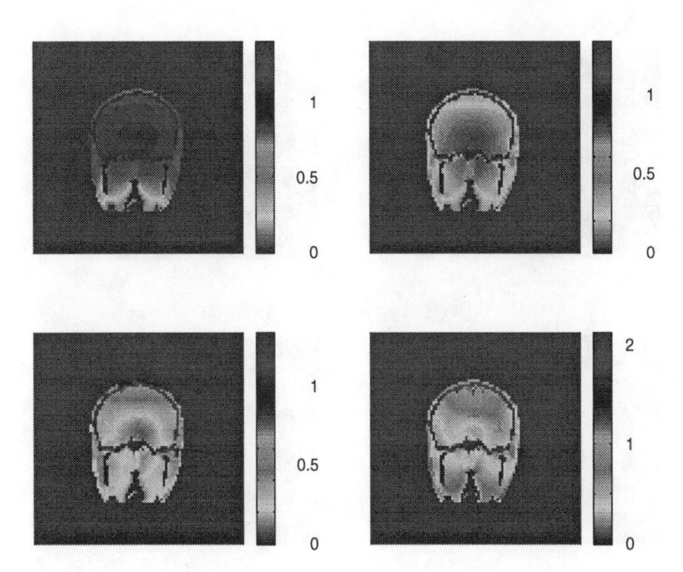


**Figure 5.30.** SAR (W/Kg) distribution in the coronal slice for an end-capped shielded birdcage coil. Top-left: 64 MHz. Top-right: 128 MHz. Bottom-left: 171 MHz. Bottom-right: 256 MHz.

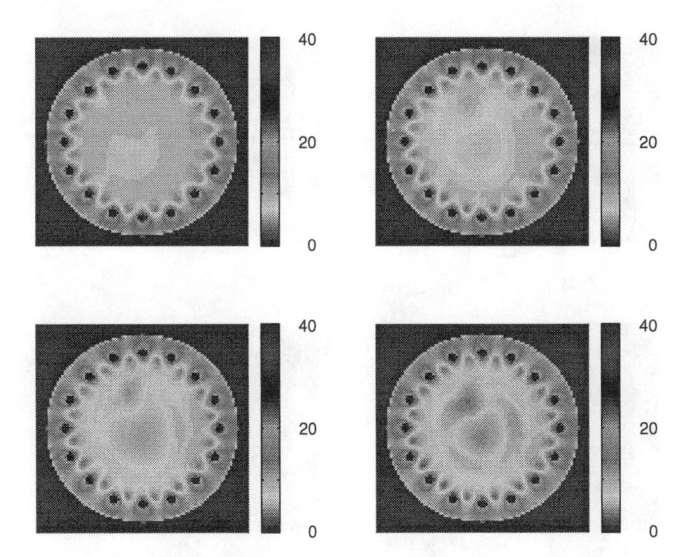


**Figure 5.31.** Magnetic field (A/m) distribution in the axial slice for an end-capped shielded birdcage coil. Top-left: 64 MHz. Top-right: 128 MHz. Bottom-left: 171 MHz. Bottom-right: 256 MHz.

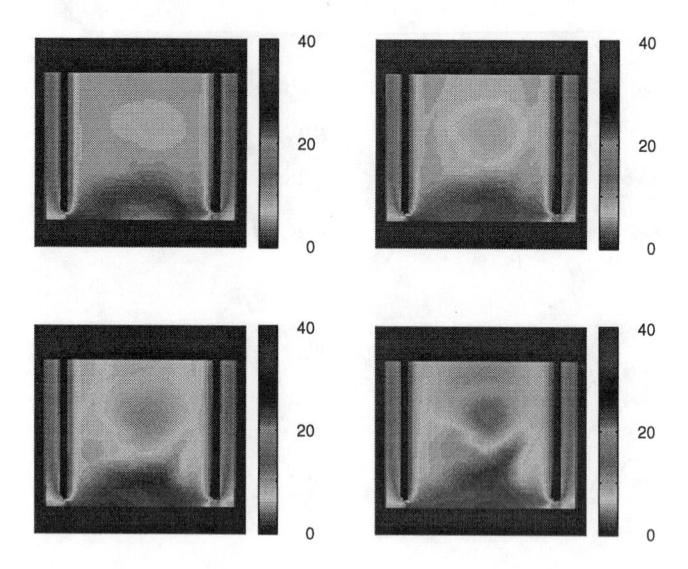


**Figure 5.32.** Magnetic field (A/m) distribution in the sagittal slice for an end-capped shielded birdcage coil. Top-left: 64 MHz. Top-right: 128 MHz. Bottom-left: 171 MHz. Bottom-right: 256 MHz.

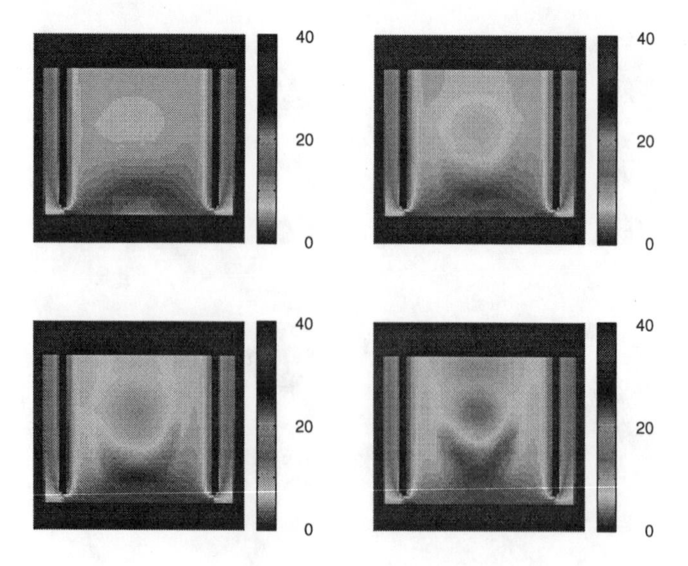


**Figure 5.33.** Magnetic field (A/m) distribution in the coronal slice for an end-capped shielded birdcage coil. Top-left: 64 MHz. Top-right: 128 MHz. Bottom-left: 171 MHz. Bottom-right: 256 MHz.

which is called Bessel's equation. They can be expressed explicitly as

$$J_n(z) = \sum_{m=0}^{\infty} (-1)^m \frac{(z/2)^{2m+n}}{m!\,(m+n)!} \tag{5.137}$$

and

$$Y_n(z) = \frac{1}{\pi}\left[\sum_{m=0}^{\infty} \frac{(-1)^m}{m!\,(m+n)!}\left(\frac{z}{2}\right)^{2m+n}\left(2\ln\frac{z}{2} + 2\gamma - \sum_{k=1}^{n+m}\frac{1}{k} - \sum_{k=1}^{m}\frac{1}{k}\right)\right.$$
$$\left. - \sum_{m=0}^{n-1} \frac{(n-m-1)!}{m!}\left(\frac{z}{2}\right)^{2m-n}\right] \tag{5.138}$$

where $\gamma \approx 0.57721566490153286$ denotes Euler's constant.

The Bessel functions have many mathematical properties, which are summarized in Abramowitz and Stegun (1964). For example, for a fixed $n$, when $z \to 0$,

$$J_0(z) \sim 1, \qquad J_n(z) \sim \frac{(z/2)^n}{n!} \quad (n > 0)$$
$$Y_0(z) \sim \frac{2}{\pi}\ln z, \qquad Y_n(z) \sim -\frac{n!}{\pi n}\left(\frac{z}{2}\right)^{-n} \quad (n > 0). \tag{5.139}$$

For a fixed $n$, when $|z| \to \infty$,

$$J_n(z) \sim \sqrt{\frac{2}{\pi z}}\cos(z - n\pi/2 - \pi/4) \qquad (|\arg z| < \pi) \tag{5.140}$$

$$Y_n(z) \sim \sqrt{\frac{2}{\pi z}}\sin(z - n\pi/2 - \pi/4) \qquad (|\arg z| < \pi). \tag{5.141}$$

For a fixed $z$, when $n \to \infty$,

$$J_n(z) \sim \frac{1}{\sqrt{2\pi n}}\left(\frac{ez}{2n}\right)^n, \qquad Y_n(z) \sim -\sqrt{\frac{2}{\pi n}}\left(\frac{ez}{2n}\right)^{-n}. \tag{5.142}$$

The Bessel functions satisfy the recurrence and differentiation relations

$$B_{n+1}(z) = \frac{2n}{z}B_n(z) - B_{n-1}(z) \tag{5.143}$$

$$B_n'(z) = B_{n-1}(z) - \frac{n}{z}B_n(z) \tag{5.144}$$

$$B_n'(z) = \frac{n}{z}B_n(z) - B_{n+1}(z) \tag{5.145}$$

$$B_n'(z) = \frac{1}{2}\left[B_{n-1}(z) - B_{n+1}(z)\right] \tag{5.146}$$

where $B_n(z)$ denotes an arbitrary solution to Bessel's equation (5.136). In other words, $B_n(z)$ can either be $J_n(z)$ and $Y_n(z)$ or their linear combination. In the special case of $n = 0$, Eq. (5.145) becomes

$$B_0'(z) = -B_1(z). \tag{5.147}$$

The Wronskian relation for the Bessel function is

$$W\left[J_n(z), Y_n(z)\right] = J_{n+1}(z)Y_n(z) - J_n(z)Y_{n+1}(z) = \frac{2}{\pi z}. \tag{5.148}$$

The numerical evaluation of the Bessel functions is described in Zhang and Jin (1996). The following is a FORTRAN program for computing $J_n(z)$ and $Y_n(z)$ and their first derivative. Two subroutines, MSTA1 and MSTA2, used in this program are given in Appendix 3.A.

```
        SUBROUTINE JYNZ(N,Z,NM,CBJ,CDJ,CBY,CDY)
C
C       =======================================================
C       Purpose: Compute Bessel functions Jn(z), Yn(z) and
C                their derivatives for a complex argument
C       Input :  z --- Complex argument of Jn(z) and Yn(z)
C                n --- Order of Jn(z) and Yn(z)
C       Output:  CBJ(n) --- Jn(z)
C                CDJ(n) --- Jn'(z)
C                CBY(n) --- Yn(z)
C                CDY(n) --- Yn'(z)
C                NM --- Highest order computed
C       Routines called:
C                MSTA1 and MSTA2 to calculate the starting
C                point for backward recurrence
C       =======================================================
C
        IMPLICIT DOUBLE PRECISION (A,B,D-H,O-Y)
        IMPLICIT COMPLEX*16 (C,Z)
        DIMENSION CBJ(0:N),CDJ(0:N),CBY(0:N),CDY(0:N),
     &            A(4),B(4),A1(4),B1(4)
        EL=0.5772156649015329D0
        PI=3.141592653589793D0
        R2P=0.63661977236758D0
        Y0=DABS(DIMAG(Z))
        A0=CDABS(Z)
        NM=N
        IF (A0.LT.1.0D-100) THEN
           DO 10 K=0,N
              CBJ(K)=(0.0D0,0.0D0)
```

```
              CDJ(K)=(0.0D0,0.0D0)
              CBY(K)=(-1.0D+300,0.0D0)
10            CDY(K)=(1.0D+300,0.0D0)
           CBJ(0)=(1.0D0,0.0D0)
           CDJ(1)=(0.5D0,0.0D0)
           RETURN
        ENDIF
        IF (A0.LE.300.0D0.OR.N.GT.INT(0.25*A0)) THEN
           IF (N.EQ.0) NM=1
           M=MSTA1(A0,200)
           IF (M.LT.NM) THEN
              NM=M
           ELSE
              M=MSTA2(A0,NM,15)
           ENDIF
           CBS=(0.0D0,0.0D0)
           CSU=(0.0D0,0.0D0)
           CSV=(0.0D0,0.0D0)
           CF2=(0.0D0,0.0D0)
           CF1=(1.0D-100,0.0D0)
           DO 15 K=M,0,-1
              CF=2.0D0*(K+1.0D0)/Z*CF1-CF2
              IF (K.LE.NM) CBJ(K)=CF
              IF (K.EQ.2*INT(K/2).AND.K.NE.0) THEN
                 IF (Y0.LE.1.0D0) THEN
                    CBS=CBS+2.0D0*CF
                 ELSE
                    CBS=CBS+(-1)**(K/2)*2.0D0*CF
                 ENDIF
                 CSU=CSU+(-1)**(K/2)*CF/K
              ELSE IF (K.GT.1) THEN
                 CSV=CSV+(-1)**(K/2)*K/(K*K-1.0)*CF
              ENDIF
              CF2=CF1
15            CF1=CF
           IF (Y0.LE.1.0D0) THEN
              CS0=CBS+CF
           ELSE
              CS0=(CBS+CF)/CDCOS(Z)
           ENDIF
           DO 20 K=0,NM
20            CBJ(K)=CBJ(K)/CS0
           CE=CDLOG(Z/2.0D0)+EL
           CBY(0)=R2P*(CE*CBJ(0)-4.0D0*CSU/CS0)
           CBY(1)=R2P*(-CBJ(0)/Z+(CE-1.0D0)*CBJ(1)-4.0D0*CSV/CS0)
```

```
      ELSE
         DATA A/-.7031250000000000D-01,.1121520996093750D+00,
     &          -.5725014209747314D+00,.6074042001273483D+01/
         DATA B/ .7324218750000000D-01,-.2271080017089844D+00,
     &           .1727727502584457D+01,-.2438052969955606D+02/
         DATA A1/.1171875000000000D+00,-.1441955566406250D+00,
     &           .6765925884246826D+00,-.6883914268109947D+01/
         DATA B1/-.1025390625000000D+00,.2775764465332031D+00,
     &           -.1993531733751297D+01,.2724882731126854D+02/
         CT1=Z-0.25D0*PI
         CP0=(1.0D0,0.0D0)
         DO 25 K=1,4
25          CP0=CP0+A(K)*Z**(-2*K)
         CQ0=-0.125D0/Z
         DO 30 K=1,4
30          CQ0=CQ0+B(K)*Z**(-2*K-1)
         CU=CDSQRT(R2P/Z)
         CBJ0=CU*(CP0*CDCOS(CT1)-CQ0*CDSIN(CT1))
         CBY0=CU*(CP0*CDSIN(CT1)+CQ0*CDCOS(CT1))
         CBJ(0)=CBJ0
         CBY(0)=CBY0
         CT2=Z-0.75D0*PI
         CP1=(1.0D0,0.0D0)
         DO 35 K=1,4
35          CP1=CP1+A1(K)*Z**(-2*K)
         CQ1=0.375D0/Z
         DO 40 K=1,4
40          CQ1=CQ1+B1(K)*Z**(-2*K-1)
         CBJ1=CU*(CP1*CDCOS(CT2)-CQ1*CDSIN(CT2))
         CBY1=CU*(CP1*CDSIN(CT2)+CQ1*CDCOS(CT2))
         CBJ(1)=CBJ1
         CBY(1)=CBY1
         DO 45 K=2,N
            CBJK=2.0D0*(K-1.0D0)/Z*CBJ1-CBJ0
            CBJ(K)=CBJK
            CBJ0=CBJ1
45          CBJ1=CBJK
      ENDIF
      CDJ(0)=-CBJ(1)
      DO 50 K=1,NM
50       CDJ(K)=CBJ(K-1)-K/Z*CBJ(K)
      IF(CDABS(CBJ(0)).GT.1.0D0) THEN
         CBY(1)=(CBJ(1)*CBY(0)-2.0D0/(PI*Z))/CBJ(0)
      ENDIF
      DO 55 K=2,NM
```

```
        IF (CDABS(CBJ(K-1)).GE.CDABS(CBJ(K-2))) THEN
           CYY=(CBJ(K)*CBY(K-1)-2.0D0/(PI*Z))/CBJ(K-1)
        ELSE
           CYY=(CBJ(K)*CBY(K-2)-4.0D0*(K-1.0D0)/(PI*Z*Z))/CBJ(K-2)
        ENDIF
        CBY(K)=CYY
55   CONTINUE
     CDY(0)=-CBY(1)
     DO 60 K=1,NM
60      CDY(K)=CBY(K-1)-K/Z*CBY(K)
     RETURN
     END
```

## 5.B Spherical Bessel Functions

The spherical Bessel functions of the first and second kinds, denoted by $j_n(z)$ and $y_n(z)$, respectively, are the two linearly independent solutions to the second-order differential equation

$$z^2\frac{d^2W}{dz^2}+2z\frac{dW}{dz}+\left[z^2-n(n+1)\right]W=0 \qquad (n=0,\pm1,\pm2,\ldots) \tag{5.149}$$

which is called the spherical Bessel's equation. The spherical Hankel functions of the first and second kinds are defined by

$$h_n^{(1)}(z)=j_n(z)+i\,y_n(z) \tag{5.150}$$

$$h_n^{(2)}(z)=j_n(z)-i\,y_n(z). \tag{5.151}$$

The series expressions for $j_n(z)$ and $y_n(z)$ are given by

$$j_n(z)=\frac{z^n}{1\cdot3\cdot5\cdots(2n+1)}\times\left[1-\frac{(z/2)^2}{1!\,(n+3/2)}+\frac{(z/2)^4}{2!\,(n+3/2)(n+5/2)}-\cdots\right] \tag{5.152}$$

$$y_n(z)=-\frac{1\cdot3\cdot5\cdots(2n-1)}{z^{n+1}}\times\left[1-\frac{(z/2)^2}{1!\,(1/2-n)}+\frac{(z/2)^4}{2!\,(1/2-n)(3/2-n)}-\cdots\right] \tag{5.153}$$

where $n=0,1,2,\ldots$. They are related to elementary functions by

$$j_0(z)=\frac{\sin z}{z}, \qquad y_0(z)=-\frac{\cos z}{z}$$

$$j_1(z) = \frac{\sin z}{z^2} - \frac{\cos z}{z}, \qquad y_1(z) = -\frac{\cos z}{z^2} - \frac{\sin z}{z}. \tag{5.154}$$

Higher-order functions can be computed conveniently using the recurrence formula

$$b_{n-1}(z) + b_{n+1}(z) = \frac{2n+1}{z} b_n(z) \tag{5.155}$$

where $b_n(z)$ represents $j_n(z)$, $y_n(z)$, $h_n^{(1)}(z)$, $h_n^{(2)}(z)$, or their linear combinations. Their derivatives are given by

$$b_n'(z) = -\frac{n+1}{z} b_n(z) + b_{n-1}(z) \tag{5.156}$$

$$b_n'(z) = -b_{n+1}(z) + \frac{n}{z} b_n(z) \tag{5.157}$$

$$b_n'(z) = \frac{1}{2n+1}\left[-(n+1)b_{n+1}(z) + nb_{n-1}(z)\right]. \tag{5.158}$$

The Wronskian relations for the spherical Bessel functions are

$$\begin{aligned} W[j_n(z),\, y_n(z)] &= j_n(z)y_n'(z) - y_n(z)j_n'(z) \\ &= j_n(z)y_{n-1}(z) - y_n(z)j_{n-1}(z) \\ &= j_{n+1}(z)y_n(z) - y_{n+1}(z)j_n(z) \\ &= \frac{z}{2n+1}\left[j_{n+1}(z)y_{n-1}(z) - y_{n+1}(z)j_{n-1}(z)\right] \\ &= z^{-2}. \end{aligned} \tag{5.159}$$

The numerical evaluation of the spherical Bessel functions is described in Zhang and Jin (1996). The following is a FORTRAN program for computing $j_n(z)$ and $y_n(z)$ and their first derivative.

```
        SUBROUTINE CSPHJY(N,Z,NM,CSJ,CDJ,CSY,CDY)
C
C       ===========================================================
C       Purpose: Compute spherical Bessel functions jn(z) & yn(z)
C                and their derivatives with a complex argument
C       Input :  z --- Complex argument
C                n --- Order of jn(z) & yn(z) ( n = 0,1,2,... )
C       Output:  CSJ(n) --- jn(z)
C                CDJ(n) --- jn'(z)
C                CSY(n) --- yn(z)
C                CDY(n) --- yn'(z)
C                NM --- Highest order computed
C       Routines called:
```

```
C             MSTA1 and MSTA2 to calculate the starting
C             point for backward recurrence
C       ==============================================================
C
        IMPLICIT COMPLEX*16 (C,Z)
        DOUBLE PRECISION A0
        DIMENSION CSJ(0:N),CDJ(0:N),CSY(0:N),CDY(0:N)
        A0=CDABS(Z)
        NM=N
        IF (A0.LT.1.0D-60) THEN
           DO 10 K=0,N
              CSJ(K)=0.0D0
              CDJ(K)=0.0D0
              CSY(K)=-1.0D+300
10            CDY(K)=1.0D+300
           CSJ(0)=(1.0D0,0.0D0)
           CDJ(1)=(.3333333333333333D0,0.0D0)
           RETURN
        ENDIF
        CSJ(0)=CDSIN(Z)/Z
        CSJ(1)=(CSJ(0)-CDCOS(Z))/Z
        IF(N.GE.2) THEN
           CSA=CSJ(0)
           CSB=CSJ(1)
           M=MSTA1(A0,200)
           IF (M.LT.N) THEN
              NM=M
           ELSE
              M=MSTA2(A0,N,15)
           ENDIF
           CF0=0.0D0
           CF1=1.0D0-100
           DO 15 K=M,0,-1
              CF=(2.0D0*K+3.0D0)*CF1/Z-CF0
              IF (K.LE.NM) CSJ(K)=CF
              CF0=CF1
15            CF1=CF
           IF (CDABS(CSA).GT.CDABS(CSB)) CS=CSA/CF
           IF (CDABS(CSA).LE.CDABS(CSB)) CS=CSB/CF0
           DO 20 K=0,NM
20            CSJ(K)=CS*CSJ(K)
        ENDIF
        CDJ(0)=(CDCOS(Z)-CDSIN(Z)/Z)/Z
        DO 25 K=1,NM
25         CDJ(K)=CSJ(K-1)-(K+1.0D0)*CSJ(K)/Z
```

```
      CSY(0)=-CDCOS(Z)/Z
      CSY(1)=(CSY(0)-CDSIN(Z))/Z
      CDY(0)=(CDSIN(Z)+CDCOS(Z)/Z)/Z
      CDY(1)=(2.0D0*CDY(0)-CDCOS(Z))/Z
      DO 30 K=2,NM
         IF (CDABS(CSJ(K-1)).GT.CDABS(CSJ(K-2))) THEN
            CSY(K)=(CSJ(K)*CSY(K-1)-1.0D0/(Z*Z))/CSJ(K-1)
         ELSE
            CSY(K)=(CSJ(K)*CSY(K-2)-(2.0D0*K-1.0D0)/Z**3)/CSJ(K-2)
         ENDIF
30    CONTINUE
      DO 35 K=2,NM
35       CDY(K)=CSY(K-1)-(K+1.0D0)*CSY(K)/Z
      RETURN
      END
```

## Problems

5.1 Based on the formulation described in Section 5.2 and using the subroutine given in Appendix 5.A, write a computer program to calculate the electric and magnetic fields inside a dielectric cylinder.

5.2 Assume $a = 10$ cm, $b = 12.5$ cm, $c = 15$ cm, $\epsilon_r = 70$, and $\sigma = 0.5$ S/m$^2$ in Fig. 5.1. Calculate the electric and magnetic fields inside a dielectric cylinder at 64, 128, and 256 MHz. Compare the results.

5.3 Assume that the current in Fig. 5.1 is given by

$$J_z(\phi) = J_0 \sin\phi.$$

Find the solution of the electric and magnetic fields inside a dielectric cylinder. Show that the magnetic field is uniform at a low frequency.

5.4 Using the results in Section 5.2 and Problem 5.3, find the solution of the electric and magnetic fields inside a dielectric cylinder when the current is given by

$$J_z(\phi) = J_0 \exp(i\phi).$$

Discuss the properties of the electric and magnetic fields.

5.5 Repeat Problem 5.2 for the current given Problem 5.4. Compare the homogeneity of the magnetic field to that obtained in Problem 5.2.

5.6 If the cylindrical surface current in Fig. 5.1 is replaced by a number of discrete wire currents, would it still be possible to derive an analytical solution to the problem? If yes, describe the basic steps.

5.7 Write a computer program based on the 2D finite difference formulation described in Section 5.3.1 to calculate the electric and magnetic fields. Validate the program using the result calculated in Problem 5.2.

5.8 Build a 2D model for a leg using an MR image or an anatomical picture given in Eycleshymer and Schoemaker (1911). Using the computer program developed in Problem 5.7 to calculate the $B_1$ field generated by a shielded birdcage coil. Consider both linear and quadrature excitations.

5.9 Apply the finite difference to Eqs. (5.54) and (5.55) to derive Eqs. (5.58) and (5.59).

5.10 Write a computer program based on the 2D finite element formulation described in Section 5.3.2 to calculate the electric and magnetic fields. Validate the program using the result calculated in Problem 5.2.

5.11 Apply the finite difference method to Eqs. (5.76) and (5.79), respectively, and derive Eqs. (5.82) and (5.85).

5.12 By approximating a rectangular cell of size $\Delta x \times \Delta y \times \Delta z$ as a sphere of the same volume, derive the result in Eq. (5.126), that is, show that

$$\int_{-\Delta x/2}^{\Delta x/2} \int_{-\Delta y/2}^{\Delta y/2} \int_{-\Delta z/2}^{\Delta z/2} \frac{\exp(ik_0 R)}{4\pi R} dx''dy''dz'' \approx \left( \frac{1}{k_0^2} - i\frac{r_0}{k_0} \right) e^{ik_0 r_0} - \frac{1}{k_0^2}.$$

Hint: Perform the integration in the spherical coordinates.

## References

M. Abramowitz and I. Stegun, Eds. (1964), *Handbook of Mathematical Functions.* Washington: National Bureau of Standards. Reprinted by Dover Publications, New York, 1968.

J.-P. Berenger (1994), "A perfectly matched layer for the absorption of electromagnetic waves," *J. Computational Phys.*, vol. 114, pp. 185–200.

N. N. Bojarski (1971), "$k$-space formulation of the electromagnetic scattering problems," *Air Force Avionic Lab. Tech. Rep. AFAL-TR-71-75.*

D. T. Borup and O. P. Gandhi (1984), "Fast-Fourier transform method for calculation of SAR distribution in finely discretized inhomogeneous models of biological bodies," *IEEE Trans. Microwave Theory Tech.*, vol. 32, pp. 355–360.

P. A. Bottomley and E. R. Andrew (1978), "RF magnetic field penetration, phase shift and power dissipation in biological tissue: Implications for NMR imaging," *Phys. Med. Biol.*, vol. 23, pp. 630–643.

P. A. Bottomley, R. W. Redington, W. A. Edlestein, and J. F. Schenck (1985), "Estimating radiofrequency power deposition in body NMR imaging," *Magn. Reson. Med.*, vol. 2, pp. 336–349.

M. F. Catedra, E. Gago, and L. Nuno (1989), "A numerical scheme to obtain the RCS of three-dimensional bodies of resonant size using the conjugate gradient method and the fast fourier transform," *IEEE Trans. Antennas Propagat.*, vol. 37, pp. 528–537.

J. Y. Chen and O. P. Gandhi (1991), "Currents induced in an anatomically based model of a human for exposure to vertically polarized electromagnetic pulses," *IEEE Trans. Microwave Theory Tech.*, vol. 39, pp. 31–39.

J. Chen, Z. Feng, and J. M. Jin (1998), "Numerical simulation of SAR and $B_1$-field inhomogeneity of shielded RF coils loaded with the human head," *IEEE Trans. Biomed. Eng.*, vol. 45, pp. 650–659.

W. C. Chew (1995), *Waves and Fields in Inhomogeneous Media.* New York: IEEE Press.

W. C. Chew and W. Weedon (1994), "A 3D perfectly matched medium from modified Maxwell's equations with stretched coordinates," *Microwave Opt. Tech. Lett.*, vol. 7, pp. 599–604.

P. J. Dimbylow and S. M. Mann (1994), "SAR calculations in an anatomically realistic model of the head for mobile communication transceivers at 900 MHz and 1.8 GHz," *Phys. Med. Biol.*, vol. 39, pp. 361–368.

A. C. Eycleshymer and D. M. Schoemaker (1911), *A Cross-Section Anatomy.* New York: D. Appleton.

T. K. Foo, C. E. Hayes, and Y. W. Kang (1991), "An analytical model for the design of RF resonators for MR body imaging," *Magn. Reson. Med.*, vol. 21, pp. 165–177.

R. W. Freund (1993), "A transpose-free quasi-minimal residual algorithm for non-hermitian linear systems," *SIAM J. Sci. Comput.*, vol. 14, pp. 470–482.

C. Gabriel, S. Gabriel, and E. Corthout (1996a), "The dielectric properties of biological tissues: I. Literature survey," *Phys. Med. Biol.*, vol. 41, pp. 2231–2249.

S. Gabriel, R. W. Lau, and C. Gabriel (1996b), "The dielectric properties of biological tissues: III. Parametric models for the dielectric spectrum of tissues," *Phys. Med. Biol.*, vol. 41, pp. 2271–2293.

H. Gan and W. C. Chew (1995), "A discrete BCG-FFT algorithm for solving 3D inhomogeneous scatterer problems," *J. Electromagn. Waves Appl.*, vol. 9, pp. 1339–1357.

O. P. Gandhi, B. Q. Gao, and J. Y. Chen (1992), "A frequency-dependent finite difference time-domain formulation for induced current calculations in human beings," *Bioelectromagn.*, vol. 13, pp. 543–555.

G. H. Glover, C. E. Hayes, N. J. Pelc, W. A. Edelstein, O. M. Mueller, H. R. Hart, C. J. Hardy, M. O'Donnell, and W. D. Barber (1985), "Comparison of linear and circular polarization for magnetic resonance imaging," *J. Magn. Reson.*, vol. 64, pp. 255–270.

M. Grandolfo, P. Vecchia, and O. P. Gandhi (1990), "Calculation of rates of energy absorption by a human-torso model," *Bioelectromagn.*, vol. 11, pp. 117–128.

Y. Han and S. M. Wright (1993), "Analysis of RF penetration effects in MRI using finite-difference time-domain method," *Proc. 12th Annu. Sci. Mtg. Soc. Magn. Reson. Med.*, p. 1327.

J. G. Harrison and J. T. Vaughan (1996), "Finite element modeling of head coils for high-frequency magnetic resonance imaging applications," *12th Annu. Rev. Prog. Appl. Comput. Electromag.*, pp. 1220–1226.

J. M. Jin (1993), *The Finite Element Method in Electromagnetics.* New York: Wiley.

J. M. Jin and J. Chen (1997), "On the SAR and field inhomogeneity of birdcage coils loaded with the human head," *Magn. Reson. Med.*, vol. 38, pp. 953–963.

J. M. Jin, J. Chen, H. Gan, W. C. Chew, R. L. Magin, and P. J. Dimbylow (1996), "Computation of electromagnetic fields for high-frequency magnetic resonance imaging applications," *Phys. Med. Biol.*, vol. 41, pp. 2719–2738.

J. R. Keltner, J. W. Carlson, M. S. Roos, S. T. Wong, T. L. Wong, and T. F. Budinger (1991), "Electromagnetic fields of surface coil in vivo NMR at high frequencies," *Magn. Reson. Med.*, vol. 22, pp. 467–480.

K. S. Kunz and R. J. Luebbers (1994), *The Finite Difference Time Domain Method for Electromagnetics.* Boca Raton: CRC Press, Inc.

J. S. Leigh (1990), "FDA safety guidlines for MRI devices," *Reson. Newslett. SMRM*, vol. 20, no. 9.

D. E. Livesay and K. M. Chen (1974), "Electromagnetic fields induced inside arbitrarily shaped biological bodies," *IEEE Trans. Microwave Theory Tech.*, vol. 22, pp. 1273–1280.

P. Mansfield and P. G. Morris (1982), "Advances in Magnetic Resonance," Suppl. 2, *NMR Imaging in Biomedicine.* New York: Academic Press.

H. Ochi, E. Yamamoto, K. Sawaya, and S. Adachi (1992), "Calculation of electromagnetic field of an MRI antenna loaded by a body," *Proc. 12th Annu. Sci. Mtg. Soc. Magn. Reson. Med.*, p. 4021.

H. Ochi, E. Yamamoto, K. Sawaya, and S. Adachi (1995), "Analysis of radio frequency magnetic field penetration in a body within magnetic resonance imaging antenna," *Syst. Comp. Japan*, vol. 26, pp. 81–88.

K. D. Paulsen, X. Jia, and J. M. Sullivan (1993), "Finite element computations of specific absorption rates in anatomically conforming full-body models for hyperthermia treatment analysis," *IEEE Trans. Biomed. Eng.*, vol. 40, pp. 933–945.

P. Roeschmann (1987), "Radiofrequency penetration and absorption in the human body: Limitations to high-field whole-body nuclear magnetic resonance imaging," *Med. Phys.*, vol. 14, pp. 922–931.

Z. S. Sacks, D. M. Kingsland, R. Lee, and J. F. Lee (1995), "A perfectly matched anisotropic absorber for use as an absorbing boundary condition," *IEEE Trans. Antenna Propagat.*, vol. 43, pp. 1460–1463.

D. H. Schaubert, D. R. Wilton, and A. W. Glisson (1984), "A tetrahedral modeling method for electromagnetic scattering by arbitrarily shaped inhomogeneous dielectric bodies," *IEEE Trans. Antennas Propagat.*, vol. 32, pp. 77–85.

C. Y. Shen, K. J. Glover, M. I. Sancer, and A. D. Varvatsis (1989), "The discrete Fourier transform method of solving differential-integral equations in scattering theory," *IEEE Trans. Antennas Propagat.*, vol. 37, pp. 1032–1041.

D. Simunic, P. Wach, W. Renhart, and R. Stollberger (1996), "Spatial distribution of high-frequency electromagnetic energy in human head during MRI: Numerical results and measurements," *IEEE Trans. Biomed. Eng.*, vol. 43, pp. 88–94.

M. A. Stuchly and S. S. Stuchly (1980), "Dielectric properties of biological substances—Tabulated," *J. Microwave Power*, vol. 15, pp. 19–26.

D. M. Sullivan (1992), "A frequency dependent FDTD method for biological applications," *IEEE Trans. Microwave Theory Tech.*, vol. 40, pp. 532–539.

A. Taflove (1995), *Computational Electrodynamics: The Finite Difference Time Domain Method.* Boston: Artech House.

C. F. Wang and J. M. Jin (1998), "Simple and efficient computation of electromagnetic fields in arbitrarily-shaped, inhomogeneous dielectric bodies using transpose-free QMR and FFT," *IEEE Trans. Microwave Theory Tech.*, vol. 46, pp. 553–558.

Q. X. Yang, C. S. Li, and M. B. Smith (1993), "The effect of sample loading on the radio frequency magnetic field distribution in high field: contributions of dielectric resonance," *Proc. 12th Annu. Sci. Mtg. Soc. Magn. Reson. Med.*, p. 1367.

Q. X. Yang, H. Maramis, C. S. Li, and M. B. Smith (1994), "Three-dimensional full wave solution of MRI radio frequency resonator," *Proc. 2nd Mtg. Soc. Magn. Reson.*, p. 1110.

K. S. Yee (1966), "Numerical solution of initial boundary vlaue problems involving Maxwell's equations in isotropic media," *IEEE Trans. Antennas Propagat.*, vol. 14, pp. 302–307.

S. Zhang and J. Jin (1996), *Computation of Special Functions.* New York: Wiley.

P. Zwamborn and P. M. van den Berg (1992), "The three-dimensional weak form of the conjugate gradient FFT method for solving scattering problems," *IEEE Trans. Microwave Theory Tech.*, vol. 40, pp. 1757–1766.

# Appendix A

# About the Software

## A.1 Introduction

To help the reader understand the basic characteristics of radiofrequency (RF) coils and the electromagnetic fields inside a biological object, we developed a software program called MRIEM, which can be downloaded from my homepage at *http://www.ece.uiuc.edu/fachtml/jin.html.* This software program can be used to demonstrate the analysis of a variety of RF coils and the calculation of the RF fields and the specific absorption rate (SAR) in the human head. However, the software is not intended for the design of RF coils. Therefore, we make no warranties of any kind, either express or implied, including but not limited to the implied warranty of merchantability and fitness for a particular purpose. Neither the author nor the publisher assumes any liability of any alleged or actual damages arising from the use of or the inability to use this software.

The software product is protected by copyright and all rights are reserved by the author and the publisher. You are licensed to use this software on a single computer. Copying the software to another medium or format for use on a single computer does not violate the U.S. Copyright Law. Copying the software for any other purpose is a violation of the U.S. Copyright Law.

To facilitate the use of the software, the computer programs are written in MATLAB. Therefore, the software can be used only on a computer installed with the MATLAB software. To use the software, you should first make a directory, say mriem.dir, in your computer and then copy all the programs into this directory. In this directory, start MATLAB and then type MRIEM. The software opens a window and displays three choices:

1. RF coil analysis
2. EM interaction simulation (2D)
3. EM interaction simulation (3D)

In the following, we describe each of the three functions. Note that in each step, there is a "main menu" bar and clicking this bar returns you back to this main page.

## A.2 RF Coil Analysis

For RF coil analysis, click the bar containing this choice. The window displays four choices for coil type:

1. Highpass birdcage coil
2. Lowpass birdcage coil
3. Highpass open coil
4. Lowpass open coil

Click a bar containing your choice, say "Highpass birdcage coil." The window displays the input page for the analysis, which includes

1. Input the number of strips (that is, the rungs or the legs)
2. Input the width of strips (inch)
3. Input the length of strips (inch)
4. Input the radius of coil (inch)
5. Input the radius of shield (inch)
6. Input the capacitance (pF)

Type in all the numbers in the corresponding boxes. If your coil is made of wires instead of strips, use the following formula to find the equivalent width:

$$w = 4.482a$$

where $a$ denotes the radius of the wires in inch. After that, click the "submit" bar. The program performs the analysis and displays the frequency of the resonant modes. The number of resonant modes equals the number of rungs in the coil. However, the end-ring resonant mode, which has the highest resonant frequency, does not support any current in the rungs. Hence, this mode is not displayed in the window. The modes having the same resonant frequency are the degenerate modes whose fields are orthogonal to each other.

To display the $B_1$ field in the axial plane, first select the display format. There are two choices: one is "image" that is actually a color density plot and the other is a "contour" plot. The default is "image." Then, select the resonant frequency and click. The window displays the $B_1$ field of the corresponding resonant mode. The value of the $B_1$ field is normalized and its absolute value is meaningless since the current strength in the coil is not specified. There are two ways to print the field plot:

1. Print from screen
2. Print to file

In the latter, you can save the $B_1$ field plot as a postscript (PS) file, or an encapsulated postscript (EPS) file, or a GIF file.

The procedure for the analysis of a lowpass birdcage coil is similar. Again, the end-ring resonant mode, which has the lowest resonant frequency, is not displayed since its current is zero in the rungs.

The procedure for the analysis of open coils is also similar. The only difference is that, in addition to the inputs described above, there is one more input item: "Input the width of the coil (inch)." This width must be less or equal to the diameter of the coil. For the latter, the cross section of the coil is a half-circle. Note that there is no end-ring resonance in an open coil and all the resonant modes are displayed in the window.

In RF coil analysis, all the self- and mutual inductances are included except for the mutual inductances between the segments comprising the end-rings. This results in a slight inaccuracy in the calculated resonant frequencies while the calculation of the $B_1$ field is basically not compromised. However, the inclusion of the mutual inductances between the segments comprising the end-rings is described in Section 4.3.

## A.3 RF Field Analysis

For RF field and SAR analysis using an approximated two-dimensional (2D) model, click the bar containing "EM interaction simulation (2D)" in the main menu. The window then displays four electromagnetic models:

1. High resolution model 1
2. High resolution model 2
3. Low resolution model 1
4. Low resolution model 2

Model 1 is a slice passing through the eyes and model 2 is a slice passing through the middle of the brain. The high resolution model is made of 2 mm cells and the low one is made of 4 mm cells. Usually, the low resolution model is sufficient and its simulation is much faster. Click the "Model selection" bar and select a model. The window displays three choices for the head size: "a large head," "a medium head," and "a small head." Make a selection by clicking the corresponding bar. The window displays the input page which contains:

1. Number of coil wires (rungs or legs of the birdcage coil)
2. Operating frequency (MHz)
3. Radius of the birdcage coil (inch)
4. Radius of the shield (inch)
5. Excitation: Linear (H-pol), Linear (V-pol), Quadrature

"Linear (H-pol)" refers to the linear excitation that produces a horizontally directed $B_1$ field and, likewise, "Linear (V-pol)" refers to the linear excitation that produces a vertically directed $B_1$ field. "Quadrature" refers to the quadrature excitation that produces a circularly polarized $B_1$ field. Type in all the numbers and select an excitation mode. Then, click the "Show geometry" bar. The window displays the position of the head, the rungs of the coil, and the shield. Click "Run Matlab" or "Run Fortran" to start the calculation using the finite-element method. If your computer does not have a Fortran compiler, click "Run Matlab." Otherwise, click "Run Fortran" because it is much faster to calculate using the Fortran program. When the calculation ends, the window displays the results of the calculation in terms of the electric field, the magnetic $B_1$ field, and the SAR. You can either print the pictures from your screen or save them as a postscript (PS) file, or an encapsulated postscript (EPS) file, or a GIF file.

Because of the extremely high complexity of the problem, the three-dimensional (3D) simulation is both memory intensive and time consuming. It usually takes several hours on a workstation. For this reason, our 3D simulation programs are not included in this software. Instead, we include some pre-computed data for display in the software. To display these data, click the bar containing "EM interaction simulation (3D)" in the main menu. The window displays three choices:

1. Shielded birdcage coil with linear excitation
2. Shielded birdcage coil with quadrature excitation

Make a selection by clicking the corresponding bar. Following the simple instructions, you can display the $B_1$ field and the SAR in the axial, sagittal, and coronal slices at several different frequencies. You can either print the pictures from the screen or save them into a file as described before.

Additional computer programs for the analysis and design of gradient and RF coils may be added to this software program in the future.

# Index